Gesell and Amatruda's

Developmental
Diagnosis

Editors

Hilda Knobloch, M.D.

Medical Specialist, New York State Department
of Mental Hygiene; Professor of Pediatrics,
Albany Medical College of Union University,
Albany, New York

Benjamin Pasamanick, M.D.

Associate Commissioner, New York State Department
of Mental Hygiene, Albany; Aubrey and Hilda Lewis Professor
of Social Psychiatry, New York School of Psychiatry,
New York; Adjunct Professor of Pediatrics, Albany Medical
College of Union University, Albany; Adjunct Professor
of Psychology, New York University; Adjunct Professor
of Epidemiology, Columbia University, New York, New York

Gesell and Amatruda's

Developmental Diagnosis

The Evaluation and Management
of Normal and Abnormal
Neuropsychologic Development
in Infancy and Early Childhood

Third Edition
Revised and Enlarged

Medical Department
HARPER & ROW, PUBLISHERS
Hagerstown, Maryland
New York, Evanston, San Francisco, London

Library of Congress Cataloging in Publication Data

Gesell, Arnold Lucius, 1880–1961.
   Gesell and Amatruda's Developmental Diagnosis. The Evaluation and Management of Normal and Abnormal Neuropsychologic Development in Infancy and Early Childhood
   Bibliography: p.
   1. Developmental psychobiology. 2. Child development deviations.
I. Amatruda, Catherine Strunk, 1903–   joint author. II. Knobloch, Hilda, 1915–   ed. III. Pasamanick, Benjamin, ed. IV. Title. V. Title: Developmental diagnosis. [DNLM: 1. Child development. 2. Child development deviations. WS350 G389d]
RJ131.G46   1975   618.9'28'588   74–9517
ISBN 0-06-141438-7

Contents

Preface

to the Third Edition

The second edition of this classic volume appeared just over a quarter century ago in 1947. The work was a pioneering venture for the instruction of pediatricians in the diagnosis and management of developmental problems. Pediatrics was to undergo a major revolution, chronic diseases becoming its chief focus of concentration. The discovery and use of chemotherapeutic agents and antibiotics removed the acute infectious diseases from their position of highest priority, and there have been dramatic advances in surgical correction of congenital malformations. Thus the central nervous system and its disorders has become one of the most important areas requiring attention.

Gesell and Amatruda foresaw this revolution. They began the application of Gesell's decades of research in normal child development to the abnormal. This endeavor was chiefly the work of Catherine Amatruda, a gifted and devoted clinician; her collaboration with Arnold Gessell resulted in a new specialty, *developmental diagnosis,* or what could better be termed *infant neuropsychiatry.* They brought together for the first time the tremendously fruitful concepts of development, neuroanatomy, neurophysiology, central nervous system syndromes and diseases, and pertinent portions of psychology, sociology, anthropology and psychiatry. So certain were they of their ground and of the future that they included methods of instruction for medical students and physicians.

It is an illuminating study in the history and practice of medicine to review what has occurred in the last three decades. The six years which intervened between the first and second editions brought more clinical experience and a few scientific discoveries for inclusion in the textbook. However, Catherine Amatruda died in the full bloom of her clinical activities shortly after the second edition was published; had she lived, she undoubtedly would be writing this preface. Left without his collaborator and having passed the University retirement age, Gesell resigned his academic and clinical titles and duties, but spent additional fruitful years before his death at age 80. The clinicians whom they had trained literally could be counted on the fingers of one hand; two of them are the editors of this revision. Unfortunately, this handful has not increased the number of developmental diagnosticians geometrically, so desirable in view of the great need. Instead, the subsequent period has been one of maturation and research.

The clinical applications were developed by Gesell and Amatruda in a short period of time from previous research on normal children. The longterm procedures of testing reliability—the reproducibility of observations by other clinicians—and then of validity was done and then replicated, to a large extent, by the current editors. Gesell and Amatruda's original observations have been supplemented by our own clinical and research studies of seven or eight thousand additional infants and children. These findings and their implications are discussed here; we believe they have added new meaning to the interpretation of both diagnosis, care and prognosis of pediatric, neurologic and psychiatric conditions.

As might have been expected, the last twenty-five years have added immeasurably to the observations of Gesell and Amatruda and in some places, have changed completely prognosis and management. The results of the fantastic burgeoning in scientific activities have been considered wherever possible in this edition. These included molecular biology and its illumination of the etiology and treatment of some developmental disorders. Basic and applied attempts at social, psychologic, public health, and educational methods—whose vistas were seen only dimly in the first two editions—also have been brought up to date and the hopes as well as disappointments discussed. Finally, the role of developmental diagnosis in public health administration, and the methods and instruments which have been developed and tested within the last decade, will be included.

Gesell and Amatruda foresaw the social need for developmental diagnosis and we have attempted to rewrite this edition so that, despite many highly technical aspects, it will be useful for as many people who work with children as possible, including general practitioners, pediatricians, psychiatrists, neurologists, nurses, social workers, psychologists and teachers. Although much of the volume has been rewritten, much of it still stands as a credit to the genius of two great pioneering investigators and acute, sensitive clinicians.

We wish to encourage the use of the materials in this volume. Professionals engaged in the evaluation and care of infants and young children may reproduce the developmental schedules and the other forms used in developmental evaluation (except those taken from other sources, which is indicated in those cases) without requesting the permission of either Harper & Row or the editors of this book, provided the use is on a nonprofit basis and the editors and source of the material are properly acknowledged.

H.K.
B.P.

Preface
to the Second Edition

The first edition of the present volume appeared six years ago. Three printings during this interval and translations into foreign languages have evidenced a growing interest in the clinical aspects of child development. The publishers have granted us a welcome opportunity to add new materials gained chiefly through continuing clinical investigations of new and old cases seen on the diagnostic and advisory services of the Yale Clinic of Child Development.

As a result of further clinical experience we are able to present with discussion a sizeable number of additional case studies illustrating the diagnostic problems involved in amentia, convulsive disorders, cerebral injuries, blindness, deafness, infantile aphasias, congenital anomalies, and prematurity. Consideration is also given to new data concerning the developmental implications of prenatal rubella, the Rh factor, retrolental fibroplasia, and electroencephalographic findings. A total of some seventy illustrative case sketches are now presented in close association with explanatory text.

The behavior growth and behavior hygiene of the fetal-infant are discussed in a new section based on our recent volume entitled *The Embryology of Behavior*. Another new section deals with the physician's role in the increasingly important problem of child adoption.

The Appendices and Bibliography have been brought up to date and call attention to recent literature on the practical phases of developmental guidance. Appendix F projects a type of medical education necessary for professional specialization in the field of developmental diagnosis and supervision.

The concluding chapter on developmental pediatrics also is new. It outlines both present and future possibilities in the domain of developmental diagnosis. By *developmental pediatrics* we mean a form of clinical medicine which is systematically concerned with the diagnosis and supervision of child development. This phase of pediatrics has vast implications for the social aspects of medicine.

Indeed, all pediatric medicine has assumed a new importance in the period of postwar reconstruction upon which we are now entering. Instinctively it is felt that this reconstruction demands an intensified conservation of the development of infants and young children. How can we gain command of our civilization if life and growth are not cherished at their source?

Responsive to deep social forces, the American Academy of Pediatrics has organized a remarkable nationwide study of the child health services of the United States, and is currently conducting a survey of the character and scope of pediatric education in medical schools and teaching hospitals. This is a basic approach to fundamental human problems which need a medical technology rivaling atomic science in thoroughness and purposefulness.

The Clinic of Child Development   A. G.
School of Medicine, Yale University

Preface

to the First Edition

This book is the fruit of a clinical loom. For a period of years the authors have been jointly engaged with the practical problems of diagnosis and advisory guidance which have arisen in an outpatient clinic for infants and preschool children. Through fortunate circumstances this clinical service has always been conducted in close correlation with a systematic study of normal child development. One interest has reinforced the other. Observations of normal behavior threw light on maldevelopment, and the deviations of development in turn helped to expose what lay beneath a deceptive layer of "obviousness" in normal infancy. We have come to sense the identity of the developmental processes which in equal measure determine the reaction patterns of the intact and the defective child, the well endowed, the partially endowed, and those blemished by injury and disease.

It is these deep, determining developmental processes which must inevitably come within the scope of clinical medicine. In preparing this volume we have had much in mind the medical student who in private or public capacity will soon be confronted with varied and exacting problems which concern the developmental welfare both of normal and abnormal children.

Medical education has sometimes been criticized for neglecting the normal characteristics of man at the expense of the pathological. If we acknowledge that development as well as disease falls within the province of medicine and public health, the criticism has some force. The strong trend toward preventive and supervisory medicine obliges us to understand assets as well as liabilities, favorable as well as unfavorable symptoms. The pediatrician and the general practitioner have to deal increasingly with relatively well children. All this places a premium upon a broad type of developmental supervision, directed toward the realization of normal potentialities.

In the present volume we have given equal weight to the normal, the atypical and the abnormal expressions of early child development. The outline of normal development is abundantly illustrated with photo-tracings based on cinema records. We hope that the concreteness of this outline will give clinical status to normality, and will serve as a background for interpreting both typical and atypical manifestations of growth.

The chapters on developmental defects and deviations are especially directed to the practitioner who faces a host of problems in every complex case of developmental failure which comes to his attention. We have considered not only the technical but the commonplace and human aspects of these problems.

The concluding chapters suggest practical avenues of application both present and impending. New social forces are slowly altering the techniques of medicine. There is a mounting demand for periodic health examinations and for consecutive individualized supervision. The state of the world is troubled, but society in the very impulse of self-preservation will demand increased protection for the sources of life. We can conserve those sources only through a more thoroughgoing supervision of early child development.

Diagnosis remains the fundamental task of medicine, because in last analysis intelligent treatment, guidance, and supervision must rest upon accurate diagnostic appraisal. This is peculiarly true of developmental conditions. The present volume is primarily devoted to methods of diagnosis and to the applications which rest securely on diagnosis. These methods are outlined in such a manner that the clinician can take them over by partial stages and can suit them to his needs and to increasing clinical experience. They are safe in the hands of a clinically minded user. We have attempted to simplify and to adapt the results of long research to the practical requirements of office, hospital, and institution.

The research has involved many studies which have been reported in previous publications and which amply reflect our indebtedness to co-workers. The primary investigations were supported by The Rockefeller Foundation and by Yale University.

The present volume is made possible by the timely support of The Carnegie Corporation of New York.

The Clinic of Child Development   A. G.
School of Medicine, Yale University

Acknowledgments

We would like to express our appreciation to those who have reviewed our material and offered critical and constructive advice—Martin H. Greenberg, M.D., for the chapter on the low birth weight infant; Earl S. Sherard, Jr., M.D., chapters on convulsive seizure disorders and neuromotor dysfunction; Ian H. Porter, M.D., and Ernest B. Hook, M.D., the section on genetics; Mark Degnan, M.D., Doris M. Greenberg, M.D., Judith Miller and Bertrand G. Winsberg, M.D., for patiently reading almost the entire manuscript and helping to clarify meaning. Ruth Nowell and Danette Odom assisted with the editing process. Frances Stevens ably filled her role of research assistant and also struggled successfully with the typewriter. Jeanne Boni paid meticulous attention to details in typing the many forms and tables, as well as the narrative text. We also are indebted to both of them for collating the bits and pieces into a single manuscript. Most authors give credit to their wives or husbands for patient endurance; we must give thanks that we have succeeded in putting up with each other. Finally, we express our gratitude to our teachers, Arnold Gesell and Catherine S. Amatruda, and for the opportunity to add some of our own experiences to what they taught us.

H. K.
B. P.

Gesell and Amatruda's

Developmental
Diagnosis

Introduction

The contents of this book can be understood only in the historic context of how society has regarded and treated children and childhood over the ages. It has been assumed incorrectly that prior to the industrial revolution children had always been thought of as little adults and treated accordingly. The idea that they are different and developing organisms is supposed to have arisen only in recent times. When examined closely, this naive concept is untenable. Historically, all societies *had* to treat children differently from adults. No infant could be expected to obtain his own food, nor could he learn the customs, mores and all else that civilization connotes without assistance or teaching, explicit or implicit. Certainly the Greek philosophers had involved theories of child development, and the countries and societies in which they lived had systematic methods for rearing and reacting to children.

We might conjecture that the stereotype of the psychosocial homunculus arose in full bloom in the Reformation, with its emphasis upon original sin and the responsibility of each person for his own relationship to God and the cosmos, the mystical underpinnings of mercantile economic structure. In such a commercial society, economic success was an indication of God's favor and a measure of one's predetermined salvation. Unbaptized children were liable to eternal damnation, and only a few chosen adults who adhered strictly to faith were excepted from this fate. In counterposition, the closely knit, largely rural family valued the work of the child and the child himself as soon as he was able to help in maintaining the life needs of its members. In a society primarily rural and agricultural, children had ultimate long-enduring productive value; even the aged and crippled could contribute their mite. The family had to be maintained, no matter how helpless some of its members became, or the entire social structure fell apart.

The industrial revolution changed this. The religious substructure was retained and strengthened by the emphasis upon individual salvation through reinforcement of individual success. Success was proved additionally by burgeoning productive capacity, and the child became a tool to be used in the changing relationship of man to nature. In Great Britain particularly, locus of the epitome of the western industrial revolution, the demands of the juggernaut of industrial productivity threw entire families off the land, which was turned to more profitable use as animal pasture. The dislocated population was used to feed the maws of the mines and mills with the labor needed to keep them in operation. Living under the most appalling circumstances in cities and mine and mill villages, where there was utter disregard for their age, children either died young or were cast upon the scrap heap.

Thus, the children were regarded no differently from adults, except perhaps as less efficient or less durable machines.

The inevitable revulsion at these practices was partially reinforced by the obvious fact that the productive population was dying from hard labor or the terribly crowded unsanitary living conditions, and not reproducing itself. The humanitarians, in conjunction with the more pragmatic industrialists, began to place brakes upon the completely laissez-faire activities of the followers of Adam Smith. This changed viewpoint made it possible to look at what had happened and to consider the poor, both children and adults, as individuals rather than as an amorphous mass whose existence was a stench.

The political and legal changes took a number of forms—female and child labor laws, poor laws, prison reforms, free education and others. Some reforms were institutionalized in totally rigid forms which in turn became handicaps, as other social concepts crept in to reshape them. For the children, orphan asylums, asylums for the retarded and brain damaged, alms houses, hospitals and indentured apprenticeships were established. In contrast to what had existed before, there was an atmosphere of light and hope in the early stages of these institutions. It became possible to distinguish individuals within the mass. Simultaneously, sanitary reforms made it possible not only to maintain those who needed congregate living but also to think of what the future growth of these children might be. This era was the time when the child was more fully differentiated from the adult, and when knowledge about functioning and the provision of remediation became possible.

At the outset, few individuals involved in these changes were concerned with children alone. Rousseau wrote not only about child development and education, but also about the political and social changes which would be necessary to nurture them. On the continent, Pinel, Esquirol, Itard, Goethe and Gall also were involved in establishing bases for scientific and political understanding and change. The early 19th century was a time of great social and scientific turmoil. On library shelves in the United States were a heterogeneous group like Jefferson, Amariah Brigham, Horace Mann and Dorothea Dix. Later, the activities became more specialized and directed toward distinctive groups. Edouard Seguin was read not only in both France and the United States, but was one of the founders of scientific diagnosis and remediation of child cerebral dysfunction and psychologic functioning.

Even greater specialization occurred with the establishment of the first psychologic laboratories. Researchers such as Wundt wanted not only to establish simple norms of psychologic functioning in the areas of perception, sensation, motor performance and their interactions, but also expected that they might provide clues to various impairments in the nervous system. It was hoped that all these could be related to that complex called "intelligence"—although written about for centuries, it was in large part still an empirical mystery. It was possible to conceive that qualitative differences in any one complex area of function would be measurable in simple components, reflecting the "black box" of the brain, from which "mind" or reactivity on the psychologic level must stem.

At the same time, it became clear that all was not utopian in the sociopolitical sphere and in the institutions which had been established. While the most gross kinds of mistreatment and exploitation had been alleviated, nations were still governed by the profit motive, and exploitation had spread to far countries and colonies. The ideological bases, which rarely if ever changed, took on a more scientific tone—social salvation through power. Ironically, its motto was the biologic statement of "survival of the fittest" applied to the sociocultural sphere by such thinkers as Spencer, Sumner and others. Darwin never meant this to be applied socially, and probably not even biologically to man, but his entire meaning of the phrase was distorted. Darwin and others like him began to write about their observations of children, usually their own. Not until the end of the 19th century were consciously systematic and longitudinal efforts made to record the behavioral development of one or more children, exemplified by the volumes published by Wilhelm Preyer.

Ultimately, it is social forces which cause change. The need for an educated and technically trained population probably played the strongest role leading to universal education in industrialized countries; in turn, the study of child functioning became a respectable academic discipline. The desire to weed out those thought unworthy of having time wasted on them in the schools led to the first validated tests of intelligence by Wilhelm Stern; even better known and still in use are those by Binet and Simon. The latter knew accurately what their instruments were meant to do and what their limitations were. Binet stated specifically that the tests were intended to predict school performance and the items were oriented primarily to educational achievement. There was no intent to determine some mystical inherent force later to be reified and called "intelligence." Binet would not have been surprised by recent findings that the tests he devised did nothing more than what he originally intended, in spite of the proliferating modifications and additions in the three-quarters of a century which followed. These tests were successful in accomplishing what they set out to do—selecting a sample of the population, largely from the middle class, most apt to learn those attributes necessary to advance a technically developing society. The tests did not predict material success after schooling or identify those who would eventually own or manage the means of production; these achievements rest upon social status and familial, primarily paternal, aid. Binet might even have predicted that society would associate innate inferiority with those who did not achieve high scores on his tests, and high social status and innate superiority with those who did. Social needs have always been more powerful than the studies and findings they set in motion, contradicting or ignoring data if they stand in the way.

Historical changes followed practically the same paths in the United States as abroad. After his European experience, Stanley Hall, the pioneer of academic studies in child development, established the first center at Clark University. There Lewis Terman received his training; with his students at Stanford University he translated, modified and standardized the Binet—Simon tests for American use. He established the long tradition of intelligence testing with which such names as Kuhlman, Goddard, Porteus and later Bayley, Cattell, Wechsler and innumerable others were associated.

Arnold Gesell, who came to Clark during Hall's last years almost contemporaneously with Terman, returned to education after graduation. He was drawn into research by exciting developments in the new field, particularly after he had followed his friend Terman to California. He chose as his area of concentration one that hardly had been touched—the unexplored, difficult, exciting and rapidly changing area of infancy. The concept of development as a unifying basis upon which to construct theories of the origins of behavior began to churn in his mind. Later he was to combine these foundations of knowledge about behavioral growth with findings by others of associated anatomic and physiologic development in the central nervous system; outline, describe and test the patterns over time; and finally establish methods for their use in clinical pediatric neuropsychiatry. In his own words, "But with all my training I lacked a realistic familiarity with the physical basis and the physiological processes of life and growth. To make good this deficit I would have to study medicine."[25] Gesell encountered the intellectual dilemmas with which Wundt and other 19th century and recent neurophysiologic workers had to struggle. All these investigators began with restricted aims "to establish the simplest norms of physiological functioning in such areas as sensation, perception, motor activity and their interactions" but also hoped that "they might offer clues to the various impairments of the nervous system . . ."[25] George Coghill later was to experience these same intellectual problems, and to parallel Gesell in founding a new field of development which attempted to integrate chemical, physiologic, anatomic, embryologic, pathologic and social and cultural variables into a psychology of normal and abnormal behavior.

Gesell went to medical school, first at Wisconsin and then at Yale, where he received his degree approximately a half-century ago and where he was to remain for the rest of his enormously productive life. Studying a large number of normal children and supplementing these observations with those of an even greater number of infants and children who presented developmental deviations and defects, he began the mapping of fetal, infant and early child behavior, establishing and standardizing stages, constructing hypotheses and theories to explain the sequences of behavioral change, and clarifying the assumptions underlying maturation and achievement.

As most scientists before him, Gesell was ever alert to new instrumentation and the assistance it might offer his research, and cinema became a powerful tool for him. Using hundreds of thousands of feet of film over the years, he demonstrated that behavior could be sectioned like a developing embryo, and tested for reliability and then predictability. Development ceased to be a vague abstraction; instead it was an organic process which yielded to scientific analysis and to diagnostic appraisal. He poured forth hundreds of papers, monographs and books, far too numerous to discuss here. His work probably was summarized best in one of his last books, *The Embryology of Behavior,* [26] the theoretical basis for the applied text which follows.

Gesell always was concerned with the welfare of children, both sick and well. He began with one aspect of child care, education, even before his graduate training and research, and expanded his efforts on behalf of children to the areas of mental subnormality, adoption, guidance and justice. When he thought the time and knowledge ripe to apply what he had accumulated for clinical infant and preschool neuropsychiatry, he recruited an outstanding pediatrician, Catherine Amatruda. and together they established a clinical service to use this knowledge for the diagnosis, guidance and teaching of child development. The first edition of *Developmental Diagnosis* was one of their cooperative efforts.

Social forces now are placing a premium upon a periodic appraisal of the developmental assets and liabilities of the growing child. Medical schools, reflecting this trend, are giving increasing attention to the study of the normal organism. Pediatrics in particular is concerned with normal development as well as disease, with prevention as well as cure, and with periodic supervision as well as emergency diagnosis. Infant welfare supervision by organized and integrated services requires a broadened type of protection of the child's growth, attained only through the application of diagnostic, therapeutic and supervisory medicine, and psychologic, social and other applied sciences.

In the United States, the relatively minor progress we have made in behalf of children is being threatened by antiintellectual attitudes and slashes in funding; it cannot be emphasized too strongly that progress is not inevitable and decadence may occur in any field. Pediatrics and neuropsychiatry are largely individualistically oriented and disorganized portions of the social institution of medicine. Child health workers, in their beginning attempts to integrate their efforts with public health preventive, curative and rehabilitative programs, must recognize current trends as retrogressive historic processes. It is incumbent upon them to redouble their efforts to organize and work against these sad changes, to help marshall the educational and political forces of the people they serve in order to reverse the interruption, and to proceed to establish the coordinated health and social service program for children which is so badly needed in this country. In the most affluent nation of the world, and in the history of the planet, infant survival rates have fallen; the United States has dropped in world standing on this crucial criterion of child health and welfare. Equally stunning is the fact that during one year of this decade life expectancy for males in this country decreased. These are but two of the indicators that the funds and priorities of our government have changed.

Both Gesell and Amatruda, with whom we had discussed the organization of child care at length, would have subscribed to the above sentiments. They themselves had felt the need for organized health service, from which they were largely excluded, even in the medical center in which they worked. It is no secret that they were isolated from their colleagues and that they lost sustaining funds from the Rockefeller Foundation long before Gesell retired and Amatruda died.

They knew the terrible pressures of seeking funds to continue their work, and of working under the threat of losing even what they had.

It is in the context of this need for a comprehensive reorganization of health services that the present extension of Gesell and Amatruda's work has been undertaken. In spite of the lip service that has been paid to the importance of development, there has been little advance in its practical incorporation into pediatric training and practice. Pediatric neuropsychiatry has suffered from an overemphasis on psychodynamic formulations which are only beginning to yield to the results of technical advances in the study of nervous system function. Developmental diagnosis is one aspect of medicine which will help establish a scientific behavioral neuropsychiatry that can serve as a core of preventive and therapeutic care.

The present volume is primarily a book on the diagnosis, prognosis and care of developmental problems in infancy. It is in no sense a handbook for intelligence testing or "IQ measurements." It presents the behavioral aspects of developmental maturity from an objective standpoint, comparable to that of clinical neurology. It is the maturity and organization of the central nervous system with which we are concerned, under the rubric of developmental sociopsychoneurology.

To round out the clinical problems, etiologic discussions, particularly of the more common deficits, will be offered; however, it should be clear that this volume is not a general textbook of clinical pediatrics and still less one in metabolism, genetics, embryology, neurophysiology, neuropsychology or neuropsychopharmacology. All of these subjects will be touched upon to the degree necessary to clarify developmental aspects of neuropsychologic disorders. Some etiologic discussions will be at a highly technical level, others at much simpler levels. In all, the clinician will benefit by referral to the technical literature, some of which will be specified in the bibliography.

Another matter of importance to the reader which may prove disconcerting and confusing is usage of words which, like the developing organisms we will discuss, undergo constant change. At times he will encounter words such as "injury" or "damage" when the more general terms "impaired" or "dysfunction" would be more proper. We are not always successful in using the most precise and accurate term possible, but the context usually will indicate the correct meaning. The reader should remember that we are attempting not only changes of addition and subtraction brought about by more than thirty scientifically hectic years, but also a translation of old terms to new ones.

PLAN OF THE VOLUME

A brief statement of the organization of the volume may prove helpful for the preliminary orientation of the reader. The text cleaves consistently to the central problem of diagnosis. Theory helps in understanding developmental changes in both normal and abnormal behavior, but there is no academic elaboration of theory for its own sake.

Part I outlines basic principles and methods, and affords a panoramic view of early child development. The nature of behavior and its development is discussed in Chapter 1. Chapter 3 is the longest and most basic in the book, because it integrates the developmental measures, the behavior characteristics, and the growth trends of the behavior patterns for the period from 4 weeks to 3 years. It describes the stages and procedures in condensed and simplified form to make them available to all students and practitioners. This chapter is organized for convenient reference and is illustrated with over 100 phototracings of scheduled behavior patterns.*

Part II is concerned with the etiology and differential diagnosis of defects and deviations of development, which are interpreted in terms of normal healthy criteria. Basic attention is given to the problem of mental subnormality because of its prime importance in the differential diagnosis of brain dysfunction. We give special attention to the neuromotor aspects of developmental diagnosis in Chapters 9, 10 and 11. They afford an introduction to that vast territory of infant neurology which is not reached by ordinary clinical neurologic methods. Significant differences in clinical manifestations determined separate chapters for low birth weight, seizure disorders, sensory impairments and psychotic behavior. Consideration is given to the effect of these conditions on performance, on trends of development and on personality organization. Illustrative case sketches are included in all these chapters, but the emphasis is varied to do justice to the special problems of diagnosis.

Part III deals with methods of protecting early child development, through organized medical care and public health measures.

The Appendices are virtually a condensed manual of directions for the various developmental evaluation procedures and for setting up examination arrangements. The comprehensive growth trend chart covers a score of age intervals in great detail and is intended as a guide for interpretation of cases which require special study. The application of cinematography and videotape to the recording and analysis of neurologic and developmental conditions also is summarized. Films and videotape are not indispensable, but for the student who wishes to perfect his diagnostic skill, an ideal program of intensive self-instruction would consist of a combination of printed text, clinical experience, videotape recording and review of his own examinations, and cinematic and videotape case studies.

The most effective teachers of all are the infants and children themselves, and healthy subjects are available in abundance for purposeful, systematic observation. The present volume is designed to encourage such observation and make it clinically productive.

*A great debt is owed to Ralph D. Alley for his skillful rendering of these drawings. They were made directly from photographic projections of cinema recordings and had the benefit of Mr. Alley's special interest as a student of medicine at Yale. Dr. Alley now is Clinical Professor of Surgery at the Albany Medical College. Because the original plates were badly worn, his drawings were traced and every attempt made to retain their form intact.

Part I

Principles and Methods

1

The Development
of Behavior

This book deals with problems of development and maturation—with the process and products of growth. Maturation produces progressive changes in structure and closely correlated changes in function. The embryologist is concerned with the formation of bodily organs and systems. The physiologist is concerned with the functioning of these organs and organ systems. The clinician is interested in the individual as a whole—in his total integrated functioning and behavior at all stages of development, in the context of society and its institutions.

§1. BEHAVIOR PATTERNS AND BEHAVIORAL DEVELOPMENT

Behavior is rooted in the brain and in the sensory and motor systems. The timing, smoothness and integration at one age foretell behavior at a later age. An infant with an intact cerebral cortex will continue to have healthy development, providing no noxious organic, psychologic or social events intervene.

Behavior is a convenient term for all the child's reactions, whether reflex, voluntary, spontaneous or learned. He blinks: this is a form of behavior. He reaches for a dangling object: this is behavior. He turns his head to the sound of the human voice: likewise, this is behavior.

A child's body grows, his behavior grows; he comes by his "mind" in the same way that he comes by his body—through the processes of development. As his nervous system undergoes growth differentiations, the forms of his behavior also differentiate. At one age he seizes with his whole hand; at a later age, he plucks with neat opposition of thumb and index finger—neural differentiation produces specialization of function and new behavior.

Development is a patterning process. There is nothing mysterious about this concept; a *behavior pattern* is simply a defined response of the neuromotor system to a specific situation. An eye blink, a knee jerk and a reflex grasp are examples. In postural adjustments and locomotion, such as sitting, creeping, standing and

3

walking, the whole body reacts in behavior patterns. A young baby follows a dangled object with his eyes—this is a behavior pattern. He closes in upon the object with both hands—another pattern with considerable significance at a certain stage of development. An older baby reaches with only one hand; a yet older baby pokes a small object with his extended index finger. Each is a well-defined response of the neuromotor system to a specific situation, each a behavior pattern indicative of a stage of maturity.

Development is subject to diagnosis, because the construction of the action system of the infant and child is an orderly process. Behavior patterns are not whimsical or accidental by-products. The human fetus becomes the human infant; the human infant, the human child and adult. This orderly sequence represents the human genetic endowment. The behavioral end-products of the total developmental process are a consequence of continuing reciprocal interaction between the genetic endowment and the environment. No matter how damaged his developmental potential or how abnormal his function, a child remains uniquely and recognizably human. His behavior patterns take shape in the same manner that the underlying structures take shape. They begin to assume characteristic forms even in the fetal period, for the same reasons that the bodily organs themselves assume characteristic forms. For example, in the 4th week of gestation, limb buds make their appearance. Cells proliferate to form the skeleton, muscles, blood vessels and nerves of arm, forearm and hand. The paddlelike hand transforms into a five-finger hand. At 11 weeks the fingers flex in a reflex grasp. Connections have been formed between nerve fibers and muscle fibers, and a behavior pattern has taken shape.

All behavior patterns, both in prenatal and postnatal life, evolve in a comparable manner. At about the 18th prenatal week the fetal hand grips as well as flexes. At the 40th postnatal week the infant hand extends its index finger to poke and pry. Throughout all infancy this same morphogenesis is at work, creating new forms of behavior, new and more advanced patterns. These patterns are the indices of the maturity and integrity of the infant's nervous system.

§2. THE FIVE FIELDS OF BEHAVIOR

A single behavior pattern, such as prying with the index finger, may have a high degree of diagnostic import. However, the human organism is a complicated action system; adequate developmental diagnosis requires examination of the quality and integration of five fields of behavior, each representing a different aspect of growth. These five major fields are (1) adaptive behavior, (2) gross motor behavior, (3) fine motor behavior, (4) language behavior and (5) personal—social behavior.

ADAPTIVE BEHAVIOR, the most important field, is concerned with the organization of stimuli, the perception of relationships, the dissection of wholes into their component parts and the reintegration of these parts in a meaningful fashion. Included in this field are finer sensorimotor adjustments to objects and situations: the coordination of eyes and hands in reaching and manipulation; the ability to utilize motor equipment appropriately in the solution of practical problems; the capacity to initiate new adjustments in the presence of simple problem situations. Significant behavior patterns will be displayed even in an infant's exploitation of a simple object such as a hand bell. He will reveal growing resourcefulness. Adaptive behavior is the forerunner of later "intelligence," which utilizes previous experience in the solution of new problems.

GROSS MOTOR BEHAVIOR includes postural reactions, head balance, sitting, standing, creeping and walking.

FINE MOTOR BEHAVIOR consists of the use of the hands and fingers in the prehensory approach to, grasping and manipulation of an object. Each field of motor behavior is of special interest to the physician because it has so many neurologic implications. The motor capacities of a child constitute a natural starting point for an estimate of his maturity; however, too often they constitute the only parameters which are evaluated. Motor and adaptive behavior—in fact, all forms of behavior—are intimately interrelated, but they can and must be separated in diagnostic usage.

LANGUAGE BEHAVIOR likewise assumes distinctive patterns which furnish clues to the organization of the child's central nervous system. We use the term broadly to include all visible and audible forms of communication, whether by facial expression, gesture, postural movements, vocalizations, words, phrases or sentences. Language behavior, moreover, includes mimicry and comprehension of the communications of others. Articulate speech is a function which depends upon a social milieu, but which also requires the readiness of sensorimotor and cortical structures. Preverbal phases prepare for the verbal phases. Inarticulate vocalizations and vocal signs precede words, which are learned from and reinforced by others in the environment. The underlying stages, in the absence of distorting neurologic or environmental factors, are as orderly as those observed in the fields of adaptive and motor behavior.

PERSONAL—SOCIAL BEHAVIOR comprises the child's personal reactions to the social culture in which he lives. These reactions are so multitudinous, variegated and contingent upon environment that they might seem to be beyond the reach of developmental diagnosis. But as in the other four fields, these behavior patterns are determined by intrinsic growth factors. Bladder and bowel control, for example, are cultural requirements, shaped by social demands, but their attainment depends upon the child's neuromotor maturity. This relationship obtains for many of the child's abilities and attitudes: feeding abilities, self-dependence in play, cooperation and responsiveness to training and social conventions. Even though personal—social behavior is particularly subject to societal goals and individual variations, the variations have normal limits and diagnostic implications.

These five areas of behavior form the basic fabric of his behavior repertoire, but equally important is *how* he demonstrates his developmental maturity. Are his sensory modalities of sight, hearing and touch intact? If he has motor or sensory handicaps, has he developed alternate pathways for the expression of his comprehension of the world? How organized and integrated are his responses, his attention and his discrimination? Is he thoughtful, or impulsive and haphazard? Are his emotional responses stable or fragile? Are they appropriate to the situation and his age? What is his level of tolerance to frustration? Finally, are convulsive seizures or specific disease entities or syndromes present?

The task of behavioral observation entails both quantitative and qualitative evaluation; moreover, behavioral observation *always* must be supplemented by adequate social and medical history and appropriate laboratory investigations.

§3. THE DEVELOPMENTAL DIAGNOSIS OF BEHAVIOR

Behavior develops. Normal behavior assumes characteristic patterns as it develops. The principles and practice of developmental diagnosis rest on these simple far-reaching propositions. Developmental diagnosis consists of a discriminating observation of behavior patterns and their appraisal by comparison with normal behavior patterns; A *normal behavior pattern* is a criterion of maturity which has been defined by systematic studies of the average healthy course of behavioral development. Study of thousands of healthy infants and young children has enabled us to ascertain the average trends of their behavioral development. We find that (a) the sequences of development, i.e., the order in which behavior patterns appear, and (b) the chronologic age at which each pattern appears, are significantly uniform. Of course, we also have noted the ranges of individual variation, but these variations cling closely to a central mean. With few exceptions, the term *normal* is used in its connotation of *healthy* in this volume.

We cannot measure a child's development with absolute precision, because there is no absolute unit. However, a series of such stages of maturity can serve as a measuring rod or calibrated scale. Consequently, we can think of behavior in terms of age, and age in terms of behavior. Developmental diagnosis translates behavior, by comparison with normal patterns, into equivalent age values.*

To illustrate these principles, we can consider a highly effective procedure for the diagnosis of fine motor coordination: A small sugar pellet is placed before a baby; he is sitting up (with support), and the pellet is in easy reach on a table surface. He rakes at the pellet with a scratchlike flexion of his fingers. Now the same behavior situation is presented to another baby. He approaches the pellet with extended index finger and plucks it forcepslike between index and thumb. How

---

*The original procedure which was used in determining the age-appropriate placement of the individual behavior patterns is discussed in the preface to Chapter 3. The correction for chronologic age necessary in case of a gestation of less than 40 weeks is discussed in Chapter 12, on low birth weight.

shall we evaluate the maturity status evidenced by each of these two behavior patterns? We can say that the raking reaction is cruder than the plucking reaction, but this tells us nothing about the actual maturity of the responses. If we consult the notches in our measuring rod, we find that the raking reaction is characteristic (typical) of a healthy 28-week infant, and that plucking is characteristic (typical) of a healthy 40-week infant. Accordingly, if the baby who raked is chronologically 40 weeks old, he certainly is *abnormal* with respect to prehensory maturity. If he is 28 weeks old, all is well for the area of behavior which is sampled by this prehension situation. Thus, developmental diagnosis is an appraisal of observed patterns in terms of normal patterns, expressed in terms of age.

In practice, diagnosis never rests on an isolated item. All areas of behavior must be sampled by a sufficient variety of procedures, and supplemented by clinical judgment. The system of developmental diagnosis will describe appropriate situations and provide detailed behavior patterns for each of the five major fields of behavior. On the average, adaptive, gross motor, fine motor, language and personal–social behavior develop abreast. The five fields are closely related and overlap, but in atypical development there are often discrepancies between fields. A child may be advanced in one field and relatively retarded in another. The first task of developmental diagnosis is to discover and to specify such imbalances in the child's behavioral repetoire. Corollary tasks are to attribute etiology and to intervene with specific therapeutic or remedial measures and general management programs. Typical behavior patterns enable us to formulate what we see in the child's total behavior picture, in terms of maturity levels; this in turn forms the basis for a diagnostic interpretation of the child's overall developmental status.

Development is a continuous process; in complicated or doubtful conditions, two or even more examinations at successive ages may be necessary to determine the tempo and trend of a child's development. If we examine him at 28 weeks and again at 40 weeks, we can see whether the two successive behavior pictures agree with each other. We compare the child with himself, or more accurately, we compare two cross-sectional determinations of his maturity at two distinct ages. Thus, developmental diagnosis also requires an orderly critical method of comparison, with matching of observations and stages. When the matching is guided and supplemented by ample clinical experience, it has the validity of true measurement.

§4. STAGES AND SEQUENCES OF DEVELOPMENT

Beginning with conception, a child's development proceeds stage by stage in orderly sequence, each stage representing a degree or level of maturity. There are so many such levels that we must select a few which will serve best as a frame of reference for diagnostic purposes. These *key ages* are 4, 16, 28, 40 and 52 weeks, 18, 24 and 36 months. They represent integrative periods and major shifts in focus and centers of organization. The key age of 52 weeks is an important chronologic milestone to parents. Developmentally, it is characterized by the incipient emergence of more mature patterns. The massive integration of these patterns comes to fruition at 15 months. The placement of 15 months in a side column rather than in a central key age position on the developmental schedules is an adventitious result of the number of ages selected for study and the number of columns in which to locate them.

To appreciate the developmental significance of these key ages, we depict their positions in the early cycle of human growth in Figs. 1-1 through 1-6. Figure 1-1 gives a comprehensive view of the entire scope of development, including the fetal period, to indicate the continuity of the growth cycle. Cognizance also should be given to preconceptional origins of development, including specific inherited disorders and a variety of environmental influences upon ova and spermatozoa.

The actual organization of behavior begins long before birth, and the general direction of this organization is simultaneously from head to foot and from proximal to distal segments. Lips and tongue are first, eye muscles follow, then neck, shoulder, arms, hands, fingers, trunk, legs and feet. Figure 1-1 reflects this law of developmental direction, and suggests that the five distinguishable fields of behavior develop conjointly in close coordination.

In brief terms, the trends of behavioral development in broad approximations of age ranges are as follows:

In the *first quarter* of the first year the infant gains control of his 12 oculomotor muscles.

In the *second quarter* (16–28 weeks) he comes into command of the muscles which support his head and upper trunk and move his arms and hands. He reaches out for, grasps, transfers and manipulates things. His head is erect and steady.

In the *third quarter* (28–40 weeks) he gains command of his trunk and fingers. He pokes and plucks, sits and creeps.

In the *fourth quarter* (40–52 weeks) he extends command to his legs and feet and discards accessory support for his hands and fingers. He plucks a pellet with adult precision. He stands and walks with support.

In the *second year* he walks and runs, articulates words and phrases, acquires bowel and bladder control and attains a rudimentary sense of personal identity.

Between the second and third years he speaks in sentences, using words as tools of thought. He shows a positive propensity to understand his environment and to comply with cultural demands. He is no longer a mere infant.

In the *fourth year* he asks innumerable questions, perceives analogies and displays an active tendency to conceptualize and generalize. He is nearly self-dependent in routines of home life.

In the *fifth year* he is well matured in motor control. He hops and skips. He talks without infantile articulation and narrates a long tale. He prefers associative play and feels socialized pride in clothes and accomplishment.

Figures 1-2 through 1-6 diagram sequences of development from birth in the adaptive, gross motor, fine motor, language and personal–social fields of behavior.

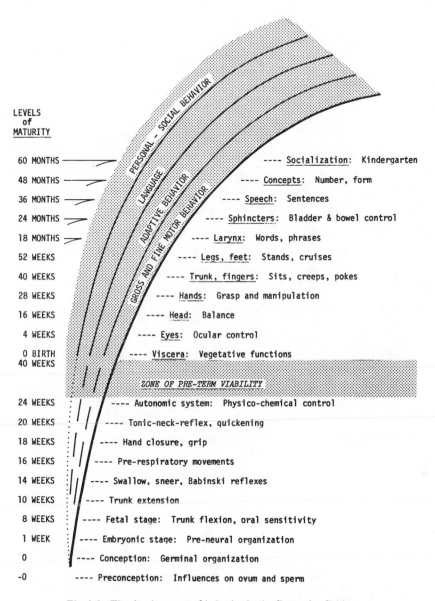

LEVELS
of
MATURITY

60 MONTHS ---- Socialization: Kindergarten

48 MONTHS ---- Concepts: Number, form

36 MONTHS ---- Speech: Sentences

24 MONTHS ---- Sphincters: Bladder & bowel control

18 MONTHS ---- Larynx: Words, phrases

52 WEEKS ---- Legs, feet: Stands, cruises

40 WEEKS ---- Trunk, fingers: Sits, creeps, pokes

28 WEEKS ---- Hands: Grasp and manipulation

16 WEEKS ---- Head: Balance

4 WEEKS ---- Eyes: Ocular control

0 BIRTH ---- Viscera: Vegetative functions
40 WEEKS

ZONE OF PRE-TERM VIABILITY

24 WEEKS ---- Autonomic system: Physico-chemical control

20 WEEKS ---- Tonic-neck-reflex, quickening

18 WEEKS ---- Hand closure, grip

16 WEEKS ---- Pre-respiratory movements

14 WEEKS ---- Swallow, sneer, Babinski reflexes

10 WEEKS ---- Trunk extension

8 WEEKS ---- Fetal stage: Trunk flexion, oral sensitivity

1 WEEK ---- Embryonic stage: Pre-neural organization

0 ---- Conception: Germinal organization

-0 ---- Preconception: Influences on ovum and sperm

Fig. 1-1. The development of behavior in the five major fields.

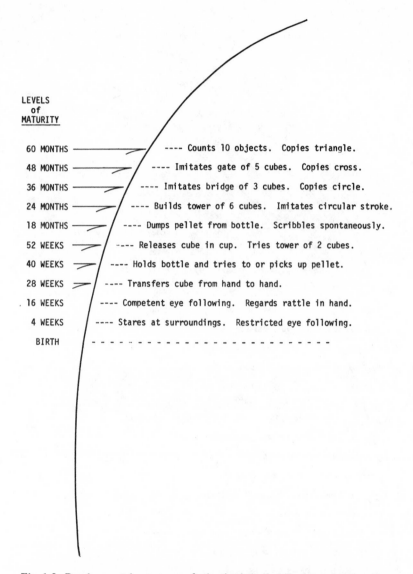

LEVELS
of
MATURITY

60 MONTHS ———————————— ---- Counts 10 objects. Copies triangle.

48 MONTHS ——————— ---- Imitates gate of 5 cubes. Copies cross.

36 MONTHS ————— ---- Imitates bridge of 3 cubes. Copies circle.

24 MONTHS ————— ---- Builds tower of 6 cubes. Imitates circular stroke.

18 MONTHS ————— ---- Dumps pellet from bottle. Scribbles spontaneously.

52 WEEKS ——— ---- Releases cube in cup. Tries tower of 2 cubes.

40 WEEKS —— ---- Holds bottle and tries to or picks up pellet.

28 WEEKS — ---- Transfers cube from hand to hand.

. 16 WEEKS   ---- Competent eye following. Regards rattle in hand.

4 WEEKS   ---- Stares at surroundings. Restricted eye following.

BIRTH   -

Fig. 1-2. Developmental sequences of adaptive behavior. To determine how the infant exploits the environment we present him with a variety of simple objects. The small one-inch cubes serve not only to test motor coordination, but also reveal the child's capacity to put his motor equipment to constructive and adaptive ends. The cube tests create an objective opportunity for the examiner to observe adaptivity in action–motor coordination combined with judgment.

Such tests illustrate the principles which also underlie the developmental diagnosis of behavior in the motor, language and personal–social fields.

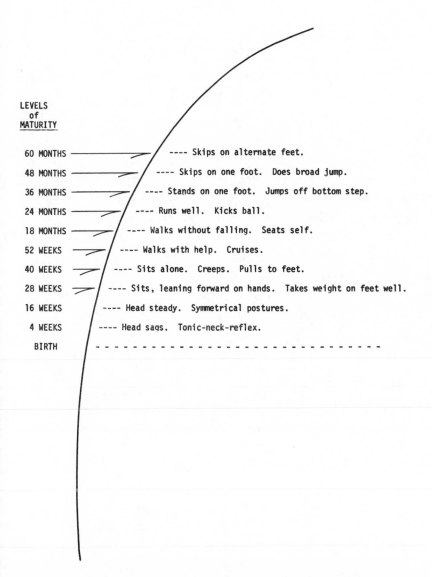

LEVELS
of
MATURITY

60 MONTHS ———————————————— ---- Skips on alternate feet.

48 MONTHS ——————————————— ---- Skips on one foot. Does broad jump.

36 MONTHS —————————————— ---- Stands on one foot. Jumps off bottom step.

24 MONTHS ———————————— ---- Runs well. Kicks ball.

18 MONTHS ——————————— ---- Walks without falling. Seats self.

52 WEEKS ————————— ---- Walks with help. Cruises.

40 WEEKS ———————— ---- Sits alone. Creeps. Pulls to feet.

28 WEEKS —————— ---- Sits, leaning forward on hands. Takes weight on feet well.

16 WEEKS ---- Head steady. Symmetrical postures.

4 WEEKS ---- Head sags. Tonic-neck-reflex.

BIRTH -

Fig. 1-3. Developmental sequences of gross motor behavior. To ascertain the maturity of postural control, we institute formal postural tests which reveal the repertoire of the infant's behavior: supine, prone, sitting and standing.

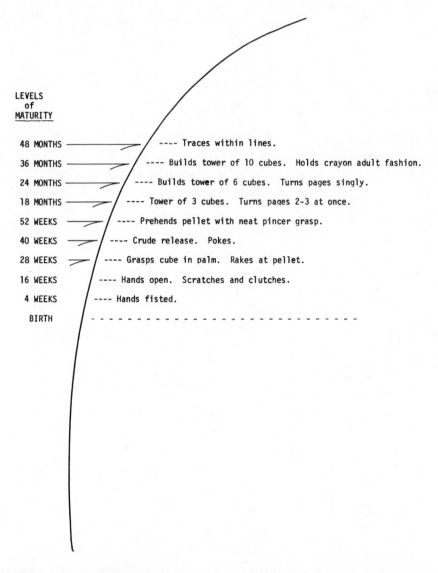

**LEVELS
of
MATURITY**

48 MONTHS ──────── ---- Traces within lines.

36 MONTHS ──────── ---- Builds tower of 10 cubes. Holds crayon adult fashion.

24 MONTHS ──────── ---- Builds tower of 6 cubes. Turns pages singly.

18 MONTHS ──────── ---- Tower of 3 cubes. Turns pages 2-3 at once.

52 WEEKS ──────── ---- Prehends pellet with neat pincer grasp.

40 WEEKS ──────── ---- Crude release. Pokes.

28 WEEKS ──────── ---- Grasps cube in palm. Rakes at pellet.

16 WEEKS ──────── ---- Hands open. Scratches and clutches.

4 WEEKS ──────── ---- Hands fisted.

BIRTH ──────── -

Fig. 1-4. Developmental sequences of fine motor behavior. Fine motor control is evaluated by using small objects such as cubes, pellet and string to elicit patterns of varying degrees of manual control.

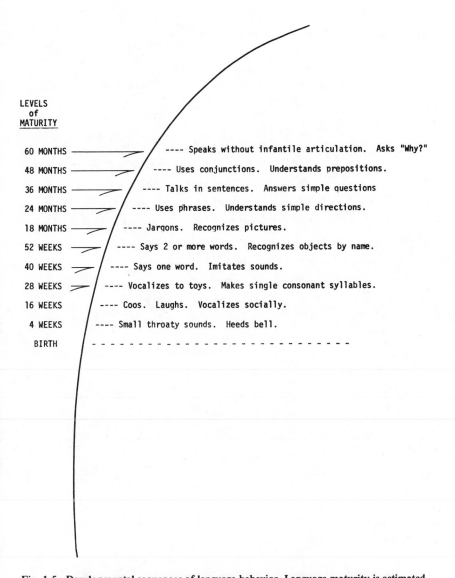

LEVELS
of
MATURITY

60 MONTHS ———————————————— ---- Speaks without infantile articulation. Asks "Why?"

48 MONTHS ———————————— ---- Uses conjunctions. Understands prepositions.

36 MONTHS ——————— ---- Talks in sentences. Answers simple questions

24 MONTHS ————— ---- Uses phrases. Understands simple directions.

18 MONTHS ——— ---- Jargons. Recognizes pictures.

52 WEEKS —— ---- Says 2 or more words. Recognizes objects by name.

40 WEEKS —— ---- Says one word. Imitates sounds.

28 WEEKS —— ---- Vocalizes to toys. Makes single consonant syllables.

16 WEEKS ---- Coos. Laughs. Vocalizes socially.

4 WEEKS ---- Small throaty sounds. Heeds bell.

BIRTH

Fig. 1-5. Developmental sequences of language behavior. Language maturity is estimated in terms of articulation, vocabulary, adaptive use and comprehension. During the course of a developmental examination, both spontaneous and responsive language behavior is observed. Valuable supplementary information also is secured by questioning the adult familiar with the child's everyday behavior at home.

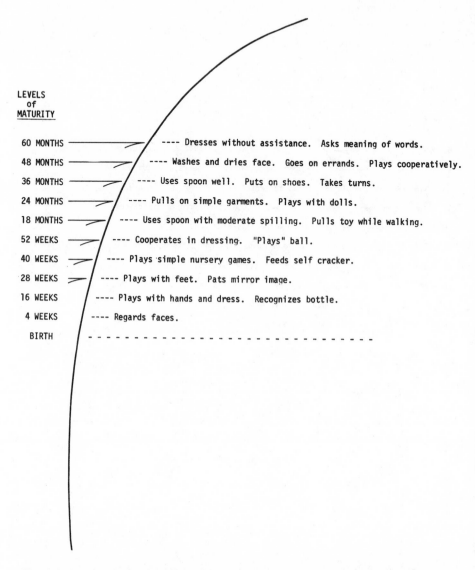

LEVELS
of
MATURITY

60 MONTHS ——————————————— ---- Dresses without assistance. Asks meaning of words.

48 MONTHS ————————————— ---- Washes and dries face. Goes on errands. Plays cooperatively.

36 MONTHS ——————————— ---- Uses spoon well. Puts on shoes. Takes turns.

24 MONTHS ——————— ---- Pulls on simple garments. Plays with dolls.

18 MONTHS —————— ---- Uses spoon with moderate spilling. Pulls toy while walking.

52 WEEKS ———— ---- Cooperates in dressing. "Plays" ball.

40 WEEKS ——— ---- Plays simple nursery games. Feeds self cracker.

28 WEEKS —— ---- Plays with feet. Pats mirror image.

16 WEEKS   ---- Plays with hands and dress. Recognizes bottle.

4 WEEKS   ---- Regards faces.

BIRTH   -

Fig. 1-6. Developmental sequences of personal—social behavior. Personal—social behavior is greatly affected by the temperament of the child and by the behavior of the parents or others by whom he is reared. The range of individual variation is wide. Nevertheless, maturity factors and the degree of intactness of the central nervous system play a role in the socialization of the child. His social conduct is ascertained by incidental observation and by inquiry. The chart illustrates types of behavior which may be considered in evaluating the interaction of environmental influences and developmental readiness.

These five fields develop interdependently, and an adequate estimate of behavioral maturity demands an appraisal of each major field. Each figure shows selected behavior patterns which illustrate the progressions of normal healthy development. These patterns also give a preliminary suggestion of the practical application of the behavioral sequences in developmental diagnosis.

2

The Developmental Assessment of Behavior

All forms of clinical pediatrics, neurology, sociopsychology and psychiatry which are concerned with the developmental welfare of infants and young children must take behavior patterns into account. Behavior patterns are indicators. A developmental assessment is essentially an appraisal of the *maturity* and *integrity* of the child's nervous system, with the aid of behavioral stages and information about past and present history.

§1. OBSERVATION OF BEHAVIORAL DEVELOPMENT

Developmental assessment has an important place in the protection and preventive care of normal children. It may be incorporated readily into the supervision of infant well-being and the periodic health examinations made by nurse, general practitioner and pediatrician. Such routine behavioral observation permits early detection of any abnormalities. In the first years of life, it is particularly important that case histories of children include concrete dated observations of behavioral capacities and development. There are three ways in which such behavioral data can be secured: by interview, by periodic screening examinations and by a detailed formal evaluation.

An interview involves brief but incisive questioning of the parent or adult familiar with the child's everyday life. Methodically undertaken, the interview will supply concrete behavior items in each of the five major fields of behavior, as well as the social context in which they developed. The interview also is a necessary preliminary to behavioral assessment. A standardized developmental inventory should be an essential and routine feature of every pediatric visit, whether done at home, in the doctor's office, in a well-baby clinic, or on a hospital ward. The techniques for conducting a productive interview are considered in detail in Chapters 4 and 17, and Appendix A-6.

When the infant is acting at or above his age level in all areas of behavior, periodic screening interviews are adequate (Chapter 17, The Developmental Screening Inventory). Usually the interviewer will be able to observe the child at the same time. When this informal observation appears to contradict the history, or when the history indicates any deviation, then direct observation of the child's behavior is necessary. The Developmental Screening Inventory examination may suffice, but a formal evaluation is indispensable in all conditions which require differential diagnosis: neurologic complications, retardation in any area of behavior, mental defect, behavior disorders, communication and visual disabilities, or problems of child adoption and institutional commitment.

Chapter 3 outlines the behavior situations and the general techniques which are used in the formal examination of infants and young children from 4 weeks to 3 years of age. Specific procedures for the individual behavior situations are detailed in Appendix A-4. Chapter 4 is a general discussion of all the aspects of conducting a developmental assessment. In some instances of developmental defect and deviation, a single examination may not always suffice; periodic screening and formal assessments which will bring a series of diagnoses into cumulative comparison may be required.

§2. THE FUNCTION OF DEVELOPMENTAL ASSESSMENT

The physician is concerned with the maturity and health of an infant or child; he has the responsibility for making a diagnosis, even if it is one of no disease. He is not asked to derive an IQ, or measure "intelligence" as such. It is his task to assess central nervous system function: to identify the presence of any neuromotor or sensory deficit, to discover the existence of treatable developmental disorders, to detect infants at risk of subsequent deterioration, and to determine pathologic conditions of the brain which preclude normal intellectual function, no matter how optimal the environmental circumstances. He is exercising his responsibility of protecting the total growth of the child under his care. To effect this protection he makes an analytic assessment of behavior.

Behavioral tests have the same logic as any of the functional tests of clinical neurology, such as the finger test for coordination, the cover test for pupillary response, and the tendon tap for a jerk reflex. They are designed to establish normality and to reveal even minor deviations in relatively healthy children. Since most of the defects and diseases of infancy and early childhood are not localized lesions occurring in an already mature central nervous system, the areas of dysfunction are not revealed by standard adult neurologic examinations. Therefore, behavioral evaluation may be more competent in disclosing significant lesions, defects, distortions, and retardations in the organization of the developing nervous system.

The situations of the developmental evaluation bring out characteristic reactions, at specific ages, which would not be forthcoming at all using more artificial procedures. Behavioral assessment in each of the five major areas—adaptive, gross motor, fine motor, language, and personal—social—open the infant to opportunistic observation. They call into play his organs of vision, hearing, touch and proprioception. They make a wide range of demands upon motor coordination, and inevitably call into requisition the higher cortical controls. For these reasons, they comprise both a maturity assessment and a neuromotor and sensory examination, and permit differentiation and detailed exploration of both normal and abnormal responses.

The *developmental, neuromotor* and *sensory* objectives of this evaluation cannot be divorced. The infant's behavior must be surveyed and appraised in terms of his true chronologic age. This behavior may prove normal, it may show general retardation in maturation, or it may show deviations which are so distinctive that they point to faults in neural structure or to impairments in central nervous system integration. There are no right or wrong behavioral responses, or successes or failures, because the examination is concerned with the infant's behavioral status. Any response in adaptive behavior is appropriate to some age or level of central nervous system function.

Because of the generally amorphous character of neonatal behavior, diagnosis and prediction of cortical integrity from this period of life are not possible. Responses at 1 and 4 weeks are essentially similar; even at 4 weeks of age, the infant's behavior has validity only for gross abnormality and group predictiveness related to high risk factors, such as low birth weight or a low Apgar score. With release from the domination of the tonic-neck-reflex by 16 weeks, adaptive behavior as an indicator of cortical intactness is already predictive of later behavior. This initial crudity is replaced by greater precision with time. The optimal period for evaluation is 40 weeks, when all parts of the body have come under some degree of voluntary control, and compensation for minor disabilities has not yet occurred. In the first year of life, behavior is for the most part uninfluenced by social environmental factors and is dependent primarily on the intactness of the infant's central nervous system—unless the environmental factors are grossly deviant (starvation or marked malnutrition, abuse, institutionalization, dysstimulation, etc.).

§3. EXAMINATION ARRANGEMENTS

Arrangements for a developmental evaluation of behavior require only a slight adaptation of conventional office furniture. The minimal physical requirements are (a) a free flat surface on which the child may display postural and other gross motor capacities, and (b) the restricted surface of a small test table on which toys may be placed to elicit adaptive and fine motor behavior. At early ages, the top of an ordinary examining table provides the flat surface on which the infant lies, sits or stands. The working surface for the presentation of the examination objects is supplied by a low portable test table, similar to a bed tray, placed on the examining table. At later ages, the child is provided with a nursery-size chair and table, and the floor becomes the arena for displaying postural control.

This statement of minimal requirements, with its emphasis on *surfaces,* indicates an important basic principle: all physical surfaces which impinge on the child are part and parcel of an examination setup. The surroundings must not be taken for granted or overlooked; they are part of the stimulating apparatus. We wish to know how the child reacts to the stimuli of horizontal and vertical surfaces, of restricted and unrestricted surfaces, and of objects in relation to surfaces. Even when we place a young infant supine, we prepare to make a behavioral assessment. We observe his spontaneous reactions to all the stimuli which arise, including the tactile pressures of the surface on which he lies. This principle applies to all stages of postural control.

Figure 2-1 shows how the examination arrangements are adapted to the ascending grades of postural control: supine, supported sitting, free sitting and chair sitting. These arrangements are simple but effective. A more elaborate setup, which includes a supportive examining chair and a special examining crib, is described in Appendix C.

For an adequate developmental evaluation, the infant or child must cooperate and participate in the examination situation. Hunger and sleepiness may interfere, particularly at the earliest ages. Fear and fragility also may negate an adequate performance. Care must be taken to allow sufficient time for acceptance of the examiner and the examining situation, without an abrupt and domineering instrusion. Patience at the beginning usually is rewarded; for most children, the examination objects have such an overwhelming appeal that sooner or later their reluctance is overcome.

§4. EXAMINATION MATERIALS

The materials required for a developmental examination also are simple, and easily contained in a kit or a table drawer. The full complement of these objects is pictured in Fig. 2-2. A detailed list of the materials also is provided in Appendix A-1. In most instances, the objects are presented on the test table singly in a prescribed order. A few are presented while the child is in the supine position, or while he is on his feet. The child reacts to these objects as though they were play materials, and they are. But for the examiner, they constitute *controlled devices* for eliciting behavior patterns indicative of developmental status. Examination materials and physical surfaces are types of stimulation which excite the infant's nervous system to characteristic responses at characteristic ages.

Each object is applied as a specialized tool charged with specific stimulus powers. Strictly speaking, it is the child who is charged with the various forms of

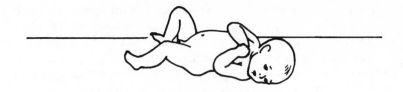

4- and 16-week zones

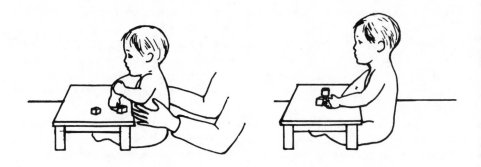

16- and 28-week zones   **40-week to 15-month zones**

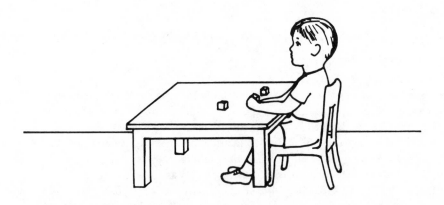

18 months and older

Fig. 2-1. Examination arrangements adapted to advancing grades of postural maturity: supine, supported sitting, free sitting and chair sitting.

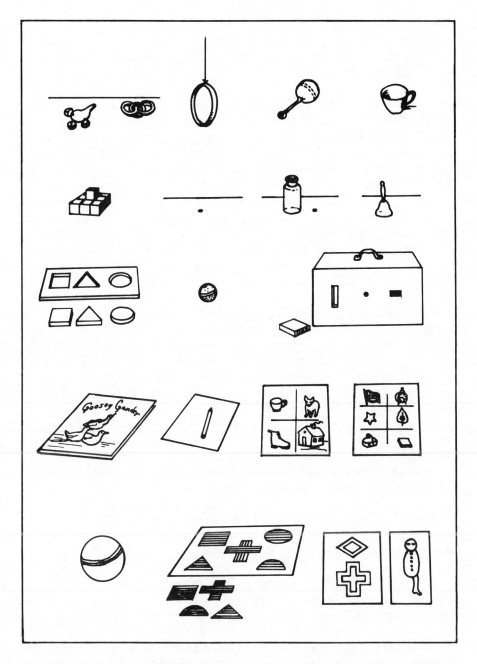

Fig. 2-2. Examination materials: Catbells and tricolored rings, dangling ring, rattle, cup, cubes, pellet, pellet and bottle, bell, formboard and 3 blocks, small ball, performance box with square block, picture book, paper and crayon, picture cards, large ball, color forms, double diamond and cross, incomplete man.

reactiveness; the examination materials are activators which release discharges of patterned and learned responses. This important principle can be illustrated by describing the stimulus values or incitements which are latent in a few typical objects and situations.

CUBES. Red wooden 1-inch cubes have almost universal appeal throughout infancy and early childhood. Their color, size, shape, weight, and texture release the very reactions which we wish to elicit: grasping when placed in the infant's hand (4 weeks); ocular fixation when placed on the table (16 weeks); prehension on sight by palmar grasp (28 weeks); prehension by digital grasp (40 weeks). The cube does not change its configuration from age to age, but it does alter the configuration of the child's reactions. The geometric shape of the cube helps us to differentiate between shapes of behavior, e.g., between gross and fine prehension as exemplified by palmar contrasted with digital grasp. Moreover, the cube is capable of exciting increasingly sophisticated exploitation, such as banging, mouthing, biting, inspection, brushing, releasing and casting. These increasing refinements of exploitation are clues to the increasing refinements in the organization of the child's nervous system.

We present the cubes singly, consecutively (1, 2, 3), in a cluster of 10, and in constructed models for imitation. Thus the stimulus values of the cubes multiply enormously and unlock the answers to many neuropsychologic questions. Can the child retain one cube and still give heed to a second? Can he retain two cubes and attend to a third? Can he bring two cubes into relationship, or does he exploit one with exclusive preoccupation? Can he place a cube in a container, the cup? Can he release it? If he has a realization of container and contained, has he also an appreciation of "on top of," and "side by side?" Does he perceive spatial relationships sufficiently to erect a tower, lay a wall and build a bridge? At 4 weeks he merely can grip a cube when it is thrust into his palm. At 3 years he can build a bridge in imitation. The cubes constitute a powerful instrument for establishing the developmental gradients which lie between 4 weeks and 3 years.

PELLET. This likewise serves to differentiate more refined ocular fixation, and to establish progressive grades of thumb opposition. Being tiny and round, it holds distinctive stimulus values.

PELLET AND BOTTLE. When we place a pellet beside a bottle, we are creating a behavior situation surcharged with rival stimuli which are bound to evoke revealing responses. These responses will evidence the child's interests and the span and course of his attention. Does his attention go exclusively to the bottle, or is he more interested in the pellet? Does he understand the relationship of container and contained? Does he comprehend the glass barrier? Does he tilt the bottle adaptively to expel the pellet? Once the examiner conceives of the objects as effective touchstones for neuropsychologic analysis, every object which the child exploits, be it cube, pellet, paper, string or cereal, will take on diagnostic significance.

BELL. This is another object which is sufficiently diversified in its physical makeup to disclose gradations of response. It comprises a cylindric handle, a conic bowl and a swinging lever, the clapper; optically, a contrast in dark handle and silvery metal; tactually, a hard rim; statically, a low center of gravity; a right-side up; and a sound effect for the ears. The very construction of the bell induces transfer from hand to hand, gross mouthing of the nipplelike end of the handle and even drinking from the bowl; it also induces inquisitive exploration by eyes and fingers. As the child matures, he pays differentiating attention to the varied components of the bell. Does he seize the bell grossly at the junction of handle and bowl, or does he grasp it digitally at the top of the handle? Does he place it vertically on the table top? Does he thrust out his index finger to investigate clapper and cavity? Does he heed sound by bodily immobilization, or by head turning? Does he initiate the sound by waving the bell spontaneously, or by imitation? To the perspicacious examiner the bell is not merely a bell. It is a complex thing of many facets, which divulges the neuropsychologic facets of the child.

BALL. Like the cube, this is a basic examination object, but it has physical properties quite unlike those of the cube; it has a minimum of stability. We capitalize upon its mobility by making it a medium of social interchange between examiner and child. In the give and take of to-and-fro ball play, a supercharged social situation is set up in which the examiner himself becomes a kind of test object. The ball thus becomes a device for revealing not only the motor aptitudes of the infant but also the maturity of his social behavior.

CRIB. This is an examination object, just as truly as is the pellet. It arouses the gross muscles rather than accessory musculature of finger and thumb; nevertheless, it is a configured entity in a physical world. It presents a circumscribed horizontal flat surface and four panels of vertical surface. Does the infant prefer the horizontal or the vertical? How does he adapt to the vertical? How does he deploy his hands and feet if he assumes an upright posture? What is his stance? What are his powers of aided and unaided locomotion?

The examination materials almost appear to have a simple intrinsic attraction. They are almost self-operative. The stimulus values of the objects are, of course, influenced by the manner in which they are presented to the child. Distractions are reduced to a minimum if the examiner takes a somewhat retired position at the child's side, so that the child's attention will favor the working surface of the test table. The examiner places the objects on this surface within easy reach for exploitation. The presentation is accomplished in a quiet, restrained manner which is calculated and timed to focus the child's attention on the object. When presented with a balance of deference, freedom and control, they give the child an ample opportunity to reveal his developmental status and his neuromotor organization. The principles and techniques of behavioral evaluation are elaborated further in Chapters 3 and 4.

In the first edition of this book, the placement of the behavior patterns presented in Chapter 3 was based on the age when approximately 50% of infants achieved success, giving consideration to whether the pattern discriminated between adjacent age levels and was increasing, decreasing or focal. The derivation of these developmental schedules differed from procedures used in establishing psychometric test norms. Children with evidence of central nervous system dysfunction were excluded. This is the approach used in the establishment of "normal" values in any area of medicine; individuals with disease are excluded. As has been stated already, the term *normal* in this volume is, with few exceptions, used in its connotation of *healthy*. The word "he" is used generically to mean "the child" or "the professional person" of either sex.

While the descriptions of behavior may read rigidly or dogmatically, all should be interpreted as meaning the usual or average behavior. A further word of caution is necessary regarding the descriptions of behavior. After the age of 15 or 18 months they apply largely to white children raised in middle- and upper-class environments. Behaviors differing from those described are not necessarily indications of developmental defects; rather they may signify differing parental or social mores. Those examination items most socially determined may be biased in favor of white middle-class populations. These social allusions are far from academic; they concern developmental diagnosis. The developmental diagnostician must distinguish the effects of brain damage or impairment, of social differences in rearing and of social and psychologic damage. He also must prescribe remediation when clinical abnormality is present. Decisions of such importance require careful consideration of individual and sociocultural variation.

In the decades since the schedules were delineated, examination of thousands of infants in different settings has indicated that acceleration in the rate of maturation has occurred. Without systematic investigation of an additional healthy population at each age, it is not possible to change arbitrarily the age placement of behavior patterns. Until such a study can be completed, the clinician must continue to relate his observations to the presently available data.

No significant violence will be done to the major function of developmental diagnosis—the clinical detection and specification of abnormalities—by the necessary reliance on the material which will be set forth. Growth trends, interrelationships and integrations have not altered. Moreover, the discussions of differential diagnosis and the variety of clinical entities in Part II of this volume will make it clear that quantification of behavior is but one aspect of diagnosis. When an infant with abnormal signs and symptoms achieves age-appropriate behavior, more weight must be given to the abnormalities in arriving at a diagnosis.

3

Stages of Development

To grasp the characteristics of child development, we must think in terms of behavior patterns, maturity stages and growth trends. The present chapter is organized to facilitate such thinking, by giving a panoramic view of the stream of *normal* development in the first 3 years of life. It also supplies a cross-sectional view of that stream at eight strategic points or key ages: 4, 16, 28, 40 and 52 weeks, 18, 24 and 36 months. There are brief added comments for 48 and 60 months. These key ages hold a prominent place in developmental diagnosis; they represent the basic stages of maturity to which observed behavior can be referred for appraisal. The discussion for each key age furnishes a guide for defining the behavioral examination, for identifying observed behavior patterns and for interpreting their developmental significance in terms of normal patterns. With these ages well in mind, the student will be oriented, and have the working knowledge of normal development necessary for an understanding of defects and deviations.

§1. ORGANIZATION OF THE CHAPTER

To emphasize the continuity of development and the essential similarity of examination methods, each key age is treated in the same manner:

ACTION DRAWINGS. Action pictures portray the behavior patterns that are diagnostically significant. The pictures are authentic tracings of film records of actual children.* These behavior patterns are representative and typical; they delineate the kinds of reactions elicited by developmental examination.

NARRATIVE TEXT. The accompanying text provides a condensed narrative picture of the developmental examination and of typical behavior for each key age. In the text, each examination situation is indicated by the words spelled in capital letters. *Italics* are used to specify all behavior which appears characteristically for

*Motion picture films available as important instructional aids are described in Appendix D.

25

the first time at each key age. The numbers which appear in the text refer to the action picture corresponding to the behavior described.

EXAMINATION SEQUENCE. For each key age, the narrative text is summarized by a tabulation of the order in which the examination situations are carried out. The situation numbers refer to the detailed description of the examination procedures found in Appendix A-4. Reference also should be made to Appendix A-3 and Section 2 of Chapter 4, where the individual sequences are collated into a single table and the general approach to the evaluation discussed.

DEVELOPMENTAL SCHEDULE. The developmental schedule codifies behavior patterns for diagnostic application. It is especially advantageous to consider a key age in relation to the two age levels immediately adjacent—the next younger and older. Accordingly, each schedule lists the behavior characteristics of the key age and its two adjacent ages in three vertical columns. The key age occupies the central position. Horizontally, the behavior characteristics are grouped by the five major behavioral fields—adaptive, gross motor, fine motor, language and personal—social. This arrangement permits ready cross-comparison in terms of kinds of behavior as well as levels of maturity.

The behavior patterns arrayed in a single age column should not be regarded as isolated "test" items. They are closely correlated and must be considered a compact organic characterization of the behavior typical for that age. These behavior patterns are the diagnositic criteria for evaluating observed behavior. Two kinds of patterns appear: (1) *permanent patterns* which come to stay or augment, and (2) *temporary patterns* which give way or transform into different and more advanced patterns at later ages. A child builds a tower of two cubes at 15 months, one of three at 18 months. This is clearly a permanent type of behavior pattern. An infant of 12 weeks sits supported with bobbing head, and one of 16 weeks sits with head steady. Steadiness supersedes the temporary pattern of bobbing and is permanent. A temporary pattern is indicated on the developmental schedules by an asterisk, followed by the age at which it is replaced by a more mature pattern of the same nature. A complete tabulation of temporary patterns and the superseding ones is found in Appendix A-7.

GLOSSARY OF BEHAVIOR PATTERNS. The items which appear on the schedules are for the most part self-explanatory. However, they are worded briefly. A glossary is necessary to clarify abbreviations of statement and to specify details. It is placed in the text rather than in a separate appendix to facilitate understanding of the precise meaning of each behavior pattern. Clarification will be enhanced further by reading the descriptions at adjacent age levels.

GROWTH TRENDS. Inasmuch as pictures and examinations provide only a cross-sectional view, it is important to recognize the growth trends which produce the behavior patterns and which alter the form of these patterns as the child matures. Accordingly, each age interval carries a brief characterization of the trends of development. Some are traced backward, others forward. The growth trends show how new behavior emerges and how one pattern of behavior is replaced by another. By following these lines of development, we are in a better position to understand the meaning of any observed behavior. A reading of the tabulation of temporary patterns in Appendix A-7, in conjunction with the growth trend chart in Appendix B, will further clarify the processes of developmental organization.

The key ages correspond to three developmental periods, or maturity zones, which indicate the usual starting position for the examination.

Key Ages	Maturity Zones
4 weeks	Supine (crib)
16 weeks	
28 weeks	Sitting (crib)
40 weeks	
52 weeks	
18 months	Locomotor (child's table and chair)
24 months	
36 months	

Three definitions will obviate repetition in the ensuing material:

Supine: lying face up.

Prone: lying face down.

Sitting: implies with support until the age of 36 or 40 weeks.

The dangling ring, rattle, and bell ringing (to elicit a response to sound) are presented in the supine position; all other objects are presented in the sitting position.

In determining the age of an infant or child at the time of examination, the following procedures should be used.

Through 59 weeks: take the midpoint of the week; e.g., 40 weeks includes the period from 39 weeks and 4 days through 40 weeks and 3 days.

Fourteen months and over: use whole and half month age intervals and include 7 days on either side of the midpoint. E.g., 18 months includes the period from 17 months and 24 days through 18 months and 7 days; 18.5 months covers the period from 18 months and 8 days through 18 months and 23 days.

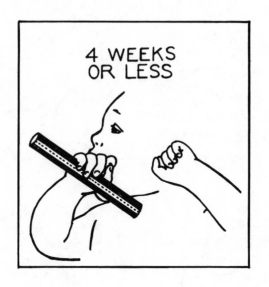

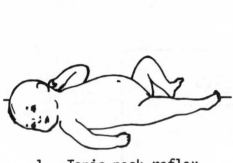

1. Tonic-neck-reflex attitude (t-n-r)

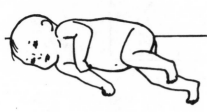

2. Rolls partway to side

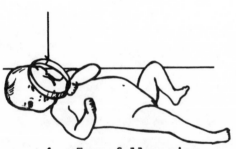

3. Disregards ring in midplane

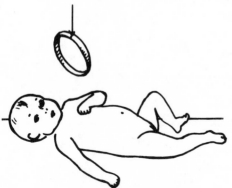

4. Eyes follow ring toward midplane

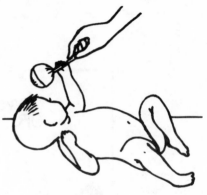

5. Hand clenches on contact

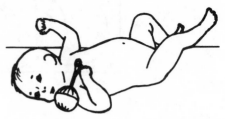

6. Drops rattle immediately

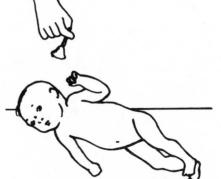

7. Attends bell; activity diminishes

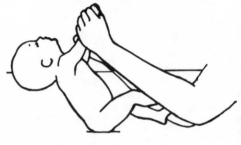

8. Marked head lag

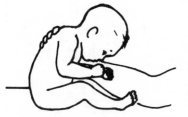

9.   Head sags forward, back evenly rounded

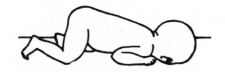

11.   Head rotation; kneeling; crawling movements

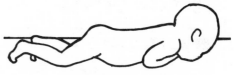

12.   Lifts head momentarily to Zone I

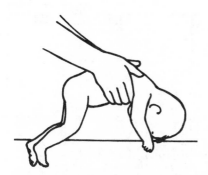

10.   Ventral suspension: head droops

§2. FOUR WEEKS OR LESS

The most opportune time to examine the 4-week infant is when he is neither drowsy nor hungry. Even so, his expression wears a remote detachment. His spontaneous *regard is staring and vague,* and remains so when he is placed on his back in the SUPINE position for observation. He lies in the *tonic-neck-reflex (t-n-r) attitude* (1): the head is turned far to the side, one arm in extension to the same (face) side, the other arm flexed close to shoulder or occiput. The face leg is also extended, the other leg flexed. At other times, both legs are flexed in external rotation with heels on the table. The *hands* are tightly *fisted;* sometimes one goes to the mouth. When active he makes more or less symmetric windmill movements, extending one or both arms sharply in the head—shoulder region. He flexes and extends the legs, lifting them an inch or two. Due to his rounded back, he may *roll partway* to the side (2).

He disregards the DANGLING RING in the midplane (3). When the ring is brought into his *line of vision* he regards it; when it is moved slowly from the side

		KEY AGE: 4 Weeks or less	H	O	8 Weeks	H	O
						H = History	
						O = Observation	

FETAL INFANCY

For developmental behavior items characteristic of the period of fetal infancy see the GROWTH TREND CHART Appendix B.

KEY AGE: 4 Weeks or less

Adaptive
Dangling Ring, Rattle: regards in line of vision only (*8w)
Dangling Ring: follows to midline
Rattle: drops immediately (*8w)
Bell-ring: attends, activity diminishes (*24w)

Gross Motor
Supine: side position head predominates (*16w)
Supine: tonic-neck-reflex (asymmetric) postures predominate (*16w)
Supine: rolls partway to side (*8w)
Pull-to-Sit: complete or marked head lag (*8w)
Sit: head predominantly sags (*8w)
Prone: head droops, ventral suspension (*8w)
Prone: placement, head rotates (*8w)
Prone: lifts head Zone I, momentarily (*8w)
Prone: crawling movements (*8w)

Fine Motor
Supine: both hands fisted (*12w)
Rattle: hand clenches on contact (*8w)

Language
Expressive: impassive face (*8w)
Expressive: vague, indirect regard (*8w)
Vocalization: small throaty noises (*8w)

Personal-Social
Social: regards examiner's face, activity diminishes (*8w)
Supine: stares indefinitely at surroundings (*8w)
Feeding: 2 night feedings (*8w)

8 Weeks

Adaptive
Dangling Ring: delayed midline regard (*12w)
D. Ring: regards examiner's hand
Dangling Ring: follows past midline
Rattle: retains briefly
Bell-ring: facial response (*24w)

Gross Motor
Sitting: head predominantly bobbingly erect (*16w)
Prone: head compensates, ventral suspension
Prone: head in midposition
Prone: lifts head Zone II, recurrently (*12w)

Language
Expressive: social smile
Expressive: alert expression
Expressive: direct, definite regard
Vocalization: single vowel sounds— ah, eh, uh (*36w)

Personal-Social
Social: facial social response
Social: follows moving person
Supine: regards examiner
Feeding: only 1 night feeding (*28w)

toward the midplane again, he *pursues it* (4) with combined eye and head movements *to the midline* and then returns the head to its preferred side position.

The RATTLE also is disregarded in the midplane and only momentarily regarded in the line of vision. When the handle of the rattle is touched to the fisted fingers he *clenches* his fist (5), and his fingers must be pried open to receive the rattle. He *drops it immediately* (6).

The examiner now confronts the baby preparatory to pull-to-sitting, shifting the baby's position if necessary. The examiner bends over and smiles and talks as a SOCIAL approach. The baby responds by *immobilizing his activity,* and he *regards the examiner's face.* The examiner then rings a hand BELL briskly, a few inches from each ear in turn; the baby heeds, and *activity ceases or lessens* (7).

By gentle maneuvers the examiner now institutes a few postural tests to determine muscular tonicity and motor response. He takes hold of the baby's hands and exerts a tentative pull toward the perpendicular sitting position to note the degree of head control. PULL-TO-SITTING is not completed if, as is usual at this age, the head falls back with *complete or marked lag* (8).

When placed in the supported SITTING position, the baby's head *prevailingly sags* forward on his chest (9), but he may erect his head momentarily. The back is evenly rounded (9).

In the STANDING position, supported at the chest in the axillary line, his legs extend briefly and the toes flex, but resistance to the table surface is slight or wanting.

The baby is then held suspended ventrally above the table in PRONE orientation. The *head droops* (10), showing *no postural compensation.* He is lowered to the table prone, and just as he is placed down, he *rotates his head* (11) so that he rests on his cheek. The arms are flexed close to the head, and the legs are in a kneeling position with the pelvis raised (11). He extends and draws up his legs in *crawling movements* (11). If the examiner gently turns the head to the midposition, the baby *rears his head* just clear of the table surface in *Zone I* (12) and then returns it to the side.

Vocalizations are confined to *small throaty sounds.* The mother reports that the baby startles easily to sudden sounds or movements, sometimes without external cause, and that he requires *two feedings* during the *night.*

Examination Sequence

Age: 0–4–8 Weeks   Situation No.
(Appendix A-4)

Supine 1
Dangling ring 2
Rattle 3
Social stimulation 4
Bell ringing 5
(Pull-to-sitting) 6
Sitting supported 50
Standing supported 51
Prone 52

( ) = situation sometimes omitted for special reasons.

(Normative behavior characteristic of the *key age: 4 weeks or less* and adjacent age levels is codified by the Developmental Schedule shown on the adjoining page.)

Glossary of Developmental Schedule Items

4 WEEKS OR LESS

Dangling Ring, Rattle: regards in line of vision only. Object not perceived until it is brought into direct line of vision at a favorable focal distance (about 12 inches).

Dangling Ring: follows to midline. As examiner moves ring to midline, infant follows with his eyes, with or without turning his head. Examiner must be certain infant is fixating upon ring, not merely making random movements which examiner then follows.

Rattle: drops immediately. After placement in hand.

Bell ringing: attends, activity diminishes. Response may be very brief; infant may inhibit respiration momentarily. Differentiate definite evidence of listening from a reflex blink response.

Supine: side position of head and tonic-neck-reflex postures predominate. Head turned to side, arm toward which face is directed (face arm) and face leg extended; other arm (occiput arm) and occiput leg flexed (fencing position). Position observed spontaneously, not elicited, but infant must be awake and lying on a surface which is firm and large enough not to restrict body movements.

Supine: rolls partway to side. Essentially, head and trunk turn passively. This position may be preferred, and flat supine impossible to maintain.

Pull-to-Sitting: complete or marked head lag. As infant is pulled toward sitting by holding his hands, head sags backwards; pull cannot be completed without support to head.

Sitting: head predominantly sags. In supported sitting head droops forward, chin on chest; may erect momentarily.

Prone: head droops, ventral suspension. When held around chest with face down, infant forms an inverted U.

Prone: placement, head rotates. As infant is placed face down in prone, he turns head to side and rests on cheek.

Prone: lifts head Zone I, momentarily. Head lifts so that face barely clears crib surface, or so that chin is about 1 inch above surface (Zone I). Examiner may turn infant's head to the midline to induce lifting.

Prone: crawling movements. Legs only; arms are inactive and tucked under chest.

Supine: both hands fisted. When infant is awake, hands primarily fisted, thumb resting outside clenched fingers.

Rattle: hand clenches on contact. Fisted hand fists more tightly when touched by rattle handle. Later, hand may open.

Expressive: impassive face. For most of examination period.

Expressive: vague, indirect regard. For most of examination period.

Vocalization: small throaty noises. Soft unformed sounds.

Social: regards examiner's face, activity diminishes. Examiner nods head and talks to infant; touching infant's face not included in social stimulation.

Supine: stares indefinitely at surroundings. Definite fixation not sustained.

Feeding: two night feedings. After early evening feeding.

8 WEEKS

Dangling Ring: delayed midline regard. When ring brought up from level of infant's feet to above his chest, he eventually turns his head, catches sight of and fixates upon ring, or upon examiner's hand holding end of string.

Dangling Ring: regards examiner's hand. When it is holding end of string.

Dangling Ring: follows past midline. Follows ring or examiner's hand; some head rotation necessary.

Rattle: retains briefly. When fingers opened by examiner and rattle placed, it is held passively and momentarily against crib surface before it drops.

Bell ringing: facial response. Eye widening, frown, smile, etc., with inhibition of activity.

Sitting: head predominantly bobbingly erect. In supported sitting head sags forward with chin on or near chest, but it lifts to erect position recurrently.

Prone: head compensates, ventral suspension. Head held in line with trunk as infant lowered into prone position.

Prone: head in midposition. When infant placed face down on crib, maintains head in midline.

Prone: lifts head Zone II, recurrently. Chin lifted 2–3 inches above crib surface; head at 45° angle to trunk (Zone II). It falls down again, without control of the movement.

Expressive: social smile. Facial brightening or smiling in response to examiner's nodding head and talking. Infant's face not touched to elicit this response.

Expressive: alert expression. Visual attention focused for most of examination.

Expressive: direct, definite regard. Visual attention focused for most of examination.

Vocalization: single vowel sounds—ah, eh, uh.

Social: facial social response. See *Expressive: social smile,* above.

Social: follows moving person. Watches as people move about.

Supine: regards examiner. Spontaneously and selectively.

Feeding: only one night feeding. After early evening feeding.

Growth Trends: Birth to Four Weeks

Infant behavior always shows developmental trends. It has a past and is advancing toward a future. The characteristics of 4-week behavior become more significant if we glance backward to its beginnings and forward to the 16-week age level.

Much of the behavior of the neonate, from birth to 4 weeks, is suggestive of earlier fetal stages. The newborn is not prepared fully for the demands of postnatal life; hence, his physiologic ineptitudes. His respiration may be irregular, his temperature regulation unsteady. Peristalsis and swallowing are under precarious directional control. He startles, sneezes or cries on slight provocation. His thresholds are low and inconstant. For such reasons his behavior seems variable, fitful and sketchy. He is not capable of those sustained postural sets which lie at the basis of sustained attention. His motor tensions are transient, partial and migratory. Even his wakefulness is not sharply differentiated from sleep. Rhythms of rest and activity are poorly defined; many of his reactions seem sporadic.

The infant fatigues readily because of his immaturity and because of the vast amount of correlation which still must be achieved between and within visceral and sensorimotor mechanisms. Crying, drowsing, irritability and fretfulness reflect the infant's difficulties. Therefore, the neonate is apt to react positively to tactile snugness and the warmth of closely wrapped blankets which possibly revive the habitudes of fetal life. His state—awake and quiet, drowsing, crying, hungry or satiated—modifies the behavior of the neonate more than at any other time of life. At this age visual and auditory responses, in terms of definite looking and listening, are indices of cortical integrity whose future evolution can be defined, but failure to elicit them is not synonymous with abnormality.

The infant makes lashing windmill movements of his arms and intensifies his grasp in a manner which appears to suggest vestiges of arboreal grasping and clinging. For 8 weeks or more he keeps his hands fisted in his waking life. Only as he grows older do his fingers begin to relax. By 12 weeks of age they are loosely closed. At 16 to 20 weeks we see the beginnings of a new kind of grasp, true prehension—a self-directed grasp on tactile and visual cues.

Prehension in the infant with vision involves a focalization of posture and a coordination of eyes and hands. The tonic-neck-reflex (t-n-r) attitude, which is one of the most conspicuous behavior patterns throughout the first 12 postnatal weeks, literally paves the way for prehension. During much of his waking life the 4-week infant lies in this position, which resembles a fencing stance. This attitude promotes and channels visual fixation on his extended hand. By gradual stages it leads to hand inspection, to active approach upon an object and to manipulation of the object. At 4 weeks the infant immediately drops a rattle inserted in his palm, but at 8 weeks he retains it briefly. At 12 weeks he both holds and glances at it. At 16 weeks he regards it prolongedly; at 20 weeks he can make a two-handed approach to the rattle merely on sight, and can prehend it if it is held near his hand.

Thus, the t-n-r attitude is not a stereotyped reaction but seemingly a scaffolding for the growth of prehension. The postural control of eyes and head is an important feature of these patterns. The 4-week infant immobilizes his roving eyes and stares indefinitely at surroundings. The range of his vision is narrowly limited by the side position of his head. However, as his head becomes emancipated, the range of his vision widens. At 8 weeks it encompasses 90°; at 12 weeks, 180°. By 16 weeks his head is beginning to prefer the midline to give him better command of the whole visual scene. Meanwhile his head station in the supported sitting position has progressed from sag, to bobbingly erect, to occasional bob, to steadily erect.

Advances in oculomotor and postural control are reflected in the scope and discrimination of his attention. At 4 weeks he gives attention by means of total reactions. He responds to the ringing of a bell by reduction of general activity. He listens massively to sounds. In the same manner, a full stomach almost absorbs his entire attention. He is very limited in his capacity to express moods and specific desires. His expressive behavior, like his perceptual behavior, has a generalized character. However, as he matures he becomes increasingly selective in his responses, and the impassive countenance of 4 weeks vanishes. Expression becomes more alert at 8 weeks, and regard for physical surroundings more direct and discriminating. His eyes may pick up an individual object like the examiner's hand.

His response to social surroundings also becomes more discriminating. At 4 weeks he reacts to social overtures by a reduction of general body activity; at 8 weeks his face animates; at 12 weeks he may vocalize in reply; at 16 weeks he initiates social play. By such tokens he registers personal and emotional growth as well as progressive neuromotor organization.

Although the newborn infant displays characteristics reminiscent of the fetus, most of the behavior of the 4-week infant has a forward reference. It is pointed toward goals. It organizes and elaborates so swiftly that by 16 weeks he appears to be penetrating his environment. At this next key age level of 16 weeks he enjoys being propped up to survey the world into which he is being incorporated. Acculturation has begun.

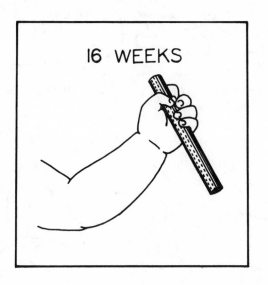

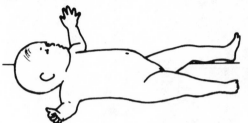

1. Symmetric posturing, head midline

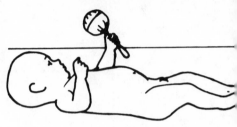

5. Regards rattle in hand

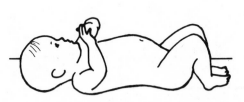

2. Hands engage at midline

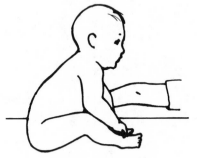

6. Head set forward, steady; lumbar curvature

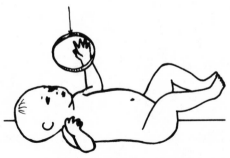

3. Regards ring immediately, arms activate

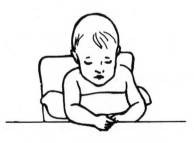

7. Looks down at table top and hands

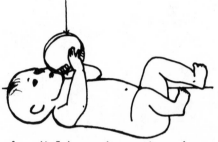

4. Holds and mouths ring, free hand approaches

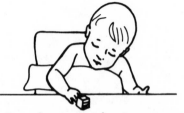

8. Arms activate; may contact cube

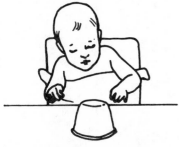

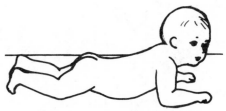

11. Holds head in
Zone III, legs extended

9. Looks from hand to
cup; arms activate

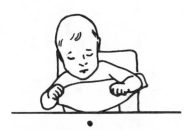

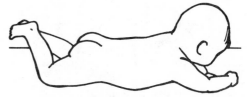

12. On verge of rolling

10. Regards pellet

§3. SIXTEEN WEEKS

The 16-week baby inspects persons and surroundings with much more alertness than the 4-week-old. This is due in part to the marked advance in eye and head control. Placed in the SUPINE position he holds his *head predominantly in the midline* (1) spontaneously. The t-n-r attitude so characteristic of 4 and 8 weeks may be seen for brief periods, but the midposition of the head reflexly favors *symmetric postures of arms* (1), so that the *hands engage* (2) near the face or over the chest or are flung out in lateral extension at shoulder level (1). Fingers are extended or only slightly flexed. He looks at the examiner and *initiates a social smile.* Spontaneous hand regard is frequent because he readily fixates any object which moves into his visual field.

He *immediately regards* (3) the DANGLING RING held over his feet *in the midplane* and follows the ring, or the examiner's hand holding the string, continuously from one side to the other through an arc of 180°. Interest in the examiner's face frequently interferes with ring following at this very social age. When the ring is held suspended over his chest, his *arms activate* (3). When it is placed in his hand he accepts it, *regards it* as he *holds* it, brings it to his *mouth* and approaches it or the midline with his *free hand* (4). His behavior with the RATTLE

H = History   O = Observation

K E Y   A G E: 16 Weeks

	12 Weeks	16 Weeks	20 Weeks
Adaptive			
	Dangling Ring: prompt midline regard (*16w)	Dangling Ring, Ra: regards immediately	Rattle, Bell: 2-hand approach (*28w)
	Dangling Ring: follows 180°	Dangling Ring, Rattle, Cube, Cup: arms activate (*24w)	Rattle, Dangling Ring: grasps only if near hand (*24w)
	Rattle: glances at in hand	Dangling Ring, Rattle: regards in hand	Rattle: visual pursuit lost rattle
	Cube, Cup: regards more than momentarily	Dangling Ring: to mouth	Cube: holds 1st regards 2nd
		D. Ring: free hand to midline (*28w)	Massed Cubes: grasps 1 on contact (*24w)
		Tabletop: looks down at table top or hands	
		Cube, Cup: looks from hand to object (*20w)	
		Pellet: regards recurrently	
Gross Motor			
	Supine: head predominantly half side (tonic-neck-reflex) (*16w)	Supine: midposition head predominates	Pull-to-Sit: no head lag
	Supine: midposition head and symmetric postures seen	Supine: symmetric postures predominate	Sit: head erect, steady
	Sit: head set forward, bobs (*16w)	Supine: hands engage (*24w)	Prone: arms extended
	Stand: small fraction weight briefly	Sit: head steady, set forward (*20w)	
	Stand: lifts foot (*28w)	Prone: head Zone III, sustainedly	
	Prone: head Zone II, sustainedly	Prone: legs extended or semi-extended (*40w)	
	Prone: on forearms (*20w)	Prone: verge of rolling (*20w)	
	Prone: hips low, legs flexed (*40w)		
Fine Motor			
	Supine: hands open or loosely closed	Dangling Ring: retains	Prone or Tabletop: scratches tabletop or platform (*28w)
	Rattle: holds actively	Supine: fingers, scratches, clutches (*24w)	Cube: precarious grasp (*24w)
	Cup: contacts		
Language			
	Vocalization: coos (*36w)	Expressive: excites, breathes heavily (*32w)	Vocalization: squeals (*36w)
	Vocalization: chuckles	Vocalization: laughs aloud	
	Social: vocal-social response		
Personal-Social			
	Social: vocal-social response	Social: spontaneous social smile	Social: smiles at mirror image
	Supine: regards examiner predominantly	Social: vocalizes or smiles, pulled to sitting (*24w)	Feeding: pats bottle, both hands (*36w)
	Play: hand regard (*16w)	Feeding: anticipates food on sight	
	Play: pulls at dress (*24w)	Play: sits propped 10-15 minutes (*40w)	
		Play: hand play, mutual fingering (*24w)	
		Play: pulls dress over face (*24w)	

(5) is similar, although because it is top-heavy, he is more likely to drop it as his hands open and close.

The examiner then confronts the baby preparatory to pull-to-sitting. The 16-week baby initiates the SOCIAL approach, smiling almost automatically in response to the examiner. The examiner then shakes the RATTLE gently a few inches from each ear in turn. The baby attends the sound by abating activity. He may blink, frown, smile or even cry. If there is no response, a hand BELL is rung briskly.

The examiner takes the baby's hands for PULL-TO-SITTING. The head lags only slightly, and he *vocalizes or smiles* pleasurably on attaining the supported SITTING position. He holds his head erect but *set forward* (6), and it is steady. He requires firm support in this position, but his back shows only a lumbar curvature (6).

Placed in a supporting chair or held seated confronting the TEST TABLE, he is interested predominantly in the examiner, but he fingers the table surface and finally *regards his own hands and the table top* (7).

When a single CUBE is presented, he follows the examiner's withdrawing hand but then spies the cube, regards it recurrently and *shifts* his *regard from hand to cube*. The *arms activate* (8), and he may contact the cube (8). The MASSED CUBES, of greater stimulus value than a single one at this age, are more likely to evoke successful contact. If they do, the cup need not be presented.

He gives the CUP immediate and prolonged attention, the *arms activate* (9), and he contacts the cup. He *looks from hand to cup (9)*.

He follows the examiner's withdrawing hand again when the PELLET is

---

Examination Sequence

Age: 12–16–20   Situation No.
     Weeks   (Appendix A-4)

Supine   1
Dangling ring   2
Rattle   3
Social stimulation   4
Bell ringing   5
Pull-to-sitting   6
Sitting supported 50
Chair–table top
Cube 1, (2) 7,8
Massed cubes 11
(Cup) 16
Pellet 18
(Bell) 22
Mirror 24
Standing supported 51
Prone 52

Italicized items appear for the first time in this sequence.
( ) = situation sometimes omitted for special reasons.

(Normative behavior characteristic of the *key age: 16 weeks* and adjacent age levels is codified by the Developmental Schedule shown on the adjoining page.)

presented, regards his own hands and finally gives the pellet *delayed, recurrent regard* (10).

The BELL also evokes prompt and prolonged regard and activation of the arms, but provides little additional information since he is unlikely to grasp it.

The test table is then removed, and the infant taken out of the chair and placed close to a large MIRROR. He may smile at his mirror image but usually just regards it.

The infant is held in the STANDING position supported at the chest in the axillary line. He sustains a small fraction of weight briefly, extending the legs recurrently and rising to his toes. He tends to flex his toes, and he may still lift his foot.

When held suspended above the table in PRONE orientation, he keeps the head in good alignment with the trunk. As he is placed down on the table he maintains the midposition of the head, holding it *sustainedly lifted* at a 90° angle in *Zone III* (11). The legs are *extended or semiextended* (11), and he props himself on his forearms. Because *one arm is flexed,* the *other more extended,* and the head position high, his prone equilibrium is unstable and he shows a *tendency to roll* (12) to the side; he may roll involuntarily to a supine position. A lure (toy) may be used to induce head lifting.

In his interest in the test toys he may *strain, breathe fast,* purse his lips and show other evidences of excitement. He is reported to coo and to *laugh aloud,* to *"recognize"* his *bottle* if bottle fed, to play with his *hands bringing them together with mutual fingering,* and to *pull his dress over his face* as his arms move up and down. He sits *propped with pillows* for 10–15 minutes.

Glossary of Developmental Schedule Items

12 WEEKS

Dangling Ring: prompt midline regard. When ring reaches chest level, infant regards ring in midline, turning his head from partly side position to do so, if necessary.

Dangling Ring: follows 180°. Eyes and head follow ring or examiner's hand to crib surface in continuous, but not necessarily smooth, arc to each side.

Rattle: glances at in hand. Examiner should be certain infant is looking at placed rattle rather than at some distant point beyond it. Infant frequently does not lift rattle from crib in this situation.

Cube, Cup: regards more than momentarily. Examiner may hold infant's head forward to favor regard. Definite fixation on object observed.

Supine: head predominantly half-side (t-n-r). Head less fully rotated than when younger; t-n-r less stereotyped and less persistent (see 4 Weeks).

Supine: midposition head and symmetric postures seen. Chin and nose in line with median line of trunk; arms symmetrically disposed. Posture not predominant, but observed.

Sitting: head set forward, bobs. In supported sitting, head primarily erect but thrust forward at an angle to trunk; it bobs forward towards chest recurrently, even when body is immobile.

Standing: small fraction of weight briefly. Infant is held at chest in axillary line; when examiner relaxes his support, infant maintains erect position for a moment before flexing at hips and knees.

Standing: lifts foot. While examiner maintains full support at chest, infant lifts one foot. A remnant of the newborn placing reflex, it is not seen if infant supports none of his weight.

Prone: head Zone II, sustainedly. Head maintained at a $45°$ angle to crib platform and put down with control.

Prone: on forearms. Elbows flexed, weight rests on elbows and forearms. Examiner may remove infant's arms caught under chest; they do not return to tucked neonatal position.

Prone: hips low, legs flexed. Upper thighs rotated inward slightly and rest on crib surface; legs still flexed at knees and abducted at hips.

Supine: hands open or loosely closed. Hands no longer need to be pried open. Fingers curl in active grasp when ring or rattle touched to them (the predominant pattern).

Rattle: holds actively. Active grasp indicated either by lifting of object from crib surface or by whitening of knuckle joints.

Cup: contacts. During regard for cup, hand brought against cup.

Vocalization: coos. Sustained single vowel sounds, "aaah . . . ., oooo . . . .," like the murmuring of a pigeon.

Vocalization: chuckles. Just short of true laughter; must be inquired about explicitly.

Social: vocal-social response. Infant vocalizes in some manner or "talks back" in response to social stimulation (see 8 Weeks, *Expressive: social smile*).

Supine: regards examiner predominantly. In preference to objects presented.

Play: hand regard. In his spontaneous play, infant brings one or both hands before his face for regard.

Play: pulls at dress. In supine position, hands close on clothes or blankets as they come in contact.

16 WEEKS

Dangling Ring, Rattle: regards immediately. Infant sees object as soon as it is brought over his feet.

Dangling Ring, Rattle, Cube, Cup: arms activate. During regard for object, infant's arms become active, though they are not necessarily brought nearer object. Activity may even be confined to tremulous poising. Response may be well-defined in only one or some of situations listed.

Dangling Ring, Rattle: regards in hand. Sustained regard of placed object; usually lifts off crib surface to look at it.

Dangling Ring, Rattle: to mouth. Object, not infant's hand, contacts mouth, even though awkwardly or recurrently.

Dangling Ring: free hand to midline. Hand approaches midline, may not reach it.

Tabletop: looks down at tabletop or hands. Spontaneously regards test table surface or own hands on table in absence of object.

Cube, Cup: looks from hand to object. Regard shifts back and forth from one to other.

Pellet: regards recurrently. Any regard that is definite. Examiner is permitted to point to pellet to attract attention to it, to move it about, etc.; infant tends to follow examiner's withdrawing hand, even if it is removed slowly.

Supine: midposition head predominates. Chin and nose held primarily in line with median line of trunk, or head may rotate freely from side to side.

Supine: symmetric postures predominate. Both arms held simultaneously either abducted or with hands together in midline; both legs either flexed or extended. Symmetric postures of the body more commonly present, while head may still prefer a side position.

Supine: hands engage. Hands come together over chest and fingers touch. May be limited by arm abduction in supine but seen in supported sitting.

Sitting: head steady, set forward. In supported sitting head held steady but thrust forward at an angle to the body; may bob forward when arms or trunk move or head turns, but not when infant is immobile.

Prone: head Zone III, sustainedly. Head lifted at 90° angle to crib platform so that plane of face vertical to crib surface and eyes look straight ahead (Zone III); put down with smooth control.

Prone: legs extended or semiextended. Anterior aspect of thighs rest on crib surface; hips not abducted although knees may flex.

Prone: verge of rolling. One arm extended or semiextended, other flexed; head in Zone III; infant shows tendency to roll passively over his extended arm.

Dangling Ring: retains. After being placed in hand, ring stays for about 1 minute even though hand opens and closes on object.

Supine: fingers, scratches, clutches. His own body, hair or dress, or he may clutch at examiner's clothes on contact; more active use of fingers than at 12 weeks.

Expressive: excites, breathes heavily. Strains during regard for an object.

Vocalization: laughs aloud. Spontaneously, or in response to social stimulation, not to tickling or roughhouse.

Social: spontaneous social smile. Infant initiates social play by a beaming smile in response to examiner's presence, without requiring social advances.

Social: vocalizes or smiles, pulled to sitting. A pleasurable response, apparently in response to translocation and new posture; sometimes almost squeals with delight. Crying not acceptable.

Feeding: anticipates food on sight. Infant becomes excited and eager when sees bottle or breast, before it is touched to his lips.

Play: sits propped 10–15 minutes. Maintains upright position when placed in corner of a sofa or his crib with aid of pillows; half-reclining in an infant carrier of some type not acceptable.

Play: hand play, mutual fingering. Hands finger each other as infant brings them together in spontaneous play.

Play: pulls dress over face. As arms move up and down, already clutched clothes or blankets come up over infant's face.

20 WEEKS

Rattle, Bell: two-hand approach. In either supine or supported sitting, both hands brought slowly towards presented object with control (see 24 Weeks: approaches and grasps).

Rattle, Dangling Ring: grasps only if near hand. If object is brought within an inch of palmar side of hand, approach completed and object grasped.

Rattle: visual pursuit lost rattle. If rattle drops within sight on crib, or examiner removes and places it while infant is regarding rattle, he turns his head to look after it.

Cube: holds first, regards second. Infant maintains contact with first cube placed in his hand, attends presentation of second at edge of tabletop and usually follows visually as it is brought towards him.

Massed Cubes: grasps one on contact. Hand falls upon or contacts a cube, with regardful approach or regard after contact, and cube is then grasped.

Pull-to-Sitting: no head lag. Head maintained in line with trunk throughout.

Sitting: head erect, steady. In supported sitting, head maintained in line with trunk; moves freely at all times without bobbing.

Prone: arms extended. Held forward as props, resting weight on hands, with entire chest off crib and elbows straight.

Prone or Tabletop: scratches tabletop or platform. Fingers scratch actively, whether or not a stimulus object is present.

Cube: precarious grasp. When placed in hand, or on spontaneous grasp. Cube held between fingers and heel of palm, usually at ulnar side. Must lift cube off table top, not merely maintain contact.

Vocalization: squeals. Infant modulates pitch of air stream to a high sound resembling a squealing pig.

Social: smiles at mirror image. Either spontaneously or when mirror is tapped to attract his attention. An occasional infant cries on seeing himself, indicating awareness of his image. Mirror must be large (cabinet or dresser) so infant cannot see around it.

Feeding: pats bottle, both hands. Infant puts both hands on bottle or breast.

Growth Trends: Sixteen Weeks

Sixteen weeks marks a turning point. The infant is graduating from the protected confines of the bassinet, and in the next 3 months he will make amazing progress. He will advance from propped sitting to the first stages of unpropped sitting; he will prehend and manipulate; he will vocalize with versatility; he will show increasing capacity to occupy himself in exploitative play. The developmental transitions from 16 to 28 weeks are not sudden, but they are unremitting.

Sixteen weeks ushers in a period of rapid cortical organization which brings about a steady transformation of sensorimotor patterns, particularly in the coordination of eyes and hands. The visual–motor system has already made enormous gains. Indeed, the 16-week infant not only can catch sight of his own hand; he can fasten his eyes on the examiner's hand, and can even fixate recurrently upon an 8-mm pellet which the examiner has placed on a table within the infant's ocular reach.

The baby can reach with his eyes before he can reach with his hand—in accordance with the cephalocaudal trend of neuromotor development. The pellet is so small that his regard for it is sketchy and comes with delay. When the larger cube is placed upon the table, his roving eyes settle immediately and his arms activate; when presented with the massed cubes he contacts one. This is prehension in the making.

The 1-inch cube has a stimulus power which lies midway between cup and pellet. The result is a developmental gradient which has some diagnostic value: 12 weeks contacts a cup; 16 weeks contacts cubes; 28 weeks contacts a pellet. The crude arm activity of 16 weeks is an embryologic *anlage* from which more refined approach, grasp and manipulation ultimately will take shape. Looking, reaching, contacting, grasping, manipulation and exploitation thus constitute a developmental sequence. One emerges from the other.

The 16-week infant is mostly limited to contacting, but it is his motor equipment rather than his dynamic vigor which is crude. The clutching and fisting so prominent in the neonatal period have not yet disappeared altogether. His hands are not completely open; they still cling near the chest. At this age, he is under the limitations of symmetry imposed by the midline position of his head. Accordingly, he brings his hands together and engages in playful mutual fingering. This fingering has a simple exploitative significance. The primitive clutch intrudes; dress and blanket are caught in the fingers and pulled up over the face. The mother may impute intention to this feat; the examiner can appreciate its neuromotor implications. The symmetric on-the-chest posture of the arms also brings the hands over the mouth, and the mouth, being a prehensory organ in its own right, often sucks the fingers or the fist. This kind of sucking has a simple sensorimotor and developmental significance and does not require elaborate psychodynamic attributions.

The 16-week infant is transcending the asymmetry of the t-n-r which threatened to make him one-sided. He is bidextrous, and tends to move his arms in unison. For the next 8 weeks he goes through a symmetric two-sided phase. Through 24 weeks of age he makes a bilateral, two-handed prehensory approach upon a toy. By 28 weeks he is transcending this phase of symmetry; his unilaterality is at a higher level of integration, and he makes a one-handed approach.

At 16 weeks there is a developmental premium on the organization of eye-and-head postures, and eye-and-hand postures. The shifting of regard from hand to cube, for example, is not a conflict between two objects in view; it is the first step toward bringing the hand into relation with the cube. The infant perceives his hands separately from the object, but he does not have sufficient control to approach and grasp it. Later the eyes direct the hand to the cube; there is immediate approach and grasp on sight. In supine the side positions of the head may still persist when the body posturing is symmetric, and the infant often brings objects to the midline or to his mouth without looking at them.

Meanwhile the rapid development of head, eye and hand coordination does not exclude development of the axial musculature. To be sure, the 16-week trunk still slumps, even with the support of the bodyband of the examining chair. In the supported sitting position the back is no longer uniformly rounded; the curvature is confined to the lumbar region; by this time the cervical region is more fully organized. At 24 weeks the trunk is "stronger"; this means that the axial musculature has attained more complete functional relationship with the central nervous system and is therefore more capable of sustained tonus. Accordingly, the 24-week baby can roll from supine to prone, and by 28 weeks he can sit for a brief moment, leaning forward on his hands for support. He is advancing from a supine to a sedentary status.

The neuromotor organization of larynx and thorax has and will continue to undergo similar differentiations. At 16 weeks his expressive behavior is still comparatively generalized. He expresses interest by straining his whole body forward, and by a heavy, rapid, excited form of breathing. He coos and laughs aloud. Later, as his vocal apparatus becomes more flexible and as his diaphragm, rib, laryngeal and palatal musculature become more sensitive to control, he utters squeals, grunts and growls. Many neuromotor differentiations must be achieved before he reaches the threshold of that highly socialized form of communication known as speech. His present vocal behavior points toward that threshold.

The second quarter of the first year proves to be almost dramatic in the scope and swiftness of its behavioral transformations. There is something prophetic in the way in which the 16-week infant relishes the sitting position. His eyes widen, pulse strengthens, breathing quickens and he smiles when he is translated from the supine horizontal to the seated perpendicular. This is more than an athletic satisfaction in his newly acquired head balance. It is more than a postural triumph. It enables a widening of horizon, a new social orientation.

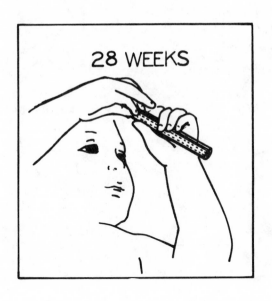

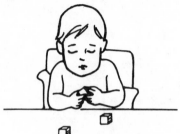

1. Transfers cube

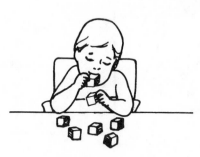

2. Holds 2 cubes more than momentarily

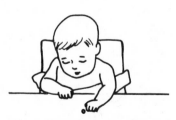

3. Rakes at pellet

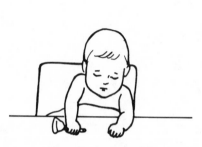

4. Bangs bell

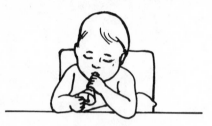

5. Transfers and mouths bell

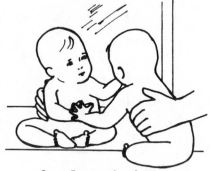

6. Regards image; pats glass

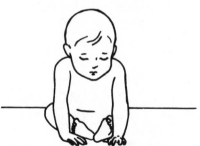

7. Sits momentarily leaning on hands

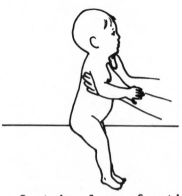

8. Sustains large fraction of weight; bounces

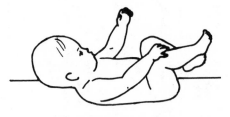

9. Lifts head

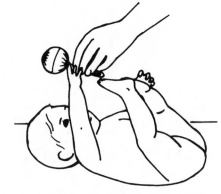

11. Reaches with one hand

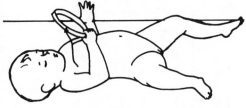

10. Transfers ring

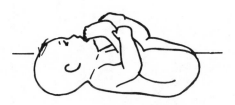

12. Feet to mouth

§4. TWENTY-EIGHT WEEKS

The 28-week infant sits with support, his trunk erect and head steady. The introductory toy is removed after a brief period, and the examiner presents the FIRST of three CUBES. The baby *reaches* with *one hand,* seizes it *immediately* with a *radial palmar* grasp and carries it to his mouth. He retains it as the SECOND CUBE is presented. He does not grasp the second cube but may approach it. As the THIRD CUBE is presented, he drops a cube. He does not grasp the third cube but mouths, *transfers* (1), drops and resecures the cube in hand.

He approaches the MASSED CUBES with both hands, grasping one cube and scattering the others. While *holding one cube he grasps another,* and he *holds two* cubes *more than momentarily* (2); he may pick up three in all. When the CUP is added while the infant is holding a CUBE, he drops the cube to grasp the cup.

He follows the examiner's hand away as the PELLET is presented; he gives delayed, intent regard to the pellet and *rakes* (3) at it with his fingers, *contacting it.*

He makes an *immediate one-handed* approach to the BELL, taking it by the bowl or junction. He *bangs* (4), mouths and *transfers* (5) the bell *adeptly, retaining* it without dropping during the course of his varied manipulation.

K E Y   A G E: 28 Weeks

H O	24 Weeks	H O	28 Weeks	H O	32 Weeks
			Adaptive		
	Dangling Ring, Rattle, Cube, Bell: approaches & grasps		Rattle, Bell: 1-hand approach & grasp		Cube: grasps 2nd cube
	Rattle: prehensile pursuit dropped rattle		Massed Cubes: holds 1, grasps another		Cube: retains 2 as 3rd presented (*36w)
	Cube: regards 3rd cube immediately		M. Cubes: holds 2 more than momentarily		Cube: holds 2 prolongedly
	Cube, Bell: to mouth (*18m)		Bell: bangs (*40w)		Cup-cube: holds cube, regards cup (*36w)
	Cube: resecures dropped cube		Rattle: shakes definitely		Ring-string: secures ring
	Massed Cubes: holds 1, approaches another (*28w)		Dangling Ring, Cube: transfers		
			Bell: transfers adeptly		
			Bell: retains		
			Gross Motor		
	Supine: lifts legs high in extension		Supine: lifts head (*40w)		Sit: 1 minute, erect, unsteady (*36w)
	Supine: rolls to prone		Sit: briefly, leans forward on hands (*32w)		Stand: maintains briefly, hands held (*36w)
	Pull-to-Sit: lifts head, assists (*40w)		Sit: erect momentarily		Prone: pivots (*40w)
	Sit in chair: trunk erect (*36w)		Stand: large fraction of weight (*32w)		
			Stand: bounces actively (*36w)		
			Fine Motor		
	Cube: grasps palmarwise (*36w)		Cube: radial palmar grasp (*36w)		Pellet: radial raking (*36w)
	Rattle: retains		Pellet: rakes with whole hand, contacts (*32w)		Pellet: unsuccessful inferior scissors (*36w)
			Language		
	Bell-ringing: turns head to bell		Vocalization: m—m—m (crying) (*40w)		Vocalization: single consonant, as da, ba, ka
	Vocalization: grunts, growls (*36w)		Vocalization: controlled polysyllabic vowel sounds (*36w)		
	Vocalization: spontaneous vocal-social (including toys)				
			Personal-Social		
	Social: discriminates strangers		Feeding: takes solids well		Play: bites, chews toys (*18m)
	Play: grasps foot, supine (*36w)		Play: feet to mouth, supine		Play: reaches persistently for toys out of reach (*40w)
	Play: sits propped 30 minutes (*40w)		Mirror: reaches, pats image		Ring-string: persistent
	Mirror: smiles and vocalizes		Ring-string: fusses or abandons effort (*32w)		

The RING AND STRING are presented, the string obliquely aligned to the right, but within reach. He reaches toward the ring, slaps and scratches the table and finally sees the string; he either *abandons the effort or fusses.*

The test table is removed. He is taken out of the chair and seated before a large MIRROR; he regards his image, smiles, vocalizes and *pats the glass* (6).

In the SITTING position he sits *briefly, leaning forward, propped* on his hands (7). He also shows some *active balance, sitting erect for a fleeting, unsteady moment.*

Held around the chest in the STANDING position, he sustains a *large fraction of weight* (8) on his extended legs as he *bounces* actively (8).

Placed PRONE, he holds the head well lifted, his weight on his abdomen and hands. He lifts one arm toward a lure and tries, unsuccessfully, to pivot.

When placed on his back on the platform, his SUPINE posturings are symmetric, with the legs lifted high in extension or semiextension. He *lifts his head* (9) as though striving to sit up. He is not very tolerant of the supine position, and this and the following three situations may have to be curtailed or omitted, if he does not quiet when offered a test object.

He grasps, *transfers* (10) and mouths the DANGLING RING, regarding it in hand. He makes an *immediate one-handed approach* to the RATTLE (11), *shakes* it vigorously, regards it and fingers it with the free hand. If it is placed on the platform at his side, he reaches for it and may roll to prone to secure it. If the infant has not already entered into SOCIAL PLAY, the examiner smiles and talks to him. (Exam procedures continued next page.)

Examination Sequence

(Normative behavior characteristic of the *key age: 28 weeks* and adjacent age levels is codified by the Developmental Schedule shown on the adjoining page.)

Age: 24–28–32 Weeks   Situation No. (Appendix A-4)

Chair–Table top

Cubes 1, 2, *3*	7,8,9
Massed cubes	11
(Cup and cubes)	17
Pellet	18
Bell	22
Ring and string	23
Mirror	24
Sitting supported	50
Standing supported	51
Prone	52
(Supine)	1
(Dangling ring)	2
(Rattle	3
Social stimulation	4
Bell ringing	5
(Pull-to-sitting)	6

Italicized items appear for the first time in this sequence.

( ) = situation sometimes omitted for special reasons.

When auditory responses are tested by shaking the RATTLE or, if necessary, by ringing a BELL opposite each ear in succession, he turns his head correctly and promptly. If the infant objects to the supine position, elicit his response to sound in sitting.

The examiner now takes his hands, and he lifts his head and assists in the PULL-TO-SITTING.

His language includes cooing, squealing and *combined vowel sounds* produced with control. He says *m-m-mum* when he cries. His mother reports that he discriminates strangers, "talks" to his toys, *takes solids well* and *brings his feet to his mouth* (12). He rolls from supine to prone position and sits propped about half an hour.

Glossary of Developmental Schedule Items

24 WEEKS

Dangling Ring, Rattle, Cube, Bell: approaches and grasps. Usually two-handed. Approach and grasp synthesized into a coordinated direct response to visual stimulus of one or some objects, in either supine or sitting (see 20 Weeks).

Rattle: prehensile pursuit dropped rattle. When rattle falls or is removed and placed in sight on crib, he reaches toward it and may roll to resecure it.

Cube: regards third cube immediately. Examiner places one or both cubes and may have to put cubes on tabletop with infant's hands on top of them to induce him to maintain contact with both cubes. Looks on presentation at table edge; regard may follow examiner's withdrawing hand, but returns at once to third cube.

Cube, Bell: to mouth. Infant secures object himself and takes *it*, not back of his hand, to his mouth.

Cube: resecures dropped cube. From massed cubes or single cube situation; analogous to but more complex than resecuring dropped rattle.

Massed Cubes: holds one, approaches another. Definitely indicates his intent to try for a second cube in mass after he secures one.

Supine: lifts legs high in extension. Or semiextension. Infant lifts legs high enough to see or grasp feet; a report to this effect accepted.

Supine: rolls to prone. Gets both arms from under his chest after rolling completely over.

Pull-to-Sitting: lifts head, assists. Flexes elbows and lifts head as soon as examiner's pull begins.

Sitting in chair: trunk erect. When securely strapped in, he does not slump to side; reerects if he leans towards tabletop in reaching.

Cube: grasps palmarwise. Whole hand grasp without radial differentiation; secures and holds cube in center of palm, fingers closed about it.

Rattle: retains. After being grasped, rattle remains in hand for about 1 minute. Hands no longer open and close automatically; if they do, top-heavy rattle falls.

Bell-ringing: turns head to bell. In response to auditory cue, he looks for source instead of merely altering his activity (see 4 and 8 Weeks).

Vocalization: grunts, growls. Modifies air stream with low-pitched sounds.

Vocalization: spontaneous vocal–socialization. Infant initiates social play by smiling and vocalizing (see 16 Weeks). He also "talks" to his toys as well as to persons.

Social: discriminates strangers. Knows difference between strangers and family. Not necessarily fearful; may simply sober and not accept strangers as quickly as familiars.

Play: grasps foot, supine. Not thighs. Must be able to lift legs in extension to do this, but converse not requisite; may lift legs and not grasp foot.

Play: sits propped 30 minutes. May succeed in high chair or infant jump seat, tied in but with less assistance from pillows (see 16 Weeks).

Mirror: smiles and vocalizes. "Talks" to his mirror image socially; may remain sober, but crying not equated with vocalizing (see 20 Weeks).

28 WEEKS

Rattle, Bell: one-hand approach and grasp. Infant freed from symmetric postures; coordinated smooth movement on sight (see 24 Weeks).

Massed Cubes: holds one, grasps another. At some point during manipulation, succeeds in securing second cube after grasping one.

Massed Cubes: holds two more than momentarily. Secures cubes by himself, without placement by examiner.

Bell: bangs. Definite up and down vertical movement in sitting; may exhibit behavior with cube or cup.

Rattle: shakes definitely. Distinguish active shaking by infant from passive sound of rattle as his arms move.

Dangling Ring, Cube: transfers. Infant exchanges grasp of object directly from one hand to other with expeditious transition, without intermediary of mouth or tabletop.

Bell: transfers adeptly. Grasping hand does not pull bell out of releasing hand, fingers don't get caught in each other.

Bell: retains. Maintains grasp during course of active banging, mouthing and transfer.

Supine: lifts head. As though straining to sit up, without aid from examiner and not from semireclining position in infant carrier.

Sitting: briefly, leans forward (on hands). Trunk straight and maintaining an angle of at least 45° with crib, arms extended as props to prevent excessive sagging forward. Surface should be *hard.*

Sitting: erect momentarily. Both arms lifted, trunk at 90° angle to crib; assumes spontaneously from forward position or may be placed. Surface should be *hard.*

Standing: large fraction of weight. Examiner supports infant around chest. Hips are extended, knees usually slightly flexed.

Standing: bounces actively. When knees flex, infant extends them again. Examiner continues to provide support around his chest.

Cube: radial palmar grasp. Cube secured in palm of hand but off-center, toward the radial side; fingers are closed about cube, thumb tending to oppose them.

Pellet: rakes with whole hand, contacts. Hand over or near pellet, all fingers flexing in a raking, scratching movement. Whole arm moves, thumb moves with fingers and acts like a finger. Infant succeeds in touching pellet.

Vocalization: mum-mum-mum (crying). First active modulation of air stream with lips, usually while crying.

Vocalization: controlled polysyllabic vowel sounds. An advance over cooing which repeats the same drawn out vowel sound; at this stage, vocalizes distinct syllables with control or diverse vowel sounds in varying combinations, e.g., "ah-ah-ah, ah-oh-oh-uh, oh-oh-oh."

Feeding: takes solids well. No longer extrudes them with the tongue; not merely willing acceptance of semisolid baby food.

Play: feet to mouth, supine. Gets foot into mouth.

Mirror: reaches, pats image. Definite regard for own face or hand, not merely random fingering of mirror itself (see 20 Weeks).

Ring and String: fusses or abandons effort. Examiner finally must place ring within reach or give it to infant.

32 WEEKS

Cube: grasps second cube. After securing first by himself, picks up second.

Cube: retains two as third presented. Retains already secured cubes, one in each hand, when third is added (see 36 Weeks).

Cube: holds two prolongedly. For more than a minute, providing he has secured them himself.

Cup and Cubes: holds cube, regards cup. Gives cup definite regard; may then drop cube when cup within reach or pick up cup while retaining cube. Be sure infant has a cube in his hand before adding cup.

Ring and String: secures ring. Hand contacts string on presentation or after reaching for ring first; in course of manipulation of string, ring comes within reach (see 44 Weeks).

Sitting: 1 minute, erect, unsteady. On *a hard* surface, maintains both hands up for 1 minute (see 28 Weeks).

Standing: maintains briefly, hands held. Examiner holds hands; infant's arms fully extended at shoulder height for balance only, not for support.

Prone: pivots. Moves in a circular manner, pivoting on abdomen, by coordinated action of arms, crossing one over other. Infant should demonstrate his capacity to pivot more than 45°; surface should be *hard.*

Pellet: radial raking. Radial side of hand definitely oriented to pellet and takes lead in raking at pellet; less arm movement than at 28 weeks.

Pellet: unsuccessful inferior scissors grasp. Infant attempts to grasp pellet by approximating thumb to side of curled or extended index finger; other fingers are curled and actively flexing simultaneously. Grasp sometimes successful (see 36 Weeks).

Vocalization: single consonant, as "da, ba, ka." Definite consonant syllable; may be preceded by vowel, e.g., "ah-da," but with stress on consonant.

Play: bites, chews toys. Distinguish from mouthing and licking only.

Play: reaches persistently for toys out of reach. May be at tabletop, in prone or in supine (usually rolls to prone).

Ring and String: persistent. Continues to pursue even if he is fussing; usually does, but may not, succeed in securing ring.

Growth Trends: Twenty-eight Weeks

One of the major goals of infant development is attaining the upright posture. The 28-week infant is chronologically and developmentally at a halfway station on the road to this goal. He is just beginning to sit alone, erecting his trunk for a brief moment. After he has doubled his age, at 56 weeks, he stands alone. When the 28-week infant is placed in supine, he lifts his head from the platform. Placed in a standing position, steadied by the trunk, his legs sustain a large fraction of weight.

His arm control is far in advance of his leg control. When placed securely in the examining chair, he delights in exercising his new powers of manipulation. At 16 weeks he sits in rather stiff bilateral symmetry. Now his trunk is more supple, and he can make an eager unilateral forward thrust to reach an object like the handbell. He is more mobile at shoulder, elbow and wrist joints. He is transcending the earlier phase of bilateral symmetry. Not only does he make a one-handed approach to the bell, he shifts the bell from one hand to the other with startling adeptness.

This shuttlelike transfer has both symmetric and asymmetric features. Nature is weaving a very complicated neuromotor fabric, laying down the warp and woof for that specialized functional asymmetry which goes by the everyday name of handedness. The neonate is unidextrous in the tonic-neck-reflex position, without selected dominance. The 16-week infant is bidextrous; the 28-week infant is bi-unidextrous, using both hands but one at a time; hence his capacity for transfer and retransfer and retransfer again. It is one of his most typical patterns. Dominance is socially determined or forced by injury to the central nervous system, which may delay its establishment. Ambidexterity is still common at 3 years, and full unilateral dominance probably is not complete until 8 or 9 years of age.

The same alternating type of action in the 32-week infant produces a circular translocation when he is placed on his abdomen. Being geared to alternating movements, he flexes and extends his arms in successional turns, causing his trunk to pivot. A few weeks later, when his arms again are geared temporarily to bilateral movements in the prone position, he pushes himself backward or crawls by dragging himself forward. Leg control is not sufficiently developed for creeping on hands and knees.

The 28-week infant is therefore far in advance of the 16-week infant in patterns of prehension, but his eyes continue to be more skillful than his fingers. Thanks to his ocular adjustments, he can pick up a string perceptually, but he is very inept at plucking it with his fingers. Likewise, he can give consistent ocular regard to a pellet, but he places his hand rather crudely over it and usually fails to secure it. Prompt, precise prehension of the pellet comes at about 40 weeks, as a result of the specialization of the radial digits—thumb and forefinger. This too is a sort of functional asymmetry developing within the hand itself. This more advanced asymmetry is already foreshadowed at 28 weeks. Even though the 28-week infant seizes the cube with a hand rather than a finger grasp, he appropriates with the *radial* side of the hand. This radial palmar grasp foretells thumb opposition, when the progression from ulnar to radial side is complete. Finger specialization occurs last for the smallest objects, just as did ocular prehension.

Although eyes are still in the lead, eyes and hands function in close interaction, each reinforcing and guiding the other. Whereas the 16-week infant is given to inspection of surroundings, the 28-week infant inspects objects. If the object is within reach, it is usually in his busy hands. The head became versatile in the previous quarter; hands become versatile in this one. As soon as he sees a cube, he grasps it, brings it to his mouth, withdraws it, looks at it on withdrawal, fingers it while he looks, looks while he rotates it, restores it to his mouth, withdraws it again for inspection, restores it again for mouthing, transfers it to the other hand, bangs it, contacts it with the free hand, retransfers, mouths it again, drops it, resecures it, mouths it yet again, repeating the cycle with variations—all in the time it takes to read this sentence. The perceptual—manipulatory behavior of the 28-week infant is highly active; it is not passive reception. It is dynamic adaptivity, fused with exploitative capacity.

His vocal behavior also is filled with forward reference. It serves little immediate social purpose, but it does serve a neurologic one. Control of lingual, labial and buccal musculature is developing, and in his diversified spontaneous vocalization he is producing vowels, consonants and even syllables and diphthongs, which in due time will eventuate in articulate communication learned from and reinforced by others. Even now an "m-m-m" utterance emerges when he cries, the first modification of the air stream by the lips.

Although he is verbally inarticulate, he is socially quite wise. He knows what is going on about the house. He expresses eagerness and impatience as he sees his mother preparing food for him. He shows familiarity and anticipation in the routines of the household. He recognizes strangers and tolerates them if they do not disappoint his expectancies. He is self-contained and will play for considerable periods by himself. Long ago he abandoned the hand play characteristic of 16 weeks. He plays with his feet instead, a cephalocaudad advance as well as part of his process of self-discovery. He is self-contained, content with his own devices. His very self-sufficiency makes him seem a more or less finished product. However, in time he will make a clearer distinction between himself as a person and other persons. He is, in fact, laying the foundations for this more socialized perceptiveness.

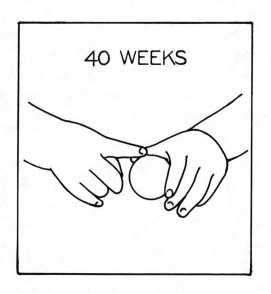

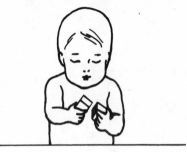

1. Matches two cubes

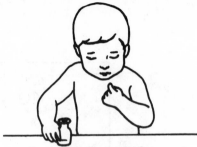

5. Holds bottle and
grasps pellet

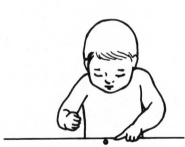

2. Fingers cube in cup

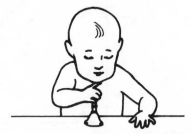

6. Grasps bell by handle

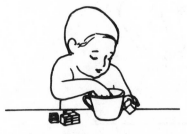

3. Approaches with
index finger

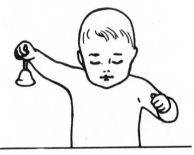

7. Waves bell

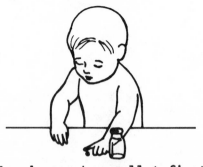

4. Approaches pellet first

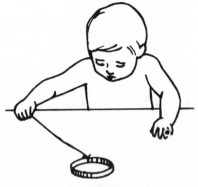

8. Plucks string easily

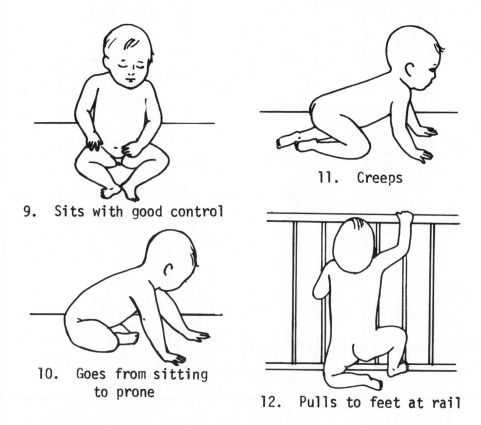

9.   Sits with good control

11.   Creeps

10.   Goes from sitting
       to prone

12.   Pulls to feet at rail

§5. FORTY WEEKS

The 40-week infant sits before the test table with good postural control, without support. He gives immediate heed to the FIRST CUBE and seizes it with a radial digital grasp. He transfers the cube and retains it as the SECOND CUBE is presented. He seizes this in a similar manner and holds the two cubes as the THIRD CUBE is presented. He drops one cube to secure the third, hitting or pushing the cube on the table with the cube in his hand, and *brings two cubes into apposition,* looking at them as he *matches* them in his hands (1).

In the MASSED CUBE situation he approaches the mass immediately with one hand and grasps a single cube, selecting a top or a corner cube. Holding one cube, he grasps another, and brings the cubes into combination. He *releases* a cube and exploits three or more in all with method and *control.*

The examiner now places the CUP at the left side of the cluster of CUBES. The baby grasps the cup by the rim; later he takes a cube and brings it against the outside of the cup. The examiner gestures and requests the infant to put the cube into the cup, but the baby is not yet able to do this. The examiner then drops a cube into the cup, and the baby reaches in and *fingers the cube in the cup* (2).

36 Weeks	KEY AGE: 40 Weeks	44 Weeks
	Adaptive	
Cube: grasps 3rd cube (*40w)	Cube: matches 2 cubes (*15m)	Cup-cube: removes cube from cup
Cube: hits, pushes cube with cube (*15m)	Cup-cube: fingers cube in cup (*44w)	Cup-cube: (demonstration) cube into cup without release (*52w)
Cup-cube: cube against cup (*44w)	Pellet: index finger approach	Pellet in bottle: points at pellet through glass (*18m)
Pellet & bottle: approaches bottle first (*40w)	Pellet & bottle: approaches pellet first	Bell: regards & pokes clapper
Ring-string: manipulates string	Pellet & bottle: grasps pellet	Ring-string: approaches string first
	Pellet in bottle: regards pellet if drops out	
	Bell: grasps by handle	
	Bell: waves or shakes	
	Gross Motor	
Sit: 10 minutes plus, steady	Sit: indefinitely, steady	Stand: at rail, lifts & replaces foot (*48w)
Sit: leans forward, reerects	Sit: goes over to prone	
Stand: holds rail, full weight (*48w)	Stand: pulls to feet at rail (*15m)	
	Prone: creeps (*15m)	
	Fine Motor	
Cube: radial digital grasp	Cube: crude release (*15m)	Bell: grasps by top of handle
Pellet: prehends, scissors grasp (*40w)	Pellet: grasps promptly	
	Pellet: inferior pincer grasp (*48w)	
	Ring-string: plucks string easily	
	Language	
Vocalization: da-da or equivalent (*40w)	Vocabulary: dada & mama, with meaning	
Vocalization: imitates sounds	Vocabulary: 1 "word"	
Comprehension: responds to name, no-no	Comprehension: bye, patacake	
	Personal-Social	
Feeding: holds bottle (*15m)	Social: waves bye, patacakes (*...)	Social: extends toy to person without release (*52w)
Feeding: feeds self cracker		Feeding: milk from cup in part (*15m)
		Mirror: reaches image of ball in mirror (*52w)

He approaches the PELLET with extended *index finger* (3). His arm rests on the table, and he prehends the pellet *promptly* with an *inferior pincer grasp.* The examiner then presents the PELLET BESIDE THE BOTTLE, the pellet on the infant's right. The baby *reaches for the pellet first* (4), *grasps the pellet,* drops it and then exploits the bottle. At some point in his exploitation, the infant *holds* the *bottle* and tries to *pick up* the *pellet at the same time* (5). Securing the baby's attention to the maneuver, the examiner drops the PELLET INTO THE BOTTLE and places the bottle on the test table. The baby watches the dropping of the pellet, but his regard for the pellet in the bottle is questionable. He grasps the bottle and mouths it. If the *pellet falls out,* he *regards it* on the table and may pick it up. If the pellet fails to fall out, the examiner can drop one surreptitiously on the table top.

He approaches the BELL and *seizes it by the handle* (6). He mouths the bell, transfers it and *waves and shakes it* (7), spontaneously or after demonstration.

The RING AND STRING, with string in oblique alignment, is placed on the test table. He reaches directly toward the ring first, then *plucks the string easily* (8), pulls the ring into reach, grasps it, transfers the ring and manipulates the string while holding the ring.

The test table is now removed and the baby turned to face a large MIRROR. He regards his image, leans forward and smiles and vocalizes as he pats the glass. He is offered the BALL, which he accepts and retains; he usually disregards the mirrored ball, but may reach for its image.

Postural behavior is now observed. He has already displayed his ability to SIT with *good control* (9). Enticed by a lure, he *goes directly from sitting to prone* (10). In prone he gets up on his *hands and knees* and CREEPS (11) forward with alternating movements. Holding a RAILING, he *pulls himself to his feet* (12),

---

Examination Sequence

Age: 36−40−44 Weeks   Situation No. (Appendix A-4)

(Normative behavior characteristic of the *key age: 40 weeks* and adjacent age levels is codified by the Developmental Schedule shown on the adjoining page.)

Table top
Cubes 1, 2, 3 7,8,9
Massed cubes 11
Cup and cubes 17
Pellet 18
Pellet beside bottle 19
Pellet in bottle 20
Bell 22
Ring and string 23
Mirror 24
Mirror and ball 25
Sitting free 53
Creeping 54
Rail 55
Cruising 56
Walking supported 57

Italicized items appear for the first time in this sequence

stands holding on, and lowers himself again. He may CRUISE at the crib railing and WALK when BOTH HANDS are HELD to provide balance.

He vocalizes *"mama"* and *"dada"* with meaning and *has one other "word."* He imitates sounds (cough, click, razz) and responds to "no-no" and his name.

He is reported to hold his bottle and to feed himself a cracker. He *patacakes,* waves *bye-bye* or engages in other *nursery tricks.* Understanding his mother's verbal requests is language behavior; requiring demonstration before imitating her gestures is personal–social behavior.

Glossary of Developmented Schedule Items

36 WEEKS

Cube: grasps third cube. Drops one of two he has picked up to secure third cube that is presented (see 32 Weeks).

Cube: hits, pushes cube with cube. Pushes cube(s) on table with one in his hand. Distinguish definite intent from accidental contact as infant bangs cubes.

Cup and Cubes: cube against cup. Hits or brings cube in hand against cup; may even contact inside of cup. Distinguish intent from accidental contact.

Pellet and Bottle: approaches bottle first. Differentiates 36- from 40-week behavior but not from less mature behavior. Any younger infant approaches bottle first and ignores pellet (see 40 Weeks), so that a positive response merely indicates less than 40-week behavior.

Ring and String: manipulates string. Holds ring in one hand and manipulates string with other; definite awareness of two parts.

Sitting: 10 minutes plus, steady. Both hands used in play. Is still apt to throw self back unexpectedly; mother unwilling to leave infant unattended.

Sitting: leans forward, reerects. Reerects completely and smoothly, without pushing up stepwise with arms.

Standing: holds rail, full weight. When placed standing at rail, holds on and maintains position without leaning chest against rail.

Cube: radial digital grasp. Cube held with ends of thumb, index and third fingers. Space visible between cube and palm (see 28 Weeks).

Pellet: prehends, scissors grasp. Successful prehension between thumb and side of curled index finger. Remaining fingers held loosely curled but do not flex and extend during prehension (see 32 Weeks).

Vocalization: "da-da" or equivalent. Definite combination of two or more consonant sounds, but without specific meaning.

Vocalization: imitates sounds. Repeats a cough, "razz," clicking of tongue, not words; initiated by mother.

Comprehension: responds to name, "no-no." Distinguishes his own name, rather than mere sound of his mother's voice; may continue what he is doing in response to "no-no" but pauses.

Feeding: holds bottle. Eight-ounce bottle with no assistance from mother; retrieves dropped bottle and completes feeding.

Feeding: feeds self cracker. Successive purposeful bites and munching, rather than simply sucking on cracker and then discarding it.

40 WEEKS

Cube: matches two cubes. Brings them into close proximity as though comparing them or brings them together patacake fashion. Both cubes are grasped and lifted, and infant watches what he is doing (to be differentiated from pushing one cube with another at 36 weeks).

Cup and Cube: fingers cube in cup. Manipulates cube examiner has dropped in without removing it from cup.

Pellet: index finger approach. Essential feature is differentiation of index finger; may be exhibited with objects other than pellet.

Pellet and Bottle: approaches pellet first. Examiner must be careful that infant fixates pellet at edge of tabletop before both objects brought within reach simultaneously. Essential feature is that smaller object is approached first, although bottle may be grasped first.

Pellet and Bottle: grasps pellet. Is aware of small object and of two objects simultaneously; tries to or does pick up pellet while holding bottle.

Pellet in Bottle: regards pellet if drops out. If pellet does not fall out within sight, examiner drops pellet on tabletop, making sure infant does not see this being done.

Bell: grasps by handle. Not by bowl *and* handle; initial approach and grasp only.

Bell: waves or shakes. Distinguish active movements to produce sound from passive ringing as arms move. Must be in sitting position, as distinct from shaking rattle in supine position (see 28 Weeks). Examiner may demonstrate finally; broad sweep of his arm is necessary.

Sitting: indefinitely, steady. Uses both hands in play. Mother knows he will not fall over if she leaves him alone in room. This is *the definition of sitting alone.*

Sitting: goes over to prone. Directly forward from steady sitting, with good control.

Standing: pulls to feet at rail. Attains fully erect position; feet remain firmly planted.

Prone: creeps. On hands and knees, or hands and feet, trunk raised. Pulling self along on abdomen (crawling) is less mature behavior than creeping; pulling self about on buttocks in sitting position (hitching) is a locomotor variant roughly equivalent to creeping in maturity value. The meaning of creeping and crawling varies with geographic locale, so precise definition necessary.

Cube: crude release. As opposed to dropping; a somewhat clumsy and exaggerated letting go. Puts cube down on table top and takes hand off, or releases cube into cup.

Pellet: grasps promptly. Independent of type of grasp, but consistently secures on first or second approach; usually not prompt if thumb and fingers not coordinated.

Pellet: inferior pincer grasp. Between ventral surface of thumb and tip of index (or middle) finger; hand and arm resting on the table surface provide accessory support (see 48 Weeks).

Ring and String: plucks string easily. Inferior pincer grasp between thumb and index (or middle) finger tip. Prompt but cruder grasp is not plucking.

Vocabulary: "dada" and "mama," with meaning. These or equivalent consonant combinations are used specifically to refer to father and mother.

Vocabulary: one "word." A sound used consistently to refer to an action, object or group of objects even if not recognizably articulated. Ask specifically if infant says something that means bye, hi, no, what (huh), etc., which are common first words.

Comprehension: "bye, patacake." Understands what mother says when she uses words, and responds appropriately. May be other nursery games such as "so big," "peek-a-boo," etc. (see below).

Social: waves bye, patacakes. Engages in nursery game if mother demonstrates it first. Social play is distinct from comprehension (above); it must also be distinguished from self-initiated stereotyped patterning unrelated to social demand.

44 WEEKS

Cup and Cube: removes cube from cup. After he sees examiner drop one in, or one falls in accidentally.

Cup and Cube: (demonstration) cube into cup without release. Thrusts hand holding cube inside cup but does not let go. Distinguish intent from accidental contact of inside of cup (see 52 Weeks).

Pellet and Bottle: points at pellet through glass. Looks at the pellet while he is poking at bottle.

Bell: regards and pokes clapper. Distinguish from accidental contact of clapper during course of manipulation; visual fixation accompanies exploration. Occasionally may clearly finger and move clapper about while looking elsewhere.

Ring and String: approaches string first. Indicates on his first approach he is aware he will obtain ring by pulling on string; watches ring come in as he pulls (see 32 Weeks).

Standing: at rail, lifts and replaces foot. In preparation for cruising, but without sidewise progression; one foot, or each alternately.

Bell: grasps by top of handle. Overhand in ends of fingers, not fist, on his first approach.

Social: extends toy to person without release. In response to extended hand and "Give it to me," "Thank you," or spontaneously.

Feeding: milk from cup (in part). Usually willing to accept water and juice from cup at earlier age than milk. Mother holds cup.

Mirror: reaches image ball in mirror. Infant holds ball in one hand, reaches into mirror with free hand for image of ball; may reach for image of his feet also, or reach for object examiner holds behind and to one side of him (a good test for visual fields, as infant often spies object itself at side of his head).

Growth Trends: Forty Weeks

The index finger comes to the fore at 40 weeks. The poking, prying, palpating, extended forefinger is itself an index of an important advance in maturity. In a neuromotor sense, the behavior patterns have become more refined and discriminating. Many of the reactions of the 28-week level are massive and crude in comparison. The 28-week infant can barely contact a pellet, and he does so with a whole-hand raking approach; the 40-week infant prehends promptly with pincer precision. Twenty-eight weeks slaps a string; 40 weeks plucks it easily. Placed on his stomach, 28 weeks stays put; 40 weeks creeps. Forty weeks sits prolongedly, 28 weeks precariously. One does not make such a comparison to the discredit of the junior infant. However, the comparison would have grave diagnostic import if it referred to a 40-week-old infant functioning at the 28-week level. For this reason, it is always pleasing to see the poking pattern come into evidence in the forties of infancy. This pattern testifies that the distal outposts of the neuromotor system—finger tip, tongue tip, feet and toes—are undergoing their normal maturation.

The increased refinements in prehension are correlated with increased discrimination in manipulation. They herald a heightened interest in small objects. A crumb on the high chair tray, as well as the pellet on the test table, provokes a tendency to poke and to palpate. Tiny objects now possess greater stimulus potency than larger ones. When the examiner places a pellet beside the bottle, he sets up two rival stimuli: large versus small object. At 36 weeks the baby reaches for the bottle first and disregards the pellet; at 40 weeks he reaches for the pellet first but then divides his attention between pellet and bottle; at 48 weeks he pays almost exclusive attention to the pellet, unless it is inside the bottle; at 52 weeks he attempts to insert the pellet in the bottle. This maturity sequence reflects the orderliness and delicacy of the developmental process: first the large object has priority; then the small object gains priority; then combination of small and large object prevails. The year-old baby usually fails in his attempt to drop the pellet into the bottle. This is due to the immaturity of prehensory release rather than a lack of perception for container and contained.

The perception of this relationship of container and content is long in the making, as indicated by the growth of behavior patterns in the cup (container) and cubes (content) situation. The infant of 28 weeks is scarcely old enough for presentation of this situation. He drops the cube to pick up the added cup. At 32 weeks he gives prior attention to the cubes, but as he holds one of the cubes he gives well-defined regard to the cup. Developmentally this presages a combination of cup and cube; in fact, it is an ocular combining. At 36 weeks it becomes a manual combining, for he literally brings the cube against the cup. But this is the limit of his combinative capacity. He will not place the cube into the cup or alter his behavior, even though the examiner plies him with gesture, command and actual demonstration. This, however, is a temporary, developmental kind of disobedience. At 40 weeks, the baby thrusts his hand into the cup after the examiner has placed a cube in it, and he fingers the cube. In another month he will extract it and rethrust his hand into the cup, retaining clenched hold of the cube. At 52 weeks he consummates the pattern by voluntarily releasing a single cube in the cup after demonstration. Further developmental elaborations of this behavior continue into the second year of life, and will be recounted later.

The 40-week infant also pulls himself to his feet at the railing of his pen, a foretoken of upright locomotion, even though for the remaining quarter of the year he will utilize the ancient method of quadrupedal progression. His creeping is one of a score of progressive stages which culminate in bipedal walking, provided that the central nervous system is intact and the environment does not interfere with this progression. The supine position so acceptable throughout the first quarter of the year now is scarcely tolerated except during sleep. The 40-week infant speedily escapes supineness by rolling or raising himself to a sitting position.

In vocalization, the 40-week infant is becoming articulate, and his sounds are acquiring meaning. He is socially responsive to demonstration; hence his nursery tricks and other engaging evidences of acculturation. At 12 and 15 months one sees how these foretokens of discriminating behavior come to their destined fulfillment.

Thus, 40 weeks marks a prophetic transition to what is almost an epoch, since there are so many new and distinctive behavior patterns emerging in the developmental complex. With inquisitive index finger the infant segregates a single detail for attention, and he reacts in a successive and combining way to two details, to two objects, to container and contained, to solid and hollow, to top and bottom, to one side and another side. His impulse to stand, albeit with support, is irrepressible. He shows a new interest in words, both as receptor and producer. Not only is he taking new social interest in the family circle, but he himself is becoming more fully adopted by that circle as a participating member. This is further evidence of important psychologic transformations to come.

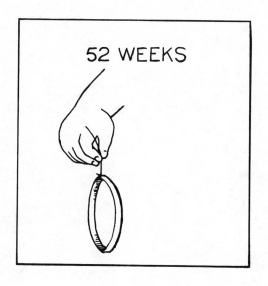

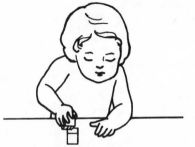

1. Applies cube on cube without release

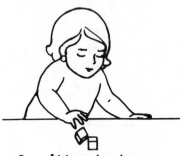

2. Attempts tower; it falls

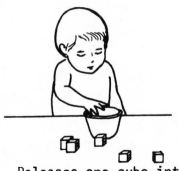

3. Releases one cube into cup after demonstration

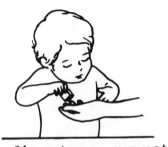

4. Gives toy on request

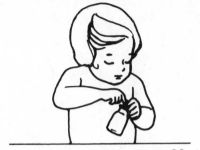

5. Tries to insert pellet

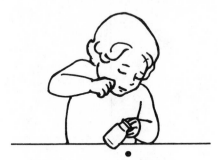

6. Pellet falls outside bottle

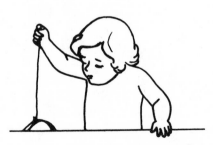

7. Dangles ring by string

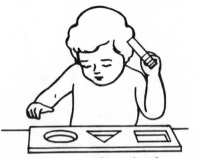

8. Looks selectively at round hole

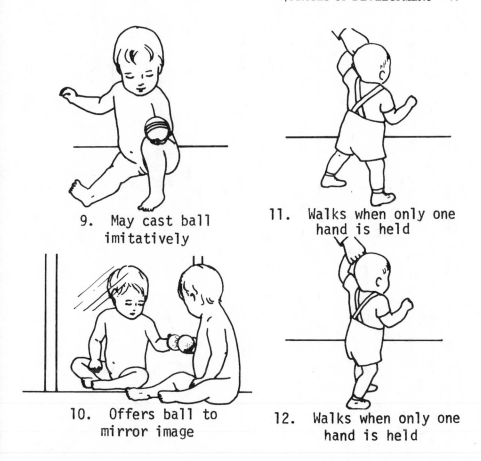

9.   May cast ball
     imitatively

11.   Walks when only one
      hand is held

10.   Offers ball to
      mirror image

12.   Walks when only one
      hand is held

§6. FIFTY-TWO WEEKS

The year-old child sits erect and unsupported before the test table, and he is quite likely to pivot in the sitting position and carry the introductory toy to the side or to the platform. The toy is removed tactfully as the FIRST, SECOND and THIRD CUBES are presented in succession. He brings the cubes together briefly, or he hits and pushes one cube with another.

The examiner builds a TOWER OF TWO cubes and tries by demonstration and gesture to induce the child to do likewise. The child manipulates the cubes, takes a cube from the model and applies *one cube upon another without release* (1). When he *attempts a tower, it falls (*2).

In the MASSED CUBES situation he takes two cubes, usually selecting the top cube and a corner cube. He exploits the cubes in a controlled manner, in combination or one-by-one sequence. He seizes and releases as many as four cubes.

The CUP is then placed to the left of the cluster of CUBES. He takes the cup,

KEY AGE: 52 Weeks

	48 Weeks		52 Weeks		56 Weeks	
	H	O	H	O	H	O
Adaptive	Cube: sequential play (*48m) Pellet & bottle: takes pellet only (*52w) Formboard: removes round block easily		Cube: (demonstration) tries tower, fails (*15m) Cup-cube: (demonstration) releases 1 cube in cup (*56w) Pellet & bottle: tries inserting, releases, fails (*15m) Ring-string: dangles ring by string Formboard: looks selectively at round hole (*56w)		Cup-cube: (no demonstration) 1 cube into cup Drawing: vigorous imitative scribble (*18m) Formboard: (demonstration) inserts round block (*15m)	
Gross Motor	Sit: pivots Stand: cruises at rail (*15m) Walks: needs 2 hands held (*52w)		Walks: needs only 1 hand held (*15m)		Stand: momentarily alone (*15m)	
Fine Motor	Pellet: neat pincer grasp				Cube: grasps 2 in 1 hand	
Language			Vocabulary: 2 "words" (besides mama, dada) Comprehension: gives a toy (request & gesture)		Vocabulary: 3-4 words Vocalization: incipient jargon (*15m) Comprehension: a few objects by name	
Personal-Social	Play: toys to side rail (*15m) Play: platform play (*15m)		Mirror: offers ball to mirror image Dressing: cooperates in dressing (*48m)		Ball: releases with slight cast toward examiner (*18m)	

and brings a cube into the cup without release. The examiner gestures and then drops a cube into the cup as a demonstration. The child immediately removes this cube, and then *releases a cube into the cup* (3). He may *give a cube* to the examiner on request and gesture (4).

Confronted with the PELLET BESIDE BOTTLE, the pellet on the right, he reaches for the pellet first and picks it up with a neat pincer grasp. The examiner points to the bottle and gently inhibits the child's taking the pellet to the mouth. After the examiner finally places the PELLET IN the BOTTLE, the child brings the pellet over the mouth of the bottle and *tries unsuccessfully to insert the pellet* (5). It *falls outside* the bottle (6).

In the RING AND STRING situation, the string in the right oblique position within reach, he reaches immediately for the end of the string, plucks it easily and secures the ring. He exploits the ring by transfer, and he *dangles the ring by the string* (7).

When the examiner DRAWS vigorously back and forth at the top of a piece of paper, and then hands the crayon to the infant, he may scribble imitatively.

He pulls at the FORMBOARD which is presented with the round hole at the right. The examiner holds the board in place and offers the child the round block. He accepts it and then *looks very selectively at the round hole* (8). The examiner inserts the round block; the child removes it easily, again looks selectively at the round hole, and bangs or releases the block near the round hole.

The test table is then removed, and the BALL is offered. He accepts the ball and on invitation extends it to the examiner. The examiner then tosses the ball so

Examination Sequence

(Normative behavior characteristic of the *key age: 52 weeks* and adjacent age levels is codified by the Developmental Schedule shown on the adjoining page.)

Age: 48–52–56 Weeks	Situation No. (Appendix A-4)
Table top	
Cubes 1, 2, 3	7,8,9
Tower 2	10
Massed cubes	11
Cup and cubes	17
Pellet beside bottle	19
Pellet in bottle	20
Ring and string	23
Drawing–scribble imitation	27
Formboard	35
Ball play	46
Mirror	24
Mirror and ball	25
Sitting free	53
Creeping	54
Rail	55
Cruising	56
Walking supported	57

Italicized items appear for the first time in this sequence.

that it rolls toward the child. After one or two demonstrations, the child *may cast the ball* imitatively (9).

Before the MIRROR he regards his own image with smiling and vocalization, leans forward and pats the glass. He accepts and retains the BALL placed in his hands, and *brings the ball against the mirror* (10), offering it to his image.

His postural behavior includes pivoting in the SITTING position, going from the sitting to the CREEPING position, creeping, pulling to his feet while holding a RAILING, CRUISING at the railing, and lowering himself again. He can WALK SUPPORTED *when only one hand is held* (11, 12).

His language includes *two "words"* in addition to "mama" and "dada." He responds to *"give it to me,"* and may look in recognition at objects named by his mother.

He is reported to drink at least some of his milk from a cup. *He cooperates in dressing* by pushing his arms through his sleeves or holding his feet up for shoes and socks.

Glossary of Developmental Schedule Items

48 WEEKS

Cube: sequential play. With definite intent, transposing one after another about on table, or from table to platform; picking up and dropping one after another, or putting several cubes into cup.

Pellet and Bottle: takes pellet only. Gives virtually exclusive attention to pellet; may pick up bottle if pellet is inside.

Formboard: removes round block easily. Usually by lifting one edge with thumb and getting underneath block; occasionally with whole hand over entire block when hand is large enough. Essential feature is awareness of how block has to be manipulated to remove it.

Sitting: pivots. Moves in a circular manner, swinging around on buttocks; uses feet only to propel himself.

Standing: cruises at rail. Sideward walking, holding rail for support, shifting hands.

Walks: needs two hands held. Trunk does not need support; child is held by his two hands for balance only and moves his legs coordinately with forward impetus.

Pellet: neat pincer grasp. The adult grasp between thumb and tip of index (or middle) finger, hand elevated above table surface; discarding accessory support of arm and hand resting on table top is what distinguishes neat from inferior pincer grasp (see 40 Weeks).

Play: toys to side rail. No longer restricted to exploitation on table top only; bangs toys on side rail of crib, or runs them along it.

Play: platform play. Carrying object to crib platform with intent or exploiting an object on platform. Does not include simple restoring of a dropped object from platform to table.

52 WEEKS

Cube: (demonstration) tries tower, fails. Tower falls when cube is released, or cube is placed on in tower fashion without release, or tower is built in hand and tower cube held on.

Cup and Cube: (demonstration) releases one cube in cup. After examiner drops cube into cup. Distinguish intent from accidental falling of cube into cup (see 44 Weeks).

Pellet and Bottle: tries inserting, releases, fails. Pellet falls outside bottle; it is not necessarily released over neck of bottle but definitely brought into relation with bottle and released, in response to demonstration, command or gesture.

Ring and String: dangles ring by string. Essential feature is awareness of relationship between ring and string. Distinguish passive dangling of ring as infant moves arm from his active exploitation.

Formboard: looks selectively at round hole. Do not credit questionable behavior. The combining by eye shifts of round block and round hole (before examiner demonstrates relationship) is very obvious when present.

Walks: needs only one hand held. Coordinated forward drive when one hand held for balance only, not support.

Vocabulary: two words (besides "mama, dada"). (See 40 Weeks for definition of a word.)

Comprehension: gives a toy (request and gesture). Places and actively releases in examiner's hand, rather than merely permitting its removal. If infant is unwilling to respond to examiner, accept a report or let mother ask child.

Mirror: offers ball to mirror image. Essential feature is offering ball to himself, rather than merely bringing it against mirror.

Dressing: cooperates in dressing. Puts foot out for shoe, completes pushing arm through sleeve, etc. May have one or two other tricks such as bringing comb to head or handkerchief to nose.

56 WEEKS

Cup and Cube: (no demonstration) one cube into cup. Spontaneously or after request and gesture. Again distinguish intent from falling (see 52 Weeks).

Drawing: vigorous imitative scribble. Reproduction of the back and forth motion demonstrated by examiner, even though no marks may appear on paper, or table top surface is utilized.

Formboard: (demonstration) inserts round block. Indicates perception of relationship after examiner inserts block; block need not be inserted completely into hole.

Standing: momentarily alone. Doesn't hold on and maintains balance briefly.

Cube: grasps two in one hand. May take two simultaneously, although intent rather than accident is clearer if secured sequentially.

Vocabulary: three–four words. In addition to "mama" and "dada" (see 40 Weeks for definition of a word).

Vocalization: incipient jargon. Jargon is distinguished from baby babbling by presence of inflections and pauses. It sounds like sentences uttered in a foreign language. At this age the jargon consists only of two or three wordlike phrases (see 15 Months).

Comprehension: a few objects by name. When mother asks "Where's the light, your shoe, the T.V.?" infant looks at object or otherwise indicates recognition. He is not required to repeat word. Includes only inanimate objects, not persons and pets.

Ball: releases with slight cast toward examiner. Encompasses both social play with examiner and ability to release ball actively.

Growth Trends: Fifty-two Weeks

Sixteen and 40 weeks were called prophetic periods. At 40 weeks the infant grasps a support and pulls himself to his feet; he plucks a string easily; he reaches his hand into a cup; he plays a nursery trick on verbal cue; he shows a growing interest in details. These are not tag-ends of behavior; they are tag-beginnings. They mark the nascent or beginning stages of patterns which come to developmental fulfillment at the age of 15 months.

Consider the advances achieved by the 15-month child. He can attain the standing position unaided; he can walk alone; he can put several cubes in and out of a cup; he can place a pellet in a bottle; he can build a tower of two cubes; he can talk in jargon; he can communicate by gesture.

The 52-week child is just at the brink of all these abilities. He can be thought of as in an "almost" stage: he almost builds a tower, almost puts the pellet into the bottle, almost puts the round block in the formboard. So much of 52-week behavior depends on an ability and willingness to release, that if the infant is a hoarder the examination can be frustrating. The infant's behavior may belie the history given by the parents, and he may even appear to be functioning below his chronologic age. For this reason, it is inadvisable to select 1 year as the age for conducting research investigations.

Speaking relatively, we may say that 40 weeks is nascent and prophetic; 52 weeks is formative and transitional; 15 months is more finished in behavioral organization. The 18-month child is still more advanced, but in turn has acquired new prophecies which point to 2 years and beyond. It helps us to understand the behavioral equipment of the 1-year child if we think of him as a 15-month child in the making. At 15 months the human infant is assuredly a biped. He prefers to walk upright like a human. He has discarded creeping, an ancient method of progression which the 1-year-old still elects. Nevertheless, we cannot regard quadrupedal locomotion as an atavism; it transforms developmentally into bipedal locomotion. Accordingly, the creeping of the 52- and 56-week infant tends to become plantigrade; the legs extend at the knees, and the soles of the feet, like the palms of the hands, are then planted on the ground. This all-fours locomotion proves to be a final step in the assumption of the erect posture. Having planted both soles on the ground, he soon rises to his feet. When feet become the fulcrum, the hands are emancipated.

The 52-week infant also displays an interesting mixture of maturity and immaturity in prehension. He can grasp a pellet or a string with almost adult precision and facility, but having grasped, he is still a mere baby in his ability to release his grasp. Sometimes he clings to an object with almost neonatal tenacity, as though he could not summon voluntary inhibition. This is particularly true in the case of small objects. Not until the age of 15 months can he release well enough to drop the pellet into the bottle, even though at 52 weeks he manages to release a cube into the cup. His repeated picking up and expulsive dropping of individual cubes in his exploitative play is an exercise of his newfound (i.e., new-grown) power of release. His tireless and apparently irresponsible casting of objects at 15 months is vigorous expression of the same but more abundant capacity. His ability at 18 months to put as many as ten cubes into a cup in an orderly manner, with little or no prompting, reflects the cultivation which comes with maturity, as well as the more sustained attention necessary for the completion of a task.

Perception of geometric form is incipient at 52 weeks. The infant at that age looks selectively at the round hole in the formboard. At 56 weeks he inserts the round block on demonstration. At 15 months he inserts it adaptively even after the examiner has reversed the position of the hole by rotating the board. The deliberate dangling of the ring by its attached string also suggests a dawning sense of form and of spatial relationships at the age of 1 year. Of similar import is the incipient, though usually unsuccessful, effort to build a tower.

The yearling is increasingly perceptive of his social as well as his physical environment. Socialized perception leads to imitation. He is responsive to demonstration; he looks intently at facial expressions; he responds to music and to primitive rhythm play; he repeats performances laughed at. He has long been capable of fear, anger, affection, jealousy, anxiety and sympathy, and these traits are now more clearly manifested. By such tokens he reveals the complexity and also the individuality of his personal—social behavior.

At 15 months, much of his behavior already reflects the impress of the social group. His actions have an outward, nonisolationist reference. He shows and offers toys to others; he says "ta-ta" on receiving, or giving, something; he helps to turn the pages of a book and begins to recognize pictures; he uses jargon; he pulls, hauls, lugs and transports, for his hands are now freed from the menial work of locomotion. Fifteen months is a time of massive integration, and more truly a key age in development.

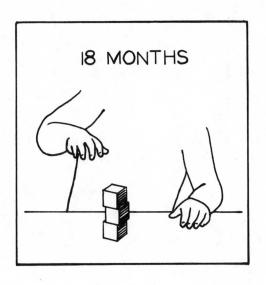

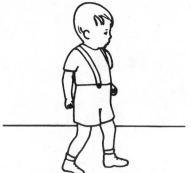

1. Walks alone; seldom falls

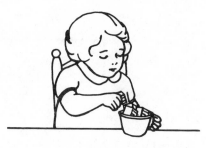

5. Fills cup with cubes

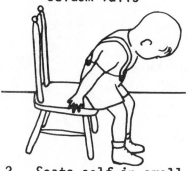

2. Seats self in small chair

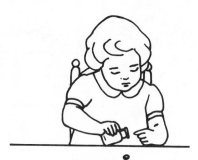

6. Dumps pellet from bottle

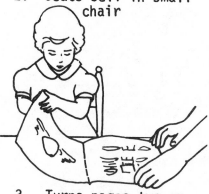

3. Turns pages two or three at a time

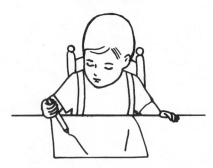

7. Imitates stroke

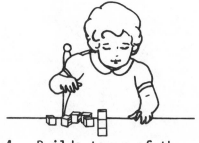

4. Builds tower of three

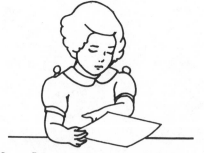

8. Identifies one picture

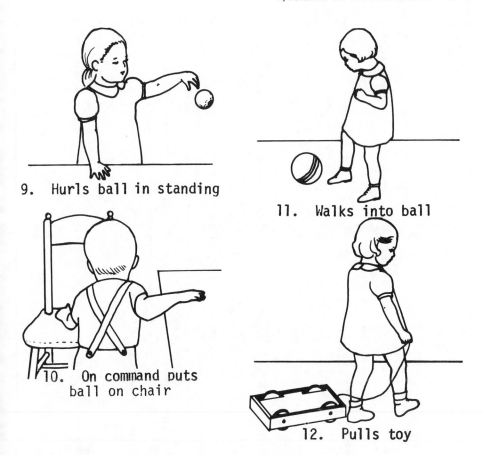

9. Hurls ball in standing

10. On command puts ball on chair

11. Walks into ball

12. Pulls toy

§7. EIGHTEEN MONTHS

The 18-month child can WALK *alone* (1), and he *seldom falls*. He *seats* himself (2) with some care in a SMALL CHAIR before the test table. The mother sits nearby and assists actively in his initial adjustment.

The PICTURE BOOK is placed on the table, and the examiner starts to turn the pages and comment on the pictures. The child *looks selectively* at the pictures and *turns the pages two or three at a time* (3).

The MASSED CUBES are then presented, and when the child has begun to manipulate them, a tower of 2–3 cubes is demonstrated and requested. The child responsively builds a *tower of 3–4 cubes* (4), the tower falling with the fourth or fifth cube. If the child has difficulty because of motor problems, succeeding cubes he tries to place may be held in position by the examiner. (See 24 Months for train demonstration.)

The CUP is then placed at the left of the cluster of CUBES. Spontaneously, or on request, the child begins to insert the cubes into the cup. If necessary, he is

K E Y A G E: 18 Months

H = History
O = Observation

H O	15 Months	H O	18 Months	H O	21 Months
			Adaptive		
	Cube: tower of 2		Massed Cubes: tower of 3-4		Massed Cubes: tower of 5-6
	Cup-cube: 6 cubes into cup (*18m)		Cup-cube: 10 into cup		Massed Cubes: imitates pushing train (*24m)
	Drawing: incipient imitation stroke (*18m)		Pellet & bottle: dumps responsively (*36m)		Formboard: places 2-3 blocks (*30m)
	Formboard: (no demonstration) places round block		Drawing: scribbles spontaneously (*36m)		Performance box: inserts corner of square (*24m)
	Formbd: adapts round block promptly		Drawing: makes stroke imitatively (*24m)		Performance box: retrieves ball
			Formboard: piles 3 blocks (*24m)		
			Gross Motor		
	Walks: few steps, starts, stops		Walks: seldom falls		Walks: squats in play (*...)
	Walks: falls by collapse (*18m)		Walks: fast, runs stiffly (*24m)		Stairs: walks down, 1 hand held (*24m)
	Walks: creeping discarded		Stairs: walks up, 1 hand held (*21m)		Stairs: walks up, holds rail (*24m)
	Stairs: creeps up (*18m)		Small chair: seats self		Large ball: (demonstration) kicks (*24m)
			Adult chair: climbs into (*...)		
			Ball: hurls (*48m)		
			Large ball: walks into (*21m)		
			Fine Motor		
	Cubes: tower of 2		Massed Cubes: tower 3-4		Massed Cubes: tower of 5-6
	Pellet: (no dem.) places in bottle		Book: turns pages, 2-3 at once (*24m)		
	Book: helps turn pages (*18m)				
			Language		
	Vocabulary: 4-6 words including names		Book: looks selectively		Vocabulary: 20 words
	Vocalization: uses jargon (*24m)		Vocabulary: 10 words including names		Speech: combines 2-3 words spontaneously (*24m)
	Book: pats pictures (*18m)		Picture card: names or points to 1		Ball: 3 directional commands
			Test object: names ball		
			Ball: 2 directional commands		
			Personal-Social		
	Feeding: bottle discarded		Feeding: hands empty dish (*...)		Feeding: handles cup well
	Feeding: inhibits grasp of dish		Feeding: feeds self in part, spills (*36m)		Communication: asks for food, toilet, drink
	Toilet: partial regulation (*24m)		Toilet: regulated daytime (*24m)		Communication: echoes 2 or more last words (*24m)
	Toilet: bowel control		Play: pulls a toy (*30m)		Communication: pulls person to show (*24m)
	Toilet: indicates wet pants (*18m)		Play: carries or hugs doll (*24m)		
	Communication: says "ta-ta" or equivalent				
	Commun: points, vocalizes wants (*21m)				
	Play: shows or offers toy (*21m)				
	Play: casts in play or refusal (*18m)				

urged to continue, or the cubes may be handed to him; he places *ten cubes in the cup* (5), filling the cup.

The PELLET AND BOTTLE are now presented, the pellet on the right. The child inserts the pellet, spontaneously or on request. When asked to get it out, he pokes into the neck of the bottle, shakes the bottle and finally *dumps the pellet out* (6) of the bottle. Demonstration may be necessary.

The DRAWING situation comes next. A blank piece of paper is placed on the table, and a crayon placed on it in a central position. The child *scribbles spontaneously;* after a decisive vertical stroke has been demonstrated, he makes an *imitative stroke* (7) without discrimination of direction. (See 24 Months for circular scribble.)

The FORMBOARD is presented with the 3 blocks on the table, each one in front of its appropriate hole. The child *piles the three blocks* on each other and may finally insert the round block. He does not adapt to rotation of the board but continues to pile and manipulate the blocks.

On presenting the PICTURE CARD, the examiner points to the dog and asks, "What's this?" (He does likewise for the shoe, cup and house.) If the child does not respond, the examiner says, "Show me the dog," etc. The child *names or points* correctly to one picture (8). He may turn the card over and hand it back.

The PERFORMANCE BOX may be presented and the child offered the square block. He brings it flat against the box and, even after demonstration, is unable to adapt the square block to the oblong hole. (Exam procedures continued next page.)

Examination Sequence

Italicized items appear for the first time in this sequence.

( ) = situation sometimes omitted for special reasons.

The child is now shown one of the TEST OBJECTS (ball) and asked to name it. He *names the ball* and is permitted to take it.

For BALL PLAY, the test table is moved slightly from its position, and the child given free access to the room. On request he *hurls the ball* (9) to the examiner and *carries out two* of the following directions: "Put it on the table . . . Put it on the chair (10). . . . Give it to mother. . . . Give it to me." The child releases the ball in the performance box and reaches into the box, but is unable to solve the problem of turning the box over and finally abandons the effort.

A LARGE BALL is placed on the floor, and a KICK of the ball is demonstrated and requested. The child responds by *walking into the ball* (11) without giving it a true kick.

He is reported to *hasten his walking steps,* but he RUNS *stiffly.* He *walks up* STAIRS *when one hand is held;* he *climbs into an adult chair.*

Language includes jargon and as many as *ten single words,* but he usually indicates his wants by pointing and vocalizing.

He has abandoned his bottle; he feeds *himself part* of his meals with a spoon, not without spilling. He *hands the empty dish* to his mother, with a sense of *fait accompli.*

His toilet *behavior is regulated during the daytime* by parental vigilance but not at night. He cooperates more fully in dressing and has some success in taking off his clothes.

In his play he *carries a doll* or teddy bear and hugs it; he walks about *pulling a toy* after himself (12).

Glossary of Developmental Schedule Items

15 MONTHS

Massed Cubes: tower of two. Demonstration may be necessary; examiner may assist by steadying bottom cube, but *at this age* it is not possible to differentiate motor disability from failure to understand cube relationships in tower building.

Cup and Cubes: six cubes into cup. Child starts to take cubes out after a few are put in, but eventually has six cubes inside cup; he cannot complete the task with all ten cubes. Consecutive cubes can be offered to the child and removal inhibited.

Drawing: incipient imitation stroke. This is judged not so much by product of crayon as by movement in air made by child in attempting to imitate stroke. Frequently he starts to respond strokewise and then scribbles instead.

Formboard: (no demonstration) places round block. Spontaneously or after command or pointing; inserts completely.

Formboard: adapts round block promptly. Makes a prompt, adaptive placement or near-placement of round block when formboard is rotated by examiner. Child's attention may or may not be sustained enough to watch and complete several rotations.

Walks: few steps, starts, stops. More is required than ability to take a few steps alone. Taking a few tottering steps from one person to another, or from one chair to another, is not sufficient. Child has enough control to get up in middle of floor by himself and stop and start again without support. This is *the definition of walking alone.*

Walks: falls by collapse. Frequent falling is characteristic of early walking; this falling is ordinarily accomplished by sitting down suddenly, without losing balance or falling forward headlong.

Walks: creeping discarded. This implies that walking is child's preferential method of locomotion and that if speed or efficiency is desired he will not revert to a more primitive method. Under stress of great fatigue he may, however, still creep occasionally.

Stairs: creeps up. Ascends at least one or two steps.

Massed Cubes: tower of two. Tower should stand without assistance from examiner. Differentiates between adaptive understanding and fine motor control.

Pellet: (no demonstration) places in bottle. On command or gesture, or spontaneously.

Book: helps turn pages. Infant completes turning of page examiner has lifted halfway by pushing it down, in proper direction.

Vocabulary: four–six words, including names. Words are beginning to acquire more specific meaning and include siblings, relatives or friends. Pronunciation need not be clear.

Vocalization: uses jargon. Richer and more elaborate, encompassing whole "sentences" (see 56 Weeks for definition).

Book: pats picture. Spontaneously or after examiner has pointed to a picture. Distinguish from indiscriminate patting without regarding.

Feeding: bottle discarded. Includes night bottle.

Feeding: inhibits grasp of dish. Mother can leave dish on feeding surface, since child no longer is apt to throw it to floor.

Toilet: partial regulation. Responds to regular placements on toilet (not invariably) but does not indicate urination needs, and does not wait to be taken to toilet if need is not correctly anticipated. Toilet "accidents" are fairly common occurrences.

Toilet: bowel control. Does not indicate toilet needs, but responds to toilet at regular hour. Toilet control is very dependent on parental demands; present trends are to delay training until later ages.

Toilet: indicates wet pants. By squirming, pulling at pants, fussing, etc.

Communication: says "ta-ta" or equivalent. For "thank you," on giving or receiving an object.

Communication: points, vocalizes wants. Indicates which specific object he desires, although vocalization may be a nondescript "uh-uh"; not merely fussing until mother guesses one desired from among many.

Play: shows, offers toy. Indicates he wants person to take it or do something with it; not merely holding it out without release (see 44 Weeks).

Play: casts in play or refusal. A very characteristic pattern at this age and one which may interfere with other examination responses. It is necessary to make a careful distinction between true casting and exaggerated release due to difficulties in motor control.

18 MONTHS

Massed Cubes: tower of three or four. May need demonstration to begin and urging to continue. For evaluation of adaptive behavior, examiner may assist with holding if child indicates his intent to build by bringing successive cubes to tower, but has a motor handicap which prevents sufficiently precise release.

Cup and Cubes: ten into cup. Puts all cubes in, spontaneously or with urging and demonstration.

Pellet: dumps responsively. In response to "get it out" or after demonstration. Hooking pellet with finger (rare) is an equivalent response. Distinguish intentional turning over of bottle from accidental dropping out of pellet as child shakes or manipulates bottle.

Drawing: scribbles spontaneously. May also do so after he is asked to "write on the paper," by pointing and/or request, but without demonstration by examiner.

Drawing: makes stroke imitatively. Without regard to direction; it may be made on tabletop. A stroke immediately obliterated by scribbling is a correct response in an overproductive child.

Formboard: piles three blocks. Stacks all three on formboard or table. Child's spontaneous behavior is observed; he is not handed successive blocks or urged to build. The less mature child becomes confused by three blocks and is unable to exploit them serially.

Walks: seldom falls. Losing balance uncommon.

Walks: fast, runs stiffly. Either pattern acceptable. Stiff running is due to very upright posture maintained. Any leaning forward in direction of the run would result in falling.

Stairs: walks up, one hand held. In erect position, not half creeping.

Small Chair: seats self. Any successful method that involves climbing in and turning around or preliminary standing with back to chair. Child often peers between legs or turns head to assure himself that his aim is accurate, or he may squat down a little to one side of chair and then slide over into position. Straddling chair is more advanced.

Adult Chair: climbs into. Child faces chair, climbs up, then turns around to sit down. Success influenced by relative sizes of child and chair.

Ball: hurls. As opposed to dropping with simple cast; also implies throwing in standing position. Younger child sits down to play ball.

Large ball: walks into. After demonstration of kicking, steps on or contacts, without foot swing. He is not permitted to hold wall, adult's hand, etc., for support.

Massed Cubes: tower of three or four. For the evaluation of fine motor behavior, tower of three should stand without assistance from examiner; it falls with fourth cube.

Book: turns pages two–three at once. Definite evidence of completing turn, in either direction, with inspection of pages. Not random manipulation for its own sake.

Book: looks selectively. At the pictures, following examiner's hand specifically. He may not point or name, but when asked, "Where is the dog?," etc., definitely looks at dog. May put finger on details of picture without accompanying verbalization.

Vocabulary: ten words including names (see 15 Months).

Picture Card: names or points to one. At this age is more apt to identify than name. Picture card is more difficult than color reproductions of picture book.

Test Object: names ball. Response may be spontaneous while child is engaging in ball play, but care must be taken to avoid using word without allowing ample time first.

Ball: two directional commands. Throwing ball at chair, table, mother or examiner is acceptable. Seating self on chair, holding ball, is not acceptable.

Feeding: hands empty dish. Gives dish for disposal when eating is completed.

Feeding: feeds self in part, spills. Eats part of meal with a spoon, not fingers, without any direct help.

Toilet: regulated, daytime. Responds to regular toilet placements. Responsibility is mother's, but she is able to keep child dry all day with only rare "accidents." He does not indicate his toilet needs but will wait a reasonable length of time for an opportunity to use toilet.

Play: pulls toy. While walking or creeping. Is not merely sitting down and using string to secure or handle to push attached toy.

Play: carries or hugs doll. Engages in active manipulation of stuffed animal or doll, not merely dragging it about after himself.

21 MONTHS

Massed Cubes: tower of five or six. May need demonstration to begin and urging to continue. Tower falls with sixth cube. (See 18 Months for distinction between adaptive and fine motor behavior.)

Massed Cubes: imitates pushing train. Pushes one or more cubes along table top. Distinguish imitation from rejection of situation by shoving cubes off table top.

Formboard: places two or three blocks. At some time during situation, after demonstration of complete task, at least two blocks inserted in proper holes.

Performance Box: inserts corner of square. Spontaneously or after demonstration of insertion achieves correct alignment of block in hole. Fails to make final adaptation for complete insertion of square block.

Performance Box: retrieves ball. Any method such as pushing box over, lifting and tilting box, creeping into box after overturning it. If performance seems highly accidental, repeat. Situation cannot be used with very tall children who are able to reach ball (rare at 21 months). This is an excellent situation in which to observe reactions of the individual child in face of difficulties—his persistence, ingenuity, emotional responses, etc.

Walks: squats in play. Implies sufficient control and balance so that this position can be maintained for several minutes while playing on floor or ground.

Stairs: walks down, one hand held. In erect position.

Stairs: walks up, holds rail. Erect.

Large Ball: (demonstration) kicks. Swings leg, foot striking ball a sharp blow; child is not permitted to hold on to any support.

Massed Cubes: tower of five or six. Tower should stand without assistance from examiner, falling with sixth cube.

Vocabulary: 20 words. (See 15 Months for definition of word.)

Speech: combines two or three words spontaneously. Implies two separate ideas. "Daddy go," "bye mama," "baby bed," are acceptable combinations; "all gone," "big boy," "oh dear," are essentially single words.

Ball: three directional commands. Throwing at correct objective is acceptable (see 18 Months).

Feeding: handles cup well. Lifts, drinks, replaces. Younger child tilts cup too far so that he spills profusely; he also is apt to drop or throw cup when finished drinking.

Communication: asks for food, toilet, drink. By words.

Communication: echoes two or more last words. Repeats end of sentence adult has said.

Communication: pulls person to show. For example, taking mother's hand or dress and leading her to kitchen sink, as compared with standing at sink, pointing and vocalizing "uh-uh" at an earlier age.

Growth Trends: Eighteen Months

The period between 1 and 2 years is extraordinarily rich from the standpoint of developmental transformations. The 18-month infant is in the very middle of this period of swift and not always easy advance. He is ceasing to be a mere baby, but he is still very dependent on a caretaker and on circumstances. It is easy to expect too much of him and to forget that he is in a critical phase of transition.

By reason of his immaturity, locomotor and otherwise, the 1-year-old is relatively protected from excessive impacts of culture, particularly if he is in the upper socioeconomic groups. However, the 18-month child is on the loose, colliding with new problems at every turn. Life is not quite so easy for him. Moreover, the relationships between the autonomic, sensorimotor and inhibitory areas of his nervous system are in a peculiarly complex state of formativeness. Larynx, legs, hands, feet and sphincters are concurrently coming under cortical control.

Therefore, the "infant—child" has an extraordinary diversity of behavior patterns to coordinate and consolidate. Because this neuromotor organization is so inclusive and intricate, he is generally limited to brief, diversified shifts of attention. At 2 years he will listen better, look longer; he will live less from moment to moment. At 3 years he is still more settled, owing to his widened attention span.

Nevertheless, the 18-month behavioral picture has more in common with 2 years than with 1 year. The 18-month child assuredly is a biped, for quadrupedal locomotion is usually abandoned by 15 months. He walks without falling and is even beginning to run, but his walk wobbles and his running gait is stiff and flat. At 2 years, ankle and knee joints are more flexible, not so much due to articular changes as due to a more advanced functional organization of the controlling neurons. Because both postural control and experience are immature, even simple acts like seating himself in a chair have their difficulties. He lacks the visual preperception and hence the judgment to perform this feat neatly. He shows the same developmental ineptitude in his manipulation of a spoon or a cup, tilting each excessively at the mouth. This gain in his skill cannot be ascribed altogether to learning through experience; it grows out of underlying postural changes determined by the maturation of the nervous system. Learning plays an increasing role with age; man is extraordinarily flexible in his capacity to learn and adapt.

Although he has scanty preperceptions and a meager memory span, his immediate perceptions are decisive. He hands you an object with a *now-that's-done* air. This trait is a key to his mentality. It accounts for the sketchy, punctuated conclusiveness of his reactions. It also makes him appear mercurial, in that his actions lack a certain margin of tentativeness which becomes more apparent at 2 and 3 years.

The language of the 18-month-old is likely to be in a jargon phase just about as well defined as his perception of persons and events. In fact, there is a close relationship between intellectual perception and command of words. Typically he shows mastery of only a dozen words. He can say "eat," and he can understand a very simple sentence if the words release a familiar motor experience, such as "Go and get your hat." However, he will become steadily more articulate. He will have a considerable vocabulary at 2 or 3 years; at 2 years he will even begin to make simple three-word sentences.

Language behavior, particularly speech, is the area most vulnerable to social experience, but becoming articulate depends upon maturity as well as on experience. Articulation signifies that discreteness is replacing diffuseness, that projection is supplementing self-absorption. These changes are more subtle, less open to inspection, than the patterns of cube behavior, but they are just as truly developmental processes. They are of the same cloth as the change from diffuse to discriminating cube manipulation, from absorbed mouthing of one cube to recognition of another cube. Step by step, the things of the physical world and the persons of the social world take on configuration for the infant—child.

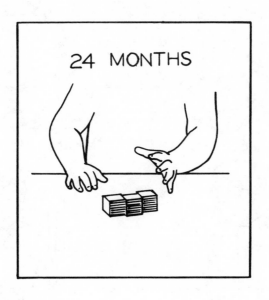

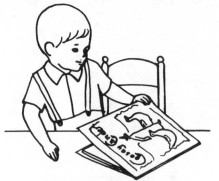

1. Turns pages singly

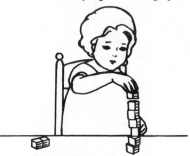

2. Builds tower of six to seven

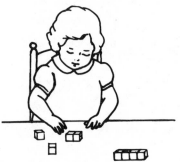

3. Aligns cubes

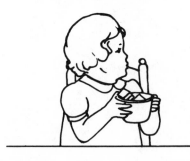

4. Hands cup of cubes to examiner

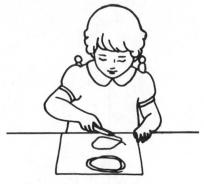

5. Imitates circular stroke

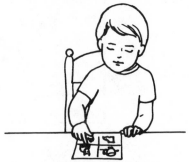

6. Identifies three to five pictures

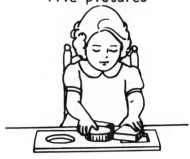

7. Places all blocks on board indiscriminately

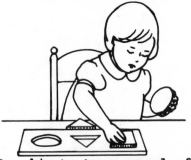

8. Adapts to reversal of board, four trials

94

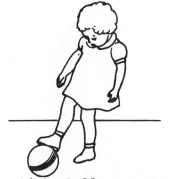

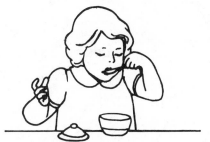

9. Kicks ball on request

11. Inhibits overturning
of spoon

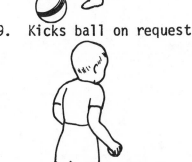

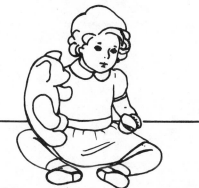

10. Runs fairly well

12. Domestic play; feeds
teddy bear

§8. TWENTY-FOUR MONTHS

The 2-year-old SEATS himself with ease and addresses himself at once to the PICTURE BOOK on the test table. He *turns the pages singly* (1) and names a few pictures.

The MASSED CUBES are then presented, and a "house" or tower is requested and demonstrated, if necessary. Responsively, the child builds a *tower of six or seven cubes* (2) which falls with the seventh or eighth. He may be urged to make the tower "high." In imitation of a four-cube train, he *aligns two or more cubes* (3). (See 36 Months for chimney demonstration.) He fills the CUP with CUBES and *hands it to the examiner* (4).

The DRAWING situation is presented. A blank piece of paper is placed on the table with a crayon in the center. The child scribbles spontaneously. When a decisive vertical stroke is demonstrated, he *imitates the vertical stroke;* however, he is unable to alter his direction in imitation of a horizontal stroke. A circular scribble is then demonstrated, and he *imitates the circular stroke* (5), differentiating it clearly from the vertical stroke.

KEY AGE: 24 Months

H = History
O = Observation

H O	21 Months	H O	24 Months	H O	30 Months
			Adaptive		
	Massed Cubes: tower of 5–6		Massed Cubes: tower of 6–7		Massed Cubes: tower of 8
	Massed Cubes: imitates pushing train (*24m)		M. Cubes: aligns 2 or more, train (*30m)		M. Cubes: adds chimney to train
	Formboard: places 2–3 blocks (*30m)		Drawing: imitates vertical stroke		**Drawing: imit. vert. & horiz. strokes**
	Performance box: inserts corner of square (*24m)		Drawing: imitates circular stroke (*36m)		**Drawing: 2 or more strokes for cross (*36m)**
	Perf. box: retrieves ball		Formbd: places single blocks on (*30m)		Color forms: places 1
			Formboard: adapts after 4 trials (*30m)		Formbd: places 3 on presentation
			Performance box: inserts square block		Formbd: adapts repeatedly, error (*36m)
					Digits: repeats 2 (1 of 3 trials)
			Gross Motor		
	Walks: squats in play (*...)		Walks: runs well, no falling		Walks: (demonstration) on tiptoe
	Stairs: walks down, 1 hand held (*24m)		Stairs: walks up & down alone		Jumps: both feet off floor
	Stairs: walks up, holds rail (*24m)		Large ball: (no demonstration) kicks		Stands: tries to stand on 1 foot
	Large ball: (dem.) kicks (*24m)				
			Fine Motor		
	Massed Cubes: tower of 5–6		Massed Cubes: tower of 6–7		Massed Cubes: tower of 8
			Book: turns pages singly		Drawing: holds crayon by fingers
			Language		
	Vocabulary: 20 words		Speech: jargon discarded		Name: gives full name
	Speech: combines 2–3 words spontaneously (*24m)		Speech: 3-word sentence		Picture cards: names 5
	Ball: 3 directional commands		Speech: uses *I, me, you*		Picture cards: identifies 7
			Picture cards: names 3 or more		Test objects: gives use
			Picture cards: identifies 5 or more		
			Test objects: names 2		
			Ball: 4 directional commands		
			Personal–Social		
	Feeding: handles cup well		Feeding: inhibits turning spoon		Communication: refers to self by pronoun rather than name
	Communication: asks for food, toilet, drink		Toilet: dry at night, taken up (*36m)		Play: pushes with good steering
	Communication: echoes 2 or more last words (*24m)		Toilet: generally verbalizes needs (*42m)		Play: helps put things away
	Communication: pulls person to show (*24m)		Dressing: pulls on simple garment		Play: can carry breakable objects
			Communication: verbalizes immediate experiences (*...)		
			Commun: refers to self by name (*30m)		
			Commun: comprehends & asks for "another"		
			Play: hands cup full of cubes		
			Play: domestic mimicry		
			Play: parallel play predominates (*42m)		

The examiner now shows the PICTURE CARDS, points to the dog and asks, "What's this?" (Likewise with the shoe, cup, house, clock, etc.) After the child has named as many as he can, the examiner continues with the rest, saying, "Show me the book," etc. The child *names three* and *identifies five pictures* (6).

The FORMBOARD is presented with each block in front of its appropriate hole. The child *places all three blocks on the board* without discriminating reference to the holes (7). After demonstration he inserts the three blocks correctly. The examiner now lifts the board and rotates it 180° to reverse the position of the holes; the square block is in front of the round hole, etc. The child tries to insert the blocks; after much trial and error, and demonstration, he finally *adapts after four trials* (8).

The PERFORMANCE BOX is next placed on the table, and the child is given the square block. He *inserts the square* in the oblong hole, making the necessary adjustments; demonstration may be necessary.

When asked, he tells his first NAME, but rarely his last name.

He is then shown the TEST OBJECTS (pencil, shoe, penny, key, ball) in rapid succession, and asked to name them. He *names* two of them, and may give their use.

He is given the BALL, and the table is moved so that he may stand and walk about. He hurls the ball on request. He *carries out all four* of the following directions: "Put it on the table . . . Put it on the chair . . . Give it to mother . . . Give it to me." (Exam procedures continued next page.)

Examination Sequence

(Normative behavior characteristic of the *key age: 24 months* and adjacent age levels is codified by the Developmental Schedule shown on the adjoining page.)

Age: 21–24–30 Months	Situation No. (Appendix A-4)
Picture book	40
Cubes: Tower	12
Train	13
(*Chimney*)	14
Cup and cubes	17
Drawing: Spontaneous	26
Vertical strokes	28
Horizontal strokes	30
Circular scribble	29
(Picture *cards*)	41
Formboard	35
Performance box	36
(*Name*)	42
(Test objects: Names)	45
Use)	45
Small ball: Throwing	46
Directions	47
(In box)	48
Kicking	58
Sitting in chair	50
Walking, running	59
Stairs	60

Italicized items appear for the first time in this sequence.

( ) = situation sometimes omitted for special reasons.

He is tall enough to reach the ball in the performance box, and the situation is omitted.

The LARGE BALL is offered, and the child is asked to KICK it. He *kicks the ball* (9) on verbal command alone, swinging his foot against it.

He is reported to RUN *fairly well* (10) without falling, and indeed habitually may run rather than walk. He *walks up and down* STAIRS *alone,* bringing both feet to one step, then both to the next, and so on. He often squats to play on the floor.

His mother estimates his vocabulary as well over 50 words, and *jargon has been replaced* by simple *three-word sentences.* He *uses the pronouns* "I," "me," and "you," though not always correctly. He soliloquizes, *verbalizing his immediate experience, referring to himself by name* ("Johnny slide . . . Johnny fall down . . ."). He asks for food, toilet and drink, and also *asks for "another,"* wanting one for each hand.

He feeds himself part of his meals, not without spilling, but he *inhibits overturning the spoon* until it is in his mouth (11). He handles a cup well.

He *verbalizes* his toilet *needs* fairly consistently during the day, and he remains *dry at night* if taken to the toilet at 10 or 11 P.M. He *pulls on a simple garment* such as socks, mittens or hat.

His play with a doll or teddy bear includes *domestic mimicry* (12), such as feeding them, and he imitates household activities. With other children he engages in *parallel play,* playing nearby and doing similar things, but without mutual cooperation.

Glossary of Developmental Schedule Items

21 MONTHS

For definitions, see glossary items in §7, Eighteen Months.

24 MONTHS

Massed Cubes: tower of six or seven. May need demonstration to start and urging to continue. Tower falls with seventh cube. (See 18 Months for distinction between adaptive and fine motor behavior.)

Massed Cubes: aligns two or more, train. After examiner demonstrates, and then dismantles train, child makes horizontal combination on table top.

Drawing: imitates vertical stroke. After demonstration, with correct directional orientation.

Drawing: imitates circular stroke. After demonstration; differentiates clearly from vertical stroke. The words "circle" and "round" are not used unless child does. May draw circular scribble spontaneously.

Formboard: places single blocks on. The spontaneous response to initial presentation without demonstration. Places on board separately, not necessarily in holes or in relation to correct holes.

Formboard: adapts after four trials. To examiner's rotation of board, by trial and error or in response to examiner's pointing.

Performance Box: inserts square block. Spontaneously or after demonstration, adapts block completely to hole.

Walks: runs well, no falling. But still not very fast; balance maintained while hurrying; stops without having to reach some barrier. Knees flex and arms alternate fairly well.

Stairs: walks up and down alone. May use banister; both feet brought to each step; erect position.

Large Ball: (no demonstration) kicks. On verbal command without demonstration. Examiner may say, "Kick it with your foot."

Massed Cubes: tower of six or seven. Tower should stand without assistance from examiner, falling with seventh cube.

Book: turns pages singly. In either direction (see 18 Months).

Speech: jargon discarded. Words may not be comprehensible but are clearly meant to be words, not merely sounds with inflection.

Speech: three-word sentence. Caution is necessary in accepting such sentences as "I don't know" or "I love you" if they are only ones used by child (see 21 Months).

Speech: uses "I, me, you." Not necessarily correctly, or all of them.

Picture Cards: names three or more. Responds to "What is this?"

Picture Cards: identifies five or more. In response to "Show me the _____ ," child points. Total includes those he already has named correctly.

Test Objects: names two. Pencil, shoes (examiner's), key, penny, ball.

Ball: four directional commands. Throwing ball at correct objective is acceptable (see 18 Months).

Feeding: inhibits turning spoon. Gets spoon to his mouth right side up.

Toilet: dry at night, taken up. All night.

Toilet: generally verbalizes needs. Asks in good time and accidents are rare. This and preceding item are highly variable, depending on parental demands.

Dress: pulls on simple garment. Socks, mittens, hat; pulls up pants.

Communication: verbalizes immediate experiences. Talks about his activities as he performs them.

Communication: refers to self by name. "Johnny wants . . .," "Johnny fall down" (see 30 Months).

Communication: comprehends and asks for "another." For example, a second cookie for his other hand, or after he eats first one.

Play: hands cup full of cubes. At completion of massed cubes situation, fills cup and hands it to examiner, spontaneously or on request. Younger child starts to take cubes out one by one or dumps them all.

Play: domestic mimicry. Puts doll to bed, pretends to feed, hammers, mops, sweeps, dusts, etc.

Play: parallel play predominates. Plays alongside another child rather than with him; often engages in same activity, but quite separately.

30 MONTHS

Massed Cubes: tower of eight. May need demonstration to start and urging to continue. (See 18 Months for distinction between adaptive and fine motor.)

Massed Cubes: adds chimney to train. The examiner may ask, "Where is the chimney?" if child responds to demonstration and dismantling only by aligning cubes.

Drawing: imitates vertical and horizontal strokes. Clearly differentiates directional orientation and usually makes only a single imitative stroke.

Drawing: two or more strokes for cross. Imitates by more than one stroke without correct orientation. Performance should be different from child's response to stroke demonstration.

Color Forms: places one. Round form may be demonstrated.

Formboard: places three on presentation. Inserts blocks into correct holes, spontaneously or in response to "Put them in."

Formboard: adapts repeatedly, error. Usually solved with error on first rotation, after examiner's comments, but subsequent trials do not eliminate an initial error.

Digits: repeats two (one of three trials). After examiner has finished a set, repeats in correct order.

Walks: (demonstration) on tiptoe. Hand may be held at first.

Jumps: both feet off floor. In place, after demonstration.

Stands: tries to stand on one foot. Examiner demonstrates, maintaining pose to encourage child to do so. Holding pants or skirt with each hand discourages holding on for support, which is not permitted. Younger child refuses this situation.

Massed Cubes: tower of eight. Tower should stand without assistance from examiner.

Drawing: holds crayon by fingers. Adult fashion, as opposed to using the fist.

Name: gives full name. Nickname permitted for first name.

Picture Cards: names five; identifies seven (see 24 Months).

Test Objects: gives use. Of one or more objects. An answer indicating comprehension is acceptable; e.g., "door" or "car" to "What do you do with the key?"

Communication: refers to self by pronoun rather than name. May confuse "I" and "me" (see 24 Months).

Play: pushes with good steering. Wagon, doll carriage or other large vehicle; backs out of corner himself.

Play: helps put things away. Generally his toys, mother working alongside him.

Play: can carry breakable objects. Mother allows him to carry glasses, dishes, ashtrays, etc.

Growth Trends: Twenty-four Months

An 18-month-old is an infant—child. At 2 years he may be considered a preschooler. He is graduating from infancy. He still has a residual stagger in his walk and spends over half of the 24-hour cycle in sleep, but he is beginning to use words for communication, and he is able to meet, at least for limited periods, the demands of playing with other children. He gives evidences of a rudimentary sense of other persons—a trait which becomes well defined by the age of 3 years.

The 24-month-old still is perfecting the fundamentals of locomotion and of postural control. He delights in running, because it is a new and formative ability. He is a runabout, preferring the novelty of running to walking. He usually manages to run without falling, but it takes him a full year more to learn to decelerate, to make sudden stops and to turn sharp corners. He has sufficient inhibitions and social responsiveness to remain seated in a chair for the examination period. Nevertheless, it takes time to acquire the motor poise and social conformability which distinguish the 3-year-old.

Fine manual coordination continues to progress at a steady rate. Accordingly, he now builds a tower of six cubes. At 18 months it was a tower of three cubes; at 36 months it will be a tower of nine or ten. The gradualness of this improvement in fine motor control reminds us that development proceeds by slow degrees. He cannot "learn" to build a tower of six cubes all at once! It seems a bit illogical that a child who has the wit to build a tower of three cubes at 18 months should, on the average, need 2 months of additional age for each additional block in his tower prior to his second birthday, and that he should need 4 months of additional age for each block added prior to his third birthday. However, such is the logic of neuromotor and attentional development.

His mastery of spatial relations depends upon his central nervous system organization, especially upon control of the complicated systems of muscles which actuate eyes, hands and fingers. An elementary command of the vertical dimension is expressed in his ability to execute a vertical stroke with a crayon and to build a tower of six cubes. His ability to arrange three cubes side-by-side denotes a comparable command of the horizontal dimension. This is evidence of increasing versatility; however, the oblique orientations between vertical and horizontal are still far beyond his ability. Even at 3 years of age he cannot crease a paper obliquely, and not until 5 years can he copy a triangle—depending, of course, upon his exposure to these materials and the instruction he may receive. This serves as another reminder that perception of forms develops by slow degrees because of the extraordinary delicacy of the requisite neuromotor equipment.

That the 2-year-old is still very much space bound and at the mercy of association by contiguity is shown in his reactions to the formboard test. He readily places a circle in its proper hole at the right. He sees the examiner rotate the board slowly through an arc of 180° so that the circular hole is now at his left instead. Valiantly he tries to press the circular block in the square hole. Three times the examiner may reverse the board before his eyes. He persists in his error. On the fourth trial he may finally adapt. The 3-year-old typically adapts at once, or with immediate correction of error.

The developmental problem of the 24-month child is to get his perceptions of the details of formed space sufficiently disengaged from their massive context so that he can use them flexibly in his adaptive thinking. He has the same problem with respect to language. His words hitherto have been closely bound up with specific actions and limited situations. He must disengage these words from their settings so that he can use them freely as his agents. The period from 2 to 3 years therefore is preeminently a period of transition, when jargon is discarded, when objects and pictures are named, when pronouns are used and when simple directions are heeded. Just as he combines three cubes in formed space to build a train, he combines three words to build a sentence. Both of these behavior patterns, one verbal, one nonverbal, have much in common. Wide individual variations are normal, but the three-word sentence is typical of the 2-year-old. Longer sentences and taller towers come later.

Sphincter control likewise takes developmental time, but it is very much socially determined by parental demands. Adult management must supplement the child's inadequacies. The 2-year-old is dry at night if he is taken up to the toilet. However, he must be taken to the toilet at special times if he is to be dry during the day. Lapses occur because the cortical controls of volition reinforced by verbalization are still immature.

In the light of all his neuromotor limitations we cannot expect too many social graces in the 2-year-old. His realization of other persons is extremely rudimentary. He may like to have others about, and may enjoy his solitary play more when other children are nearby, provided they are not too near to interfere. However, he has more capacity to snatch, scuffle and kick than to give and take—this for reasons of developmental immaturity rather than depravity. His hugging is just as ill-measured as his pushing. He does not know how to ask for help; the need for asking is not clear to him because he is incapable of envisaging another person as disengaged from his own person. Yet he is at the very threshold of accomplishing just such socializing disengagements. This is shown by many tokens: he refers to himself by his own name; he sometimes says "you"; he understands and even uses the word "another"; he is interested in dolls; he mimics domestic events.

These characteristic behavior patterns have a mixed personal and social reference. The details of personal—social patterns are determined by the environment, but the integrity of the child's own constitution plays a vital role. Therefore, even everyday manifestations of household behavior serve as indicators of the child's developmental maturity. We may not expect too much of the 2-year-old, yet we see the foretokens of socialized behavior which come to considerable and charming fulfillment at the age of 3 years.

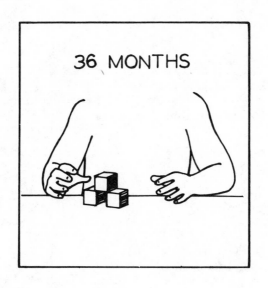

36 MONTHS

103

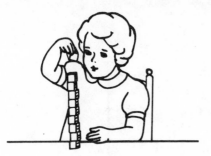

1. Builds tower of ten

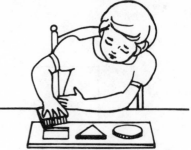

5. Adapts immediately to board reversal

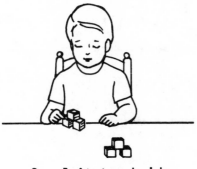

2. Imitates bridge

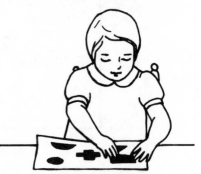

6. Matches three color forms

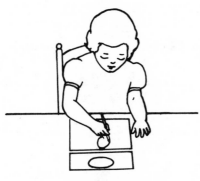

3. Copies circle

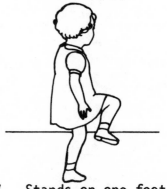

7. Stands on one foot momentarily

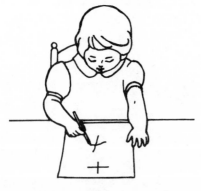

4. Imitates cross

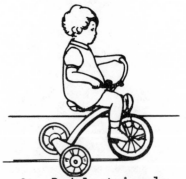

8. Pedals tricycle

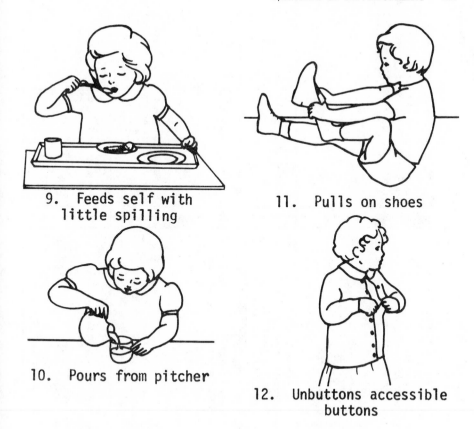

9. Feeds self with little spilling

11. Pulls on shoes

10. Pours from pitcher

12. Unbuttons accessible buttons

§9. THIRTY-SIX MONTHS

The 3-year-old accepts a chair readily and remains seated as long as the examination requires. He turns the pages of the PICTURE BOOK singly, names the pictures and on request *tells the action* delineated, e.g., the baby is sleeping. He knows a few rhymes or television commercials, and with a little encouragement may recite Little Bo-Peep, Little Miss Muffet or more contemporary rhymes, all depending upon his social environment and conditioning.

The MASSED CUBES are presented, and a "house" or tower is requested. The child *builds a tower of nine cubes,* and in three trials a successful *tower of ten cubes* (1). On demonstration of the model train, four cubes with a fifth cube superimposed as chimney, he duplicates the model, chimney and all, using the same cubes. The examiner then demonstrates with running comment the construction of a bridge with three cubes. The model is left standing, and the child is given three other cubes. He *imitates the bridge* accurately (2).

Given paper and crayon for spontaneous DRAWING, he holds the crayon with his fingers, rather than in his fist; he scribbles or scrawls, but in response to a

30 Months	K E Y A G E: 36 Months	42 Months
Adaptive	*Adaptive*	Massed Cubes: builds bridge from model
Massed Cubes: tower of 8	M. Cubes: tower of 9 (10 on 3 trials)	Geometric forms: points to 6
Massed Cubes: adds chimney to train	Massed Cubes: imitates bridge (*42m)	Digits: repeats 3 (2 of 3 trials)
Drawing: imitates vertical & horizontal strokes	Pellets: 10 into bottle in 30 seconds	Weights: gives heavy block (2 of 3 trials)
Drawing: 2 or more strokes for cross (*36m)	Drawing: names own drawing	
Color forms: places 1	Drawing: names incomplete man	
Formboard: places 3 blocks on presentation	Drawing: copies circle	
Formboard: adapts repeatedly, error (*36m)	Drawing: imitates cross (*48m)	
Digits: repeats 2 (1 of 3 trials)	Color forms: places 3	
	Geometric forms: points to 4	
	Formboard: adapts, no error, or immediate correction of error	
	Digits: repeats 3 (1 of 3 trials)	
Gross Motor	*Gross Motor*	Stands: on 1 foot, 2 seconds
Walks: (demonstration) on tiptoe	Stairs: alternates feet going up	
Jumps: both feet off floor	Jumps: from bottom stair	
Stands: tries to stand on 1 foot	Rides: tricycle using pedals	
	Stands: on 1 foot, momentary balance	
Fine Motor	*Fine Motor*	Drawing: traces diamond
Massed Cubes: tower of 8	Massed Cubes: tower 9 (10 on 3 trials)	
Drawing: holds crayon by fingers	Pellets: 10 into bottle in 30 seconds	
Language	*Language*	Picture cards: names all
Name: gives full name	Book: gives action	Pictures: enumerates 3
Picture cards: names 5	Speech: uses plurals	Comprehension Questions A: answers 2
Picture cards: identifies 7	Picture cards: names 8	Prepositions: obeys 3, ball & chair
Test objects: gives use	Sex: tells sex	
	Comprehension Questions A: answers 1	
	Prepositions: obeys 2, ball & chair	
Personal-Social	*Personal-Social*	Dressing: washes, dries hands, face
Communication: refers to self by pronoun rather than name	Feeding: feeds self, spills little	Play: associative play replaces parallel play. (*48m)
Play: pushes with good steering	Feeding: pours well from pitcher	
Play: helps put things away	Dressing: puts on shoes	
Play: can carry breakable objects	Dressing: unbuttons accessible buttons	
	Communication: understands taking turns	
	Communication: knows a few rhymes	

question, *names what he has drawn.* He imitates demonstrated vertical and horizontal strokes, differentiating them clearly. He *copies a circle* from a model without aid of demonstration (3). He cannot copy a cross from a model, but after demonstration he *imitates the cross* crudely (4). He *names the incomplete man,* but in response to the questions "What does he need?" and "What's missing?" scribbles indiscriminately even when the specific parts lacking are pointed out. Rarely does he trace the diamond within the prescribed lines.

The examiner then shows the PICTURE CARDS, asking the child to name each picture in turn. He *names eight pictures correctly.*

The FORMBOARD is now presented with each block in front of its appropriate hole. He inserts the blocks promptly. The examiner now rotates the board 180°, reversing the position of the holes; the square block is in front of the round hole, etc. The child *adapts to the reversal without error* or with *immediate spontaneous correction* of his error (5).

The placard carrying the five red COLOR FORMS is placed on the table, and the child is asked to place the circle, square, triangle, semicircle and cross, one after

Examination Sequence

(Normative behavior characteristic of the *key age: 36 months* and adjacent age levels is codified by the Developmental Schedule shown on the adjoining page.)

Age: 30–36–42 Months	Situation No. (Appendix A-4)
Picture book	40
Cubes: Tower	12
Train	13
Chimney	14
Bridge	15
Drawing: Spontaneous	26
Strokes	28,30
Circle	31
Cross	32
Incomplete man	33
Trace diamond	34
(Picture cards)	41
Formboard	35
Color forms	37
(Name, *sex*)	42
(*Comprehension*)	43
(*Digits*)	44
Geometric forms	38
Weighted blocks	39
Ten Pellets and bottle	21
(Test objects—use)	45
Small ball: Throwing	46
Prepositions	49
Kicking	58
Running	59
Walking on tiptoe	61
Standing on one foot	62
Jumping	63
Stairs	60

Italicized items appear for the first time in this sequence.

( ) = situation sometimes omitted for special reasons.

the other, where they fit. The circle may be demonstrated. He correctly *matches three color forms* (6).

On request he gives his full NAME and *tells his SEX* in response to the question, "Are you a little boy or a little girl?"

He is then asked three simple COMPREHENSION QUESTIONS A, "What do you do when you are hungry? sleepy? cold?" He *answers one question* satisfactorily.

His immediate recall is tested by asking him to repeat the DIGITS 4–2, then 6–4–1, 3–5–2, and 8–3–7. He repeats *one series of three digits* correctly.

He is now given the placard with the ten black and white GEOMETRIC FORMS from the Stanford–Binet Test. One at a time the small cards are placed on the X of the test card, and the child asked to show the examiner the matching form. He may be asked and permitted to put it where it fits. The circle may be demonstrated. The order is circle, square, triangle, oval, rectangle, hexagon, arched square, rhomboid, parallelogram and irregular. He *points to* or places four forms correctly.

He is given the lightest and heaviest of the five WEIGHTED BLOCKS, one for each hand, and asked to give the examiner the heavy block. The blocks are juggled, and the heavy one given to his other hand. He gives the heavy block on two of three trials.

The BOTTLE AND TEN PELLETS are placed before the child, in a position which favors the use of the child's preferred hand, and he is asked to put them all in the bottle, one at a time, just as fast as he can. The positions of pellets and bottle are then reversed. He *puts all ten in sequentially in 30 seconds* in the best of several trials.

He names all the TEST OBJECTS and gives the use of a few of them.

He is given the BALL, and the table is removed to one side so that he may stand and walk about. He hurls the ball and then *carries out two* of the following *prepositional* directions: "Put the ball on, under, in front of, beside, in back of the chair."

He KICKS the LARGE BALL with facility, but he can STAND *on one foot with only momentary balance* (7).

He is reported to RUN well and to *walk up* STAIRS *alternating his feet* on consecutive treads, though he still walks down by bringing both feet to the same tread. He jumps on both feet, and can JUMP *down* from a height of 6–8 inches, as from the bottom step. He squats to play on the floor, and he can WALK ON TIPTOE. He *rides a tricycle,* steering and *using the pedals* (8).

His vocabulary contains innumerable words and he speaks in well-formed simple sentences, *using plurals.* He refers to himself by pronoun.

He *feeds himself well* without help and *with little spilling* (9); he *pours well from a small pitcher* (10), gauging the capacity of the cup correctly.

He is assuming responsibility for his toilet needs and is usually dry all night. He pulls on simple garments, *puts on his shoes* (11), but not always on the correct foot, and *unbuttons accessible buttons* (12).

Glossary of Developmental Schedule Items

30 MONTHS

For definitions, see glossary items in § 8, Twenty-four Months.

36 MONTHS

Massed Cubes: tower of nine (ten on three trials). May need urging to try again. (See 18 Months for distinction between adaptive and fine motor.)

Massed Cubes: imitates bridge. Examiner demonstrates construction and leaves model standing.

Pellets: ten into bottle in 30 seconds. One at a time; younger child does not have concept and takes handful of pellets.

Drawing: names own drawing. Spontaneously, or in response to "What is it?" although only a scribble is made.

Drawing: names incomplete man. "Snowman," or any response indicating a person.

Drawing: copies circle. From model on card. Use word only if child does first. Need not be perfect sphere.

Drawing: imitates cross. Examiner demonstrates. Essential feature is recognition of different orientation of two lines. May be produced in three or four segments rather than by two strokes.

Color Forms: places three. Round form may be demonstrated.

Geometric Forms: points to four. Round form may be demonstrated. May be permitted to place, as with color forms; most 3-year-olds will not point.

Formboard: adapts to rotation without error, or immediate correction of error. Error eliminated by self-correction, if there has been one on first rotation (see 30 Months).

Digits: repeats three (one of three trials). After examiner has finished a set, repeats in correct order.

Stairs: alternates feet going up. One foot to a step, adult fashion.

Jumps: from bottom stair. Both feet together; lands erect.

Rides: tricycle using pedals. Propels and steers without assistance.

Stands: on one foot, momentary balance. Examiner demonstrates and maintains pose to encourage child to do so. He may be timed by slow counting aloud (see 30 Months).

Massed Cubes: tower of nine (ten on three trials). Tower should stand.

Pellets: ten into bottle in 30 seconds. One at a time; best time of either hand.

Picture Book: gives action. In response to question, "What is . . . doing?"

Speech: uses plurals. Says "dogs, babies, shoes," etc., if more than one.

Picture Cards: names eight. May identify the two additional ones also.

Comprehension Questions A: answers one. Single-word answers of appropriate nouns or verbs acceptable.

Sex: Tells own sex correctly.

Prepositions: obeys two with ball and chair. "On" and "under" are most commonly understood; "in back of, in front of, beside" less so. Throwing ball correctly is acceptable.

Feeding: feeds self, spills little. With a spoon without help.

Feeding: pours well from pitcher. From a small pitcher or glass into another, judging quantity correctly.

Dressing: puts on shoes. Not necessarily on correct feet. Slippers not acceptable.

Dressing: unbuttons accessible buttons. No longer merely pulls apart to open.

Communication: understands taking turns. In play with other children, or with adults. Examiner may observe during examination.

Communication: knows a few rhymes. Recites words all the way through. Television commercials are equivalent response and more common today.

42 MONTHS

Massed Cubes: builds bridge from model. Examiner builds out of sight and leaves model standing.

Geometric Forms: points to six. See 36 Months.

Digits: repeats three (two of three trials). See 36 Months.

Weights: gives heavy block (two of three trials). If child doesn't understand meaning of words "heavy" and "light," tends to give right-or left-hand block each time.

Stands: on one foot for 2 seconds. Examiner demonstrates and maintains pose to encourage child to do so. He may be timed by slow counting (see 30 Months).

Drawing: traces diamond. Manages to stay within lines of the double diamond most of time, but angles rounded.

Picture Cards: names all. Without a specific question for each picture.

Picture: enumerates three. Names three objects without prompting.

Comprehension Questions A: answers two. See 36 Months.

Prepositions: obeys three, ball and chair. See 36 Months.

Dressing: washes, dries hands, face. Without reminder to dry to prevent his playing in the water. Washing or drying may not be very efficient.

Play: associative group play replaces parallel play. Several children engage in same activity with frequent cross-references and comment.

Growth Trends: Thirty-six Months

Three years is a nodal age; it marks a kind of culmination in the processes of early development. The child is not yet completed; it will be a whole decade before he enters his teens. However, in his organization he has already achieved a full stage of preadolescence. When his developmental status at 3 years is compared with the callowness of infancy or even of 2 years, he proves to be a relatively mature being.

He also is domesticated. He washes and dries his hands. He feeds himself with a spoon without much spilling. He may sleep through the night without wetting his bed. He takes daytime responsibility for the toilet. It would be full responsibility were it not for the awkward posteriority of buttons and buttocks. He shows an interest in domestic routines.

His interest extends to events and environments outside the household. He is good company. He likes to please. He is heedful of words. He uses them as tools and builds them into sentences. His speech, to be sure, is limited largely to concrete situations. He does not deal verbally with generalizations and quasiabstractions after the manner of the 5-year-old. However, the child of 3 years does ask rhetorical questions, and frequently he asks, "Is that right?" "Do it this way?" Such questions express his matured and maturing tendency to project himself into his cultural milieu, not only at home but abroad. He shows himself to be understanding of social requirements. He wants to keep himself within proper bounds.

Such fluctuations from year to year and sometimes from week to week are part of the very physiology of development. They are like the reciprocal balancing of flexors and extensors, of left and right, of alternation and unison, of grasping and releasing, of positive and negative inhibition. How can the child learn "within bounds" if he does not make a foray into "without bounds?" By the same token, he must have limits set for him in order to learn what the boundaries are. Total permissiveness can lead only to disorganization; consistency on the part of the parents, once they have determined what the rules for their household should be, cannot be instituted suddenly at the age of 3.

Some of the social amenability of the 3-year-old is also based on his greater neuromotor maturity. He has mastered the essentials of walking, running, dodging, throwing, stop—go and turn. When he walks he goes with a destination in mind. He has a practical command of the principals of the lever. He manages a spoon. He holds a crayon adaptively, and makes it obedient to curved as well as straight lines. When he wields a paint brush, designs take shape. He has an elementary sense of order. Given four random cubes, he tends to assemble them into a neat square. He builds a bridge of three cubes. He deploys his hand with an intentfulness which in the species led to tool using and primitive art.

Thus, the 3-year-old embodies many of the fundamental behavior traits of human culture. He recognizes others and "otherness." He can wait his turn. He can bargain. He can cooperate in play with other children. He likes to participate as well as to play alone. He is achieving a dissociation of spoken words from corresponding body movements and postural sets. This will enable him, in due time, to use words as vehicles to communicate past experience, the prime behavior pattern of man as a maker and bearer of culture.

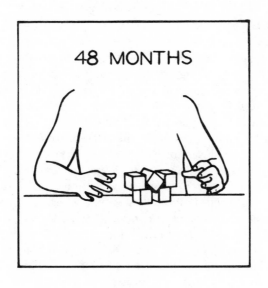

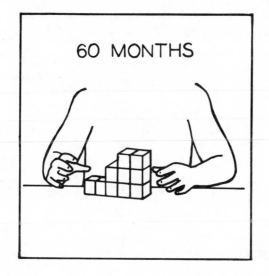

113

§ 10. FORTY-EIGHT AND SIXTY MONTHS

It is beyond the scope of this volume to enter into a detailed discussion of the later preschool years. Our emphasis here is on the early evaluation of neuropsychologic status for the detection of abnormality and the institution of remedial measures.

Parents are excellent observers of behavior, but in infancy particularly, the accuracy of their reporting hinges on the clarity with which the examiner specifies each pattern. As the child grows older, the behavior patterns evaluated are more and more part of the vocabulary of everyday life. The problems become more ones of educational planning rather than ones of differential diagnosis.

All too often, however, a physician is confronted clinically with a 4- or 5-year-old, particularly when the child's speech is lagging. The developmental schedules for 48 and 60 months are included as guides, but the reader also is referred to *The First Five Years of Life*[27] for a detailed discussion of examination procedures and growth trends. At older ages in particular, the items on the developmental schedules can be found on a variety of other psychological tests. The separation into the five areas of behavior is preserved, and as for younger ages, greatest attention is paid to adaptive behavior in the evaluation of intellectual potential. Only in this way can one make an adequate diagnosis and continue to differentiate between mental deficiency and specific motor, language or integrative handicaps associated with normal intelligence.

K E Y   A G E: 48 Months

H = History
O = Observation

42 Months	48 Months (KEY AGE)	54 Months
Adaptive	**Adaptive**	**Adaptive**
Massed Cubes: builds bridge from model	Massed Cubes: imitates gate (*54m)	Massed Cubes: makes gate from model
Geometric forms: points to 6	Drawing: man with 2 parts (*60m)	Drawing: copies square
Digits: repeats 3 (2 of 3 trials)	Drawing: copies cross	Geometric forms: points to 9
Weights: gives heavy block (2 of 3 trials)	Drawing: adds 3 parts to Incomplete Man	Counts: 4 objects & answers "how many"
	Geometric forms: points to 8	Esthetic comparison: correct
	Missing Parts: 1 correct	Missing parts: 2 correct
	Counts: 3 objects with correct pointing	Digits: repeats 4 (1 of 3 trials)
	Weights: selects heavier invariably	
Gross Motor	**Gross Motor**	
Stands: on 1 foot, 2 seconds	Stairs: walks down, 1 foot to step	Hops: on 1 foot
	Skips: on 1 foot only (*60m)	Articulation: not infantile
	Jumps: running or standing broad jump	
	Ball: throws overhand	
	Stands: on 1 foot, 4-8 seconds	
Fine Motor	**Fine Motor**	**Fine Motor**
Drawing: traces diamond	Pellets: 10 into bottle in 25 seconds	Drawing: traces cross
Language	**Language**	
Picture cards: names all	Color card: names 1	Defines: 4 in terms of use
Pictures: enumerates 3	Prepositions: obeys 4, ball & chair	Comprehension Questions B: 1 correct
Comprehension Quest. A: answers 2		
Prepositions: obeys 3, ball & chair		
Personal-Social	**Personal-Social**	
Dressing: washes, dries hands, face	Dressing: washes & dries hands & face, brushes teeth	Communication: calls attention to own performance (*60m)
Play: associative play replaces parallel play (*48m)	Dress: dresses & undresses, supervised (*60m)	Communication: relates fanciful tales (*60m)
	Dressing: laces shoes	Communication: bosses & criticizes (*60m)
	Dressing: distinguishes front & back of clothes	Play: shows off dramatically (*60m)
	Play: cooperates with children	
	Play: builds building with blocks	
	Developmental Detachment: goes on errands outside home (no crossing street)	
	Developmental Detachment: tends to go out of prescribed bounds (*60m)	

115

KEY AGE: 60 Months

H = History   O = Observation

	54 Months	60 Months	72 Months
Adaptive	Massed Cubes: makes gate from model Drawing: copies square Geometric forms: points to 9 Counts: 4 objects & answers "how many" Esthetic comparison: correct Missing parts: 2 correct Digits: repeats 4 (1 of 3 trials)	Massed Cubes: builds 2 steps Drawing: unmistakable man with body, etc. Drawing: copies triangle (Drawing: copies rectangle with diagonals 66m.) Drawing: adds 7 parts to Incomplete Man Counts: 10 objects, correct pointing (Counts: 12 objects correctly 66m.) Weights: only 1 error in 5 block test (*72m) Fingers: correct number, each hand (*72m)	Massed Cubes: builds 3 steps Drawing: man with neck, hands, clothes Drawing: man's legs are 2-dimensional Drawing: copies diamond Drawing: adds 9 parts to Incomplete Man Weights: 5 blocks, no error best trial Missing parts: all correct Digits: 4 correct (2 of 3 trials) Fingers: correct number each hand and both together Adds and subtracts: within 5
Gross Motor	Hops: on 1 foot Articulation: not infantile	Skips: using feet, alternately Stands: on 1 foot more than 8 seconds	Jumps: from height 12", lands on toes Ball: advanced throwing Stands: on each foot alternately, eyes closed
Fine Motor	Drawing: traces cross	Pellets: 10 into bottle in 20 seconds	Drawing: copies diamond
Language	Defines: 4 in terms of use Comprehension Questions B: 1 correct	Coins: names penny, nickel, dime Color card: names all four Pictures: descriptive comment with enumeration Comprehension Questions B: 2 correct Commissions: 3 in succession	Binet items to be used here
Personal-Social	Communication: calls attention to own performance (*60m) Communication: relates fanciful tales (*60m) Communication: bosses & criticizes (*60m) Play: shows off dramatically (*60m)	Dressing: dresses & undresses, no assistance Communication: asks meaning of words Play: dresses up in adult clothes (Play: prints a few letters 60–66m.)	Dressing: ties shoe laces Communication: differentiates A.M. & P.M. Commun: knows right & left (3 of 3) or complete reversal (6 of 6) Communication: recites numbers to 30

4

The Conduct of the Evaluation

The previous chapters have shown that developmental assessment is essentially a device for determining the integrity and functional maturity of the child's nervous system. As an integral part of medical practice, the developmental examination may be undertaken as a screening procedure, by a general practitioner or pediatrician in the course of routine supervision of a child under his care, or during a diagnostic consultation by the specialist physician for a suspected developmental problem. Developmental screening will be discussed in Chapter 17.

The conduct of a developmental diagnostic assessment and the beginning of management entails five steps: (1) a history and preliminary interview; (2) the formal behavioral examination, in an established order; (3) recording of the results and a diagnostic review of the evaluation as a whole; (4) a discussion of the findings and recommendations with the parents; (5) a written report for the child's record and to the referring source. This chapter provides a general discussion of these five tasks; procedural details and sample forms are given in Appendix A.

Some sections of the chapter have pertinence primarily for the consultant specialist in developmental diagnosis; for such situations the assumption is made that the examination represents the first contact with the family. Detailed information may or may not be available from the referring physician or agency, but the general nature of the problem is known.

§1. HISTORY AND PRELIMINARY INTERVIEW

As in all of medicine, an adequate history is a *sine qua non* for diagnosis. It is essential to obtain this information, preferably before examining the child. An adequate history includes information about the family, the specific pregnancy, labor, delivery and neonatal period, illnesses, convulsive seizures, past development, current behavior, and pertinent environmental and social variables. The physician providing continuous care for a child should have this information already at hand.

For the consultant, foreknowledge about the child should be gained by sending questions from the Developmental Screening Inventory (DSI) to the parents prior to an appointment (Appendix A-6). For infants under 18 months of age, these questions will focus on behavior appropriate to the child's age; for children over 18 months they should cover the details of past development. The information obtained in this manner can be transferred to the appropriate developmental schedules prior to the child's arrival.

Whenever possible, the appointment should be scheduled for the time of day which coincides with the child's period of greatest alertness and cooperation. The replies from the parents and their chief complaint will be clues to the complexity of the ensuing evaluation. Under 18 months, obtaining the needed additional history and the behavioral examination generally can be combined in a single session. After this age, the interview may be so long that the child will tire before it is completed. For most diagnostic problems after 2½ years of age, an initial history session usually is advisable, and it will be necessary in selected complex cases between 18 and 30 months. If two sessions are not possible for any reason, a child whose behavior is disturbing can be removed by one parent while the other is being interviewed.

The interview should be friendly and informal rather than inquisitorial. On the other hand, little is gained and much lost by open-ended generalities. The questions should be specific enough so that there is no confusion in the parents' minds about the information being requested. Often it will be helpful if the examiner illustrates what he means. Each examiner formulates questions in his own way, of course—the answer to one question often changing the form of the next. Rigid adherence to a standard form is neither expected nor desirable, but systematic review is vital.

The information should be recorded as it is elicited. A specific history form which contains the essential medical and social information is found in Appendix A-5. Although this form may appear formidably long, it requires a minimum of writing; the length results primarily from almost complete precoding for IBM card punching. Any necessary clarification of the replies about behavior already received from the parents follows, and information about items not included on the DSI questionnaire sent them is added to what has been transcribed already to developmental schedules. Obviously, the entire age range of behavior patterns is not covered. The examiner uses the information he has obtained already and the child's behavior he may have observed during the interview to modify his questions.

The general approach in asking the parents about behavior patterns is to cover one area of behavior at a time, exploring the upper limits in one field before proceeding to the next. Inquiry is made systematically about gross motor, language, and personal—social behavior; questions about adaptive and fine motor areas may be curtailed, since these abilities generally are exhibited by the child in the course of the examination. On each of the developmental schedules presented in Chapter 3 certain items in the history columns have been blocked out, indicating that these patterns are so precisely defined that the behavior must be observed by the examiner.

In all instances, the decision about the need for additional information on past development can be made by asking two questions to supplement the parents' chief complaint and the age of the child when they first became concerned about his development: *"Has your child ever failed to make progress?" "Has he ever lost any behavior once acquired?"* Part II, on problems of differential diagnosis, will provide further information for eliciting important historic data relative to abnormalities.

A word of caution is necessary about the reliability of the history obtained. It is extremely important to believe what the parents are telling you; parents are good observers of their child's behavior, and they do not come to you with intent to deceive. The burden of proof that they are wrong is on you, and you will get into far more difficulties in diagnosis if you discount their reports. If what the parents say is at variance with your initial impression of the child or knowledge of developmental patterns, make certain that they understand the questions you are asking and that you are asking them correctly, or look for some modifying factors. For example, the mother of a 28-week old may tell you that he is able to sit leaning forward on his hands for support, but when you ask about his head control, she says "It's terrible, doctor." Your immediate reaction is to say she is an inadequate historian, because it isn't possible at this age for the infant to support himself in sitting and yet have poor head control. However, when you see an akinetic seizure, with loss not only of head control but of all body control, her answers are understandable. You have not been specific enough in your interrogation.

With practice, the examiner will become familiar enough with the area of developmental diagnosis so that his attention will not be glued to the forms. He will be able to listen to what the parents are saying; he will not repeat questions for which information already has been given spontaneously; and he will be able to look at the child and the parents for important clues their impromptu behavior may provide. However, the examiner must be alert to the child's state, interrupt the questioning, and proceed to the behavioral evaluation if excessive restlessness supervenes. How the child tolerates the interview and what he does during it have diagnostic significance in themselves.

Rapport with the child should be established during the interview, before beginning the examination. This rapport is facilitated if the examiner wears a coat of a color other than the white usually associated with a doctor. If an infant is sensitive to strangers, or if a child is wary, it is good policy to delay any direct overtures to the young visitor and give chief attention to the mother. This seeming neglect will in itself tend to disarm the child. He will conclude that the examiner has no violent designs upon him, and as confidence takes root, you may tentatively offer him a toy during the course of the questioning. If he does not accept the proffer, he needs more time to make his initial adjustment. When he accepts the toy freely from your hands, he has accepted you. Then it usually is safe to proceed, though not too abruptly, to the examination. If there has been a separate interview with the parents, or if for any reason the interview is not conducted in the examining room, some questions should be asked again about the child's current behavior in order to establish the necessary rapport. Thus, an interview also is used as a preparatory stage for the formal behavioral examination.

Table 4-1   EXAMINATION SEQUENCES

Supine (Crib)

4 Weeks Zone 0 - 4 - 8 weeks	16 Weeks Zone 12 - 16 - 20 weeks
Situation Number* Supine-------------------------- 1 Dangling ring--------------------- 2 Rattle--------------------------- 3 Social stimulation--------------- 4 Bell-ringing--------------------- 5 (Pull-to-sitting)---------------- 6 Sitting supported----------------50 Standing supported---------------51 Prone----------------------------52	Situation Number Supine--------------------------- 1 Dangling ring--------------------- 2 Rattle--------------------------- 3 Social stimulation--------------- 4 Bell-ringing--------------------- 5 Pull-to-sitting------------------ 6 Sitting supported----------------50 *Chair--Table top*------------------- *Cube 1,(2)*----------------------7,8 *Massed cubes*--------------------11 *(Cup)*---------------------------16 *Pellet*--------------------------18 *(Bell)*--------------------------22 *Mirror*--------------------------24 Standing supported---------------51 Prone----------------------------52

Sitting (Chair)	*Sitting (Crib)*
28 Weeks Zone 24 - 28 - 32 weeks	40 Weeks Zone 36 - 40 - 44 weeks
Chair--Table top Situation Number Cube, 1,2,3----------------------7,8,9 Massed cubes---------------------11 *(Cup and cubes)*-----------------17 Pellet---------------------------18 Bell-----------------------------22 *Ring and String*-----------------23 Mirror---------------------------24 Sitting supported----------------50 Standing supported---------------51 Prone----------------------------52 (Supine)-------------------------- 1 (Dangling ring)------------------- 2 (Rattle)------------------------- 3 Social stimulation--------------- 4 Bell-ringing--------------------- 5 (Pull-to-sitting)---------------- 6	Table top Situation Number Cubes 1,2,3----------------------7,8,9 Massed cubes---------------------11 Cup and cubes--------------------17 Pellet---------------------------18 *Pellet beside bottle*------------19 *Pellet in bottle*----------------20 Bell-----------------------------22 Ring and String------------------23 Mirror---------------------------24 *Mirror and ball*-----------------25 *Sitting free*--------------------53 *Creeping*------------------------54 *Rail*----------------------------55 *Cruising*------------------------56 *Walking supported*---------------57

( ) = Situation sometimes omitted for special reasons.
Italicized items appear for first time in this sequence.
*Situation number identifies the test situation described
in Appendix A, Examination Procedures.

§2. ORDER OF THE EXAMINATION

Table 4-1 lists the recommended examination sequences for each of the eight key age zones: 4, 16, 28, 40 and 52 weeks, 18, 24 and 36 months. The sequences are graduated but flexible; no sequence differs drastically from the adjacent ones. The new behavior situations which progressively appear at each age are indicated by italics, and situations omitted in certain circumstances are in parentheses. The objective is *to learn the general progression of the sequences from age to age,* and

Table 4-1 *Continued*

Sitting (Crib)	*Locomotor (Child's Table and Chair)*
52 Weeks Zone **48 - 52 - 56 weeks**	**18 Months Zone** **15 - 18 - 21 months**

Table top   Situation Number
Cubes 1,2,3--------------------7,8,9
Tower 2------------------------10
Massed cubes---------------------11
Cup and cubes--------------------17
Pellet beside bottle-------------19
Pellet in bottle-----------------20
Ring and String------------------23
Drawing-Scribble imitation-------27
Formboard-----------------------35
Ball play-----------------------46
Mirror---------------------------24
Mirror and ball------------------25
Sitting free---------------------53
Creeping-------------------------54
Rail-----------------------------55
Cruising-------------------------56
Walking supported----------------**57**
	Situation Number
	Picture book----------------------40
	Cubes: Tower--------------------12
	        (Train)------------------13
	Cup and cubes--------------------17
	Pellet beside bottle-------------19
	Drawing: *Spontaneous*------------26
	         Scribble imitation------27
	         Vertical strokes-------28
	         (Circular scribble)-----29
	Formboard------------------------35
	(Picture card)--------------------41
	(Performance box)-----------------36
	(Test objects)--------------------45
	Small ball: Throwing------------46
	         Directions----------47
	         (In box)------------48
	Kicking------------------------58
	Sitting in chair------------------50
	Walking, running------------------59
	Stairs--------------------------60

Locomotor (Child's Table and Chair)	
24 Months Zone **21 - 24 - 30 months**	**36 Months Zone** **30 - 36 - 42 months**

Situation Number
Picture book---------------------40
Cubes: Tower--------------------12
        Train--------------------13
        (Chimney)----------------14
Cup and cubes--------------------17
Drawing: Spontaneous------------26
         Vertical strokes--------28
         Horizontal strokes------30
         Circular scribble-------29
(Picture cards)-------------------41
Formboard------------------------35
Performance box------------------36
(Name)--------------------------42
(Test objects: Names)-----------45
         Use)-----------45
Small ball: Throwing-------------46
         Directions----------47
         (In box)------------48
Kicking--------------------------58
Sitting in chair-----------------50
Walking, running-----------------59
Stairs---------------------------60
	Situation Number
	Picture book---------------------40
	Cubes: Tower--------------------12
	        Train--------------------13
	        Chimney------------------14
	        Bridge-------------------15
	Drawing: Spontaneous------------26
	         Strokes-------------28,30
	         Circle-------------------31
	         Cross--------------------32
	         Incomplete man----------33
	         Trace diamond-----------34
	(Picture cards)-------------------41
	Formboard------------------------35
	Color forms----------------------37
	(Name, *sex*)---------------------42
	(Comprehension)-------------------43
	(Digits)------------------------44
	Geometric Forms------------------38
	Weighted blocks------------------39
	10 Pellets and bottle-------------21
	(Test objects-use)---------------45
	Small ball: Throwing------------46
	         Prepositions--------49
	Kicking--------------------------58
	Running--------------------------59
	Walking on tiptoe-----------------61
	Standing on one foot-------------62
	Jumping-------------------------63
	Stairs---------------------------60

how to present the different examination objects, and then observe the responses they evoke. Often it will help in understanding the meaning of a given pattern if similar behavior at adjacent ages is surveyed. Details for conducting the examination procedures themselves are outlined in Appendix A-4.

The sequences for 4 and 16 weeks begin with supine situations. The ones for 28, 40 and 52 weeks assume a child who can sit, supported or unsupported. Those for 18, 24 and 36 months assume an ambulatory (locomotor) child who can be seated in front of a small table. To choose the proper sequence for a particular child, determine first the category in which the child fits best. If there are no contraindications, select the sequence nearest to his chronologic age. If obvious deviations, defects or retardations have been noted, make due allowances. Having selected one sequence, do not fail to shift to a more advanced or a lower one if the child's performance so demands. Adjacent sequences are so closely related that shifts generally do not entail any serious readjustments. However, the standard order of the situations within each sequence should be maintained as far as possible.

The chief point is that the child's demonstrated abilities and interests should determine the specific situations that are used. Your aim is to ascertain the maximum levels of his abilities, so it is desirable to stretch his adjustment to this maximum. For example, you may be examining a 32-week child on the 28-week sequence; he has given such an excellent performance in the Single and Massed Cubes situations that you can introduce the Cup and Cubes situation, which appears on the 28-week sequence in parentheses. You may even shift entirely to the 40-week sequence.

Conversely, do not hesitate to start at or shift to a lower sequence. Many unsuccessful examinations, particularly with deviant children, are unsuccessful because the examiner learns during the interview that there are fragments of behavior at, or close to, the child's chronologic age. Therefore, he assumes that the child's developmental age is in the normal range. As a consequence, he remains within this age range in his presentations and obtains meaningless, chaotic behavior which he then diagnoses as psychotic. By dropping abruptly, or gradually, to a much lower age range, he secures behavior revealing of the child's true capacity; those patterns necessary for making a more definitive diagnosis then can be explored.

There is a rationale to the order of presentation within each sequence. Cubes are used at or near the beginning of most of the sequences because the cubes have universal ingratiating appeal. The seriated cube presentations build up an anticipation in an infant which projects itself into ensuing situations. He soon expects you to give him something new to do. This expectation, properly guided and satisfied, imparts flow and dynamic progression to the examination. In general, postural tests are deferred to the end to reduce any possible disturbing effect and to give the child more free play in the examining crib or on the floor.

Since the examination in its entirety is a single unit, the transitions between situations are as important as the situations *per se;* they are neither to be overlooked nor regarded as impediments. It is relatively simple to make a smooth transition from the interview to the formal examination situation. The ambulatory child already has been seated at the examining table during the interview. In the case of an infant, the mother has removed his shoes and stockings during the interview; the remainder of his disrobing is best left until the postural tests are undertaken, unless the clothes interfere with performance prior to this time. The mother places the infant in the proper examining position, and the examiner remains initially at a proper distance. Once an adaptation is made, if she does not spontaneously do so, the mother is asked to remain on the side to allow the examiner full sway. (How the mother handles the child throughout, and how the child reacts to her as well as to the examiner, can also provide information which is of diagnostic import.) If the child is playing with a toy at the close of the interview, he is permitted to retain the toy, which may be removed as soon as the cubes, for example, are presented. Either he will drop it in response to the new rival toy or you may extract it gently at the moment of cube presentation. By a similar ruse, you may remove the cube before the next object, the pellet, is presented. Some children cling more tightly than others to an object in hand; however, most of them make a prompt adjustment from one object to the next, and once the examination is under way there is little difficulty in accomplishing transitions.

The tempo of the examination always should be regulated freely to meet individual requirements. It is impractical and unnecessary to allot a specified amount of time to each of the behavior situations. You will learn empirically how soon a child is ready for the next situation. Sometimes, as with the pellet, a few seconds of exploitation may suffice. However, if the infant shows great eagerness and versatility in his exploitation, for example, of the bell, you may permit him to manipulate it for several minutes. The tempo will differ greatly with each child: One may run through the whole series of situations in less than 10 minutes; another may take twice as long or more. Certain modes or cycles of exploitation also tend to repeat themselves. Such cycles are characteristic patterns of activity which afford a clue to the timing of the examination situations.

With skillful management, a child's interest in the materials will mount as the examination proceeds. No situation should be allowed to drag or exhaust itself. The examination should not be interrupted to make elaborate recordings. One situation should shift into the next with a smooth swing. If necessary, the recommended order may be altered to suit child or exigency. That tempo is best which stimulates, builds up, and sustains the child's interest.

There is one final procedural point applicable to the examination of an infant: The examiner should learn to talk about what the infant is doing as it occurs. This serves several purposes. One is to sharpen the examiner's ability to observe behavior and recall it more completely for subsequent recording. Second, a quietly dictated commentary may actually enhance an infant's performance by eliminating the void of silence.

§3. RECORDING AND DIAGNOSTIC REVIEW

A detailed record of behavior observed during the examination must be added to the historic information obtained. The examiner's commentary during an infant examination supplies especially valuable data in complicated cases requiring long supervision. When audio- or videotape recording is available, observations can be captured at the very time they are being made for immediate postexamination review. If no electronic equipment is available, the dictation may be recorded by a stenographer. Since comments by the examiner may interfere with an older child, the stenographic assistant also can be trained to observe and write out a complete account of the child's behavior. Ideally, the assistant should be seated in an inconspicuous corner of the room where no distraction to the examination is offered. Still better is stationing the stenographer behind a one-way-vision screen, described in Appendix C-4, which can be installed easily in any office. A final alternative is to recall and jot down pertinent comments immediately after the examination. It is unwise for the examiner to attempt to write any observations during the course of the examination, lest the flow of the child's behavior be interrupted.

A minimal record, which may be adequate for children without abnormalities, consists of plus and minus signs entered on the developmental schedules. In all other instances, the Developmental and Neurologic Examination form should be completed (Appendix A-5). Suffice it to say that the plus and minus signs do not automatically deliver a diagnosis. Here, as in all diagnosis, clinical judgment always must be brought to bear. Through experience and study, the examiner should have a fairly well-defined mental image of the normal behavior characteristics of a representative child at any given key age. He also has an image of the behavior characteristics he has just witnessed. He then can match the witnessed behavior picture against the normal image for the child as a whole, and separately for each of the five behavior fields. Controlled objectively by the stages embodied in the developmental schedules, such critical comparison permits determination of developmental age.

A thorough knowledge of normal central nervous system function is the basis on which detection of abnormality rests. Familiarity with changes in behavior resulting from localized or generalized dysfunction, as well as an intensive knowledge of the various neuropsychiatric clinical entities, are absolutely essential for more definitive diagnosis and treatment. After consideration of the behavioral pictures of various clinical conditions in Part II, the examiner will discover how the behavior of atypical and defective children deviates from the normal. He will recognize deviations as signs of maldevelopment and will be able to arrive at differential and descriptive diagnoses. He will have a clearer understanding of the more detailed directions for recording and evaluating behavior which are found in Appendix A-5.

§4. DISCUSSION OF THE FINDINGS AND RECOMMENDATIONS

Immediately following the recording and diagnostic review of the examination, either by the examiner alone or with students or clinical personnel who have been involved in the evaluation process, a discussion should be held with the parents. The manner in which the diagnosis is made and imparted to the parents is fundamental to successful guidance, and there are certain principles which should be followed. First, if the parents are to be satisfied with the diagnosis and prognosis given them and receptive to the necessary plans for management, they must know the basis on which the diagnosis is being made. The diagnostic process is thus an integral part of the treatment. Observation of the examination is the way in which the parents best can understand the basis for the diagnosis. It also clarifies their feelings and systematizes their own observations, permits them to see behavior and symptoms which will be important in management, and allows the physician to observe interactions between the child and the parents.

During the postexamination discussion, physician and parents should be seated comfortably and any impression of haste eliminated. If a trial of treatment or further tests are indicated before coming to firm conclusions about prognosis, preliminary findings and the reasons for further steps should be explained. If the physician will take 15 or 20 minutes to cover certain points in a structured fashion, he will find that he usually has answered most of the parents' questions, even though he may have to go over some points several times. A more detailed discussion of the content of such a conference is reserved for Chapter 18. As with recording and diagnostic review, such a discussion will have more significance following the presentation in Part II of the problems of differential diagnosis.

§5. THE WRITTEN REPORT

All the information gathered forms the basis for a written report to the referring physician or agency and for inclusion in the child's record and hospital chart. The purposes of such a report are to clarify in the examiner's mind what he has observed, to give the data on which he is basing his diagnosis, prognosis and recommendations for management, and to transmit this information in a clear and understandable way to others. Certain basic information is included for all patients, but the report should be geared toward specific description of the distinctive abilities and disabilities of the child under consideration. A general outline and illustrative specimen for this report are detailed in Appendix A-5.

Part II

Defects and Deviations of Development

5

Problems of Differential Diagnosis

Clinical manifestations of abnormal and atypical development in infancy always present problems of diagnosis and prognosis. What are the causes of deviation? What is the developmental outlook? Is there any therapy that is curative or ameliorative? Considering the outlook, the possibilities of treatment and the family situation, what is to be done?

The function of a developmental neurologic assessment is to establish a differential diagnosis. It is the physician's first and foremost responsibility, which he cannot abdicate. He must distinguish between inborn and acquired abnormalities, and between permanent deviations and those that are remediable or self-correcting. He must also recognize mixed types and partial syndromes. He has the further responsibility of discussing the diagnosis and prognosis with the parents with honesty and tact, of supervising or referring the patient for indicated medical treatment, and of referring to appropriate resources for the auxiliary health, educational, social and rehabilitative facilities necessary for ongoing management and maximizing developmental potential.

These problems are enormously complicated, since we are dealing with a growing organism, one which has a developmental past, present and future. In the normal infant in a normal environment, development is methodical, orderly and timed; it goes through a gradient that can be divided into stages which follow each other with such regularity that they are, in the main, predictable. This is the true meaning of man's genetic endowment. The *human* infant becomes a *human* adult, a person, unique, shaped by the hereditary, biopsychosocial and cultural factors which have impinged upon him since the species and individual evolved, grew and developed.

That there always is interaction between the organic constitution of an individual and his environment is implicit in any consideration of development. It is not a matter of either—or, of nature versus nurture, but of interplay between the two at all stages of development. The biologic intactness of the central nervous system depends on a multitude of factors. All available data indicate that, except for specific hereditary diseases, environmental factors are more crucial determinants of differential behavior, and are largely socioeconomically derived. The mother's antecedent life history has a vital effect on the gestation of her infant, and the interaction between host and environment continues postnatally, with sociocultural factors influencing the psychologic level of integration, not only through cultural and educational opportunities, but also through the effects of disease and malnutrition on the biologic substrate. In this manner the phenotype results from the interaction of the genotype with the environment. Consideration of this interaction is essential in diagnosis and prognosis, even though it appears to be ignored in the discussion of particular clinical entities.

§1. THE SPECTRUM OF NEUROPSYCHIATRIC DISABILITY

Even the abnormal infant follows human development: No matter how distorted, the progressions still are recognizable as characteristic of man alone. In the abnormal infant, some degree of retardation is nearly always the most obvious symptom, but not necessarily in all areas simultaneously, or to the same degree in each area of behavior. Secondly, development is distorted; behavior patterns may be deformed or hypertrophied, or they may fail to appear. The amount of retardation and distortion depends upon the nature of the etiologic factors, their severity, and the time of their occurrence in the child's life cycle.

Figure 5-1 presents schematically the components of the continuum of reproductive casualty, listing the clinical disorders associated with chronic organic brain disease.[61] Antecedent etiologic factors, particularly complications of pregnancy and low birth weight and their neuropsychiatric sequelae are found with greater frequency in lower socioeconomic strata. There is a lethal component evidenced by abortions, stillbirths and neonatal deaths. Depending on the site and

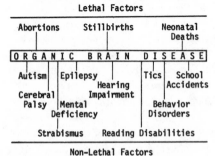

Fig. 5-1. Schematic representation of the continuum of reproductive casualty.

extent of the injury, survivors may manifest a spectrum of disorders. Severe injury results in major crippling central nervous system dysfunction, such as "cerebral palsy," epilepsy and mental deficiency; lesser degrees of damage are sufficient to disorganize behavioral development and lower thresholds to stress, resulting in all types of behavioral and learning disabilities.

Even though intimate interrelationships exist among the different facets of behavioral development, each aspect demands separate analysis and study for adequate differential diagnosis and prognosis. However, all are evaluated concurrently in the course of the developmental assessment. It is not possible to say "Now we are evaluating intellectual potential; next we will do the neuromotor examination." Both are aspects of a neurologic examination. The infant cannot be fragmented into psychometric and neurologic halves, or into any other independent subdivisions. Neuromotor integrity and maturational status are inextricably intertwined.

Using this monistic approach in Part II, we will discuss six broad aspects of neuropsychiatric disability. First, interference with intellectual function prevents full expression of those behaviors which are most uniquely human. Mental subnormality may indicate deficiency due to organic disease of the brain, or retardation secondary to suboptimal experience, or both (Chapters 6–8). Second, neuromotor abnormalities range from deviations which are of no clinical importance to major disabilities subsumed under the rubric "cerebral palsy." Motor aspects of neurologic function in infancy are the most sensitive indices of minor disturbances of central nervous system integration (Chapters 9–11). Third, convulsive disorders may appear in conjunction with other abnormalities or as the only expression of central nervous system disease; certain atypical seizures common in infancy may masquerade as intellectual inadequacy (Chapter 13). Fourth, specific sensory defects of hearing or vision, both peripheral and central, may modify the normal developmental progressions (Chapters 14, 15). Fifth, the quality of the total integration of behavior and the emotional relationship of the child to his environment is of fundamental importance in determining his functioning; the most extreme deviations in integrative ability have been labeled "autism" or infantile psychosis (Chapter 16). Finally, there is a whole host of specific syndromes associated with central nervous system dysfunction which must be identified and included in any diagnostic summary. Some are amenable to specific therapy, others have great importance for genetic counseling. For the most part, management and guidance will be discussed in Chapter 18, and will not be confined to any one neuropsychiatric disability.

Any or all of these disabilities may appear, singly or in combination, as end results of genetic defect, reproductive casualty, or postnatal insult. At later ages, a variety of learning and behavioral disabilities may appear as manifestations of cerebral dysfunction. These are cut from the same cloth, but are beyond the scope of this volume in their full detail (Chapter 11). The remainder of this chapter is devoted to a detailed discussion of etiologic factors, the use of the developmental quotient (DQ) in diagnosis, the reliability and validity of developmental assessment, and other medical diagnostic procedures.

§2. ETIOLOGIC CONSIDERATIONS

Although a great deal of our knowledge is incomplete, it is increasing rapidly. In determining etiology of abnormalities, one should think in terms of the time in the child's life cycle when the noxious agent acts; within limits, the time of action is possibly of greater importance than the nature of the agent. The developmental period extends from the time of conception to roughly 8 or 9 years, the age at which motor skills reach adult levels of integration.

The term chromosomal abnormalities which produce a distinctive complex of anatomic characteristics usually can be recognized at birth, but manifestations of most hereditary disorders vary greatly in their time of appearance and severity. Adverse influences in the first 8 weeks of fetal life, the embryonal period, usually result in gross malformations, both within and without the central nervous system. They often result in death and expulsion of the fetus. In the remainder of the prenatal period, noxious influences such as anoxia, malnutrition or infection, if not severe enough to cause fetal death, are more likely to produce the continuum of reproductive casualty, the signs and symptoms of which depend on the extent and location of the damage. Results of postnatal insults also are different for developing and mature organisms. A handicap in a developing infant imposes difficulties in integrating and learning those behavior patterns which already are present in older children and adults. Damage to the developing organism typically is diffuse rather than localized, so that more often than not a combination of disabilities results. Unfortunately, the term damage carries the connotation of a physical insult which results in the death of tissue and a visible lesion. While this may be the case, dysfunction is a preferable concept. Malfunctioning neurons, or enzymes, may well result in greater disabilities and disturbances than does the presence of nonfunctioning dead cells. Unprovoked or uncoordinated firing of a damaged cell, or its failure to fire, could lead to any of the neuropsychiatric disabilities. Thus, dysfunction attributable to central nervous system pathology can exist in the absence of demonstrable lesions. Table 5-1 presents a heuristic, if incomplete, etiologic classification of developmental defects and deviations, grouped by the time of action of the noxious agents.

Chromosomal and Hereditary Defects

Cognizance must be given to chromosomal disorders and inborn errors of metabolism, which have been the subjects of some of the most recent scientific advances. The reader is referred to Section 2 of Appendix E for selected references from the vast literature for detailed information. In spite of the large number of

Table 5-1. ETIOLOGIC CLASSIFICATION OF DEVELOPMENTAL
DEFECTS AND DEVIATIONS

GENETIC
    Chromosomal abnormalities
    Degenerative diseases
    Inborn errors of metabolism
    Malformations
PRENATAL
    External trauma
    Low birth weight
    Malformations
    Maternal infection
    Maternal irradiation
    Maternal intoxication
    Maternal malnutrition--pre- and postconception
    Other complications during pregnancy
    Placental defects--degeneration, placenta previa, premature separation
    Seasonal and geographic factors
    Socioeconomic factors
    "Stress"--emotional, overwork, others
PERINATAL
    Anoxia
    Crushing or laceration of central nervous system tissues
    Hemorrhage
    Hyperbilirubinemia--blood group incompatability, sepsis, other
    Other neonatal disorders
POSTNATAL
    Degenerative and neoplastic diseases
    Infection
    Intoxication
    Malnutrition
    "Maternal deprivation"
    Sociocultural and educational impoverishment
    Trauma

---

recognized clinical entities, such defects contribute only a small proportion to etiology, in the totality of developmental disorders.

Chromosomal disorders result from alterations in the number or structure of the chromosomes; either autosomes or sex chromosomes may be involved. While some mechanisms which produce the chromosomal abnormalities are understood, specific etiologic factors which cause the abnormal gametes to develop in any given individual have not been determined.

Autosomal trisomies produce distinctive anatomic constellations recognizable at birth, and are almost invariably associated with some degree of developmental deviation. When only some cells contain the abnormal chromosome material (mosaicism), the clinical signs are thought to be milder. Absence of an entire autosome (monosomy) is very rare and almost always incompatible with survival of the fetus. The most common autosomal abnormality in liveborn infants is trisomy 21 (Chapter 7, Section 4).

A much greater range of sex chromosome abnormalities exists. Absence of a sex chromosome or extra material has less severe effects, and the association with mental deficiency is less frequent, but sexual function is influenced. Syndromes of congenital defects usually recognizable at birth are associated with XO (Turner's syndrome) and XXXXY.

Current techniques permit identification of individual chromosomes and some individual chromosome segments. Diagnosis of the disorders can be made prenatally from cultured cells obtained by amniocentesis as early as the 12th week of pregnancy.

Hundreds of inborn errors of metabolism, involving almost every organ system and every type of metabolic substrate, also have been identified. Many are, or appear likely to be, diagnosable prenatally. Although the number of known single gene defects associated with single enzyme deficiencies is growing constantly, the incidence of most of the disorders is low, represented by only a handful of cases. Moreover, only a small proportion of these single gene disorders causes metabolic disturbances associated with or resulting in central nervous system dysfunction. Most are inherited as recessive traits; in occasional conditions the heterozygote carriers can be identified by means of enzyme assays or loading tests with the substrate they are unable to metabolize effectively. A few of the potentially treatable inborn errors can cause serious disturbances in the newborn period. In some of these conditions, dietary restriction of the substrate which cannot be metabolized is believed—but not proven—to be effective in ameliorating or preventing the associated cerebral malfunction. The prototypes of these disorders are phenylketonuria (Chapter 7, Section 5) and galactosemia.

A significant number of the disorders referred to as progressive neurologic degenerative diseases of childhood are hereditary disorders transmitted by single genes. The majority of these disorders are not necessarily manifest in early life by gross behavioral deviation, although some qualitative or quantitative developmental abnormality usually is present from birth. Specific enzyme deficits already have been demonstrated in some of these conditions, e.g., Tay-Sachs' disease and metachromatic leucodystrophy. Tuberous sclerosis and Friedreich's ataxia are among those for which a specific defect has not yet been identified.

Prenatal Factors

In the embryonic period, faulty physiologic regulation of somatic growth usually produces gross anatomic defects. Cerebral maldevelopments include anencephaly, other aplasias, encephalocele and cortical hemangiomata. Hydrocephaly, porencephaly, oxycephaly and sclerosis may evolve at this time or at subsequent stages in the life cycle. The growth disturbance may be due to gene defects, to biochemical influences, to environmental factors such as infections or drugs to which the mother is exposed, or to their interaction.

Adequate nutrition may be the most important substrate for development in the prenatal period; most other factors—e.g., socioeconomic, seasonal, and geographic—exert their influence through effects on food intake and utilization. This is now supported by pathologic studies of brain cell number and size.[80,81] Low birth weight is probably the most frequent abnormality associated with a great variety of developmental deviations. A correlation also exists between function and a birth weight above the 2500 g dividing line between "prematurity" and fullterm gestation (Chapter 12). Inadequate intrauterine growth or premature delivery may be secondary to improper placental implantation with resultant bleeding, to maternal toxemia, to heavy cigarette smoking or connected with other documented abnormalities. Certain specific infections during pregnancy such as syphilis, cytomegalic inclusion disease, rubella and toxoplasmosis adversely affect the developing nervous system. Other infections also may affect the nervous system, although they do not produce characteristic clinical syndromes. All these conditions have an increased incidence in the lower socioeconomic groups.

Maternal irradiation has been demonstrated to produce microcephaly and a variety of dysfunctions. The disastrous phocomelias from thalidomide ingestion are well known. Narcotic addiction causes neonatal withdrawal symptoms, but there is little evidence for later sequelae. Similarly, other drugs such as alcohol or LSD have not been demonstrated to have adverse effects that could not be explained by other aspects of the life style of the parents. Adverse sequelae from "emotional stress" have not been demonstrated unless associated with other factors such as low socioeconomic status, overcrowding, hard and prolonged work or multiparity.

Perinatal Factors

The time immediately around birth has its own peculiar dangers to growth potential, but the effects of "birth trauma" are greatly overemphasized today. The hazards are related to the level of obstetric care; the gross hemorrhages and crushing and lacerating injuries seen previously are relative rarities in mature infants now where sophisticated medical care is available. Nevertheless, mechanical laceration and bleeding, particularly in the low birth weight infant, still are potent causes of gross brain damage, which may be incompatible with survival. Almost all the medical literature still equates failure to breathe at birth with such "injury," placing the damage at the time of delivery. Towbin's examination of serial whole brain sections demonstrated that the major portion of central nervous system pathologic lesions had their origin prenatally, well before the onset of labor.[75] Preexisting brain damage interferes with the ability to adjust to extrauterine life and to initiate respiration; it is the previously abnormal infant who cannot withstand the anoxia and mild acidosis normally present at birth and who shows persistent neuropsychiatric defects of varying degree. The intraventricular, periventricular and multiple minute hemorrhages commonly seen most often result from hypoxia secondary to the wide variety of prenatal insults.[74]

Hyperbilirubinemia due to blood group incompatibility, while manifest in the perinatal period, has prenatal origins; at the present time the adverse effects are almost completely preventable. However, there are causes of hyperbilirubinemia other than blood group incompatibility, one of which is sepsis, to which the neonate is particularly susceptible.

Postnatal Factors

Even after independent extrauterine life is well established, the infant and child are not immune to hazards. The list of infections, general or specific malnutritions, traumas or toxic agents is almost endless. There also are degenerative processes which do not appear to be genetic and may be related to infection or toxins.

The infant's new environment exposes him to a new order of experience as well. Gross deprivation may be possible in institutional settings, and parental rejection and abuse do occur. Improperly managed blindness and hearing impairment may reduce exposure to normal experiences. Repeated illnesses and hospitalizations exact their biologic toll and may affect emotional adjustment adversely. Contrary to the accepted stereotype, they usually provide a plethora rather than a lack of sensory stimuli, pain-producing though these may be. In a lower socioeconomic milieu there may be a lack of academically oriented activity, the yardstick by which a schoolchild's function is measured. In such settings, dysstimulation is the more common pattern, resulting from bombardment by sensory stimuli of all modalities in the crowded quarters of a slum environment. The child with an intact nervous system has difficulty enough in such an environment. The injured child with impaired inhibitory, attentional and integrative capacities responds with dysfunctional reactions which make it even more difficult, if not impossible, to mature successfully (Chapter 11). Thus, there is interaction between the social causes of central nervous system dysfunction, the effects of that damage on behavior and the social context in which the injured child develops.

In all periods, damage may be great, small or selective, leaving certain growth potentials unimpaired. Developmental potentials may be impoverished to an extreme degree; growth potentials may be abiotrophic, the developmental impetus expending itself early. Deceleration or actual deterioration also may occur. However, a marked or moderate reduction of developmental potential does not rule out consistent, slow development over a long period of time.

§3. THE DEVELOPMENTAL QUOTIENT (DQ)

Diagnosis and prediction are inseparable in dealing with developmental problems. Each time a diagnosis is made, a prognosis is implied. If retardation is present, accurate diagnosis determines whether the future probabilities are in favor of deterioration, consistent progress at a reduced rate and level or improvement.

In the absence of progressive retardation, intervening biologic or sociocultural insult, specific treatment, or compensation, a relatively constant rate of development is the rule. In other words a normal infant becomes a normal child and adult; a subnormal infant, a subnormal child and adult.

Employing the assessment measures described in the preceding chapters, we can compare the developmental status of any child with the behavior appropriate to his age, and determine whether and by how much he deviates. We ascertain the completeness as well as the rate of his development; we make qualitative and quantitative comparisons.

The developmental quotient, or DQ, is the beginning and not the end of developmental diagnosis. It serves as a point of departure, and must not be oversimplified or overstretched. The DQ is a shorthand device for expressing the rate of development. The DQ is simply the relationship between maturity age (derived from the behavioral performance) and actual age, expressed as a ratio:

$$DQ = \frac{\text{Maturity age}}{\text{Chronologic age}} \times 100$$

To illustrate, the developmental stages are the points of reference derived from behavior characteristic at given ages, and represent the theoretically "perfectly average child" who consistently maintains a "perfectly average rate" of development; maturity age and chronologic age always coincide:

$$DQ = \frac{\text{Maturity age}}{\text{Chronologic age}} = \frac{8 \text{ wks}}{8 \text{ wks}} \times 100 = \frac{24 \text{ wks}}{24 \text{ wks}} \times 100 = \frac{52 \text{ wks}}{52 \text{ wks}} \times 100 =$$

$$\frac{24 \text{ mos}}{24 \text{ mos}} \times 100 = \frac{36 \text{ mos}}{36 \text{ mos}} \times 100 = 100$$

The ratio between maturity age and chronologic age is always unity or 100%; the DQ is 100.

In a situation where relatively consistent retardation is to be expected, 4 weeks of retardation at the age of 8 weeks lengthens into 12 weeks at 24 weeks, and into 1 year at 2 years of age. The child as he grows older is achieving only half his expected developmental potential:

$$DQ = \frac{4 \text{ weeks}}{8 \text{ weeks}} \times 100 = \frac{12 \text{ weeks}}{24 \text{ weeks}} \times 100 = \frac{1 \text{ year}}{2 \text{ years}} \times 100 = 50$$

Thus the DQ represents the proportion of normal development that is present at any given age. (Appendix A-5 discusses in detail how maturity ages are determined.)

§4. DIAGNOSTIC IMPORT OF AREAS OF BEHAVIOR

Developmental quotients must be assigned in each area of behavior, and the role of each area understood clearly, to approach the problems of diagnosis and prediction rationally.

One must discard the terms *sensorimotor* and *psychomotor* development, and abandon the concept that one can measure only motor behavior in infancy. Overemphasis on motor development explains in large measure why predictions from infant evaluations in the past have been poor; some psychologists have been led to conclude that intellectual growth is inherently unstable and the attributes of later intellectual function are not present in the first year of life.[4] Motor behavior is vital for an assessment of neuromotor integrity, but it is *not* the primary basis for assessing intellectual potential. Accelerated motor behavior does not indicate superior intellectual ability, and a small proportion of mentally defective children even have normal gross motor development for their age. Conversely, while mental deficiency usually is accompanied by retardation in motor function, such abnormal neuromotor development is not synonymous with intellectual defect; in fact, it is seen more often as a selective disability in the presence of normal intellectual potential.

Language behavior is used similarly, beginning about 2 years of age, as the criterion of intellectual adequacy. Although mental deficiency is the most common cause of significant language retardation, delay in language development is *not* synonymous with intellectual defect, as illustrated amply by children with hearing defects. In some children who are otherwise normal, speech production may be delayed, while language comprehension and communication through gesture and pantomime remain entirely age-appropriate. Given the minimal prerequisite of normal intellectual potential, language is socially determined: It may remain limited and simple or idiosyncratic in dialect. If the input is rich, language is elaborated and facilitates the development and expression of other cognitive abilities. A restricted language milieu may exact a developmental penalty, but the child should not be penalized for his limitations in communication. However, in contrast to motor behavior, if language development is normal or accelerated, a diagnosis of mental deficiency can be ruled out.

Personal–social behavior is most subject to variation from differences in cultural milieu, but also is dependent on both neuromotor and intellectual integrity. In certain instances of severe motor and/or sensory handicap in the early years, it may be the sole index of normal potential, which is capable of expression only at later ages.

Adaptive behavior, the forerunner of later intelligent behavior, must be the primary basis for predicting intellectual potential. Its expressions in infancy are simpler than the complex manifestations at later ages, but they are only superficially simple. For his age, the infant's integration of stimuli in a meaningful fashion is a complicated process, and is the index of the intactness of his cerebral cortex.

A general developmental level assigned is *not* an average of the five areas of behavior; motor abilities do not figure in its derivation. The general DQ is the overall prediction of intellectual potential, assuming continuing adequate environmental circumstances. It takes into account the qualitative features of the maturity and integrity of behavior and also gives weight to discrepancies. The general developmental level is usually the same as, but *never less* than, the adaptive level.

The adaptive maturity level may be raised a week or two under three circumstances: if there is a neuromotor or sensory disability which interferes with performance; if the quality of behavior is very good even though the level of achievement is not advanced; if language behavior is significantly more advanced. Since language has implications for later intellectual function, in the presence of a neuromotor handicap or marked disorganization in behavior which results in significant discrepancies between adaptive and language behavior, language may be a more valid predictor of later function when defective adaptive behavior is elicited. A general developmental level is not assigned in such circumstances.

The DQ accordingly has considerable value in clinical diagnosis; it furnishes an index of the current rate of development. In *infancy,* any adaptive DQ below 85 probably indicates organic impairment of some type. Whenever any DQs fall decisively below the two-thirds or three-fourths ratio (DQ = 65–75), there is reason to suspect serious retardation. The retardation may be permanent, or it may be inconsequential if limited only to certain areas of behavior. However, it is a clinical indication which calls for further study. It helps to define the issues which need interpretation. Further implications of specific DQ values are discussed in Chapter 6.

§5. DQ AND IQ

Although the numerical principle which underlies the DQ is similar to that of the IQ, or intelligence quotient, there are important differences in clinical application which should be indicated. Historically, the IQ can be traced most directly to the work of Alfred Binet, who drew up a measuring scale of intelligence in school children based upon age norms. Ratings on this scale are expressed in terms of mental age—mental age being equivalent to intelligence age. Stern and Terman converted this mental age into an intelligence quotient (IQ) by establishing a ratio with chronologic age, similar to the ratio between developmental maturity age and chronologic age.

The IQ does not measure intelligence in an absolute way; rather, it signifies the relative rate at which so-called intelligence is developing on the basis of a standardized psychometric scale, consisting largely of verbal and problem-solving tests. The tests are scored on an arbitrary basis of success and failure. The successes, irrespective of their distribution, are added. The sum is the mental age. From the standpoint of diagnosis this is an obvious oversimplification; in clinical usage it leads to the fallacy of regarding intelligence as a global entity, and it does not differentiate individual types of intelligence, giftedness or disability. Intelligence measured in this fashion has a very large component of socially determined functioning, modifiable to a remarkable degree by management, familial, educational and other psychosocial factors.

The Stanford–Binet and a number of other intelligence scales have been applied chiefly to children of school age.[71] The IQ does correlate highly with school performance and with other tests presumed to measure entirely different aspects of central nervous system function. Interestingly enough, Jencks' recent work has stated that the IQ does not predict various aspects of social performance, such as vocational success as measured by income.[35] The latter seems to be predicted best by the sociocultural status of the family, indicating the extremely narrow range of usefulness of most intelligence tests. The IQ has been used and misused for many social, psychologic and political purposes.

The Eighth International Classification of Diseases subdivides the degrees of subnormal intelligence on an IQ basis as follows: profound, IQ under 20; severe, IQ 20–35; moderate, IQ 36–51; mild IQ 52–67; borderline, IQ 68–85.[20] This arbitrary psychometric classification may have descriptive, administrative, statistical and communication value, but it leads to serious errors if not used with caution in clinical situations. Neither an IQ nor a DQ automatically delivers a diagnosis; both need qualification and interpretation. At no age should assignment to a broad clinical category be defined rigidly by numerical quotients–52 is mild, but 51 moderate; 94 is low average, but 95 average. A few points in a score are not the basis for deciding if a child has "just average intelligence" or higher abilities, is mildly retarded or of borderline intelligence. Quite the contrary, if a quotient is at odds with clinical impressions of the quality and integrity of behavior, the quotient is at greater risk of being wrong, particularly in infancy. In an academically oriented professional home, an older child with a measured IQ of 85, or even 95, is clearly impaired in comparison to other family members, most likely on the basis of organic brain disease. In a ghetto milieu, he probably has no significant brain pathology and would respond to an optimum environment, in its broadest sense, and an adequate educational program. In both instances the IQ of 85 has management and treatment implications, but different ones.

As noted in Chapter 2, developmental diagnosis does not attempt a direct measurement of intelligence as such, but aims at clinical estimates of intellectual potential based upon an analysis of maturity status. We are most interested in those aspects of intelligence we have called *adaptive behavior*–the capacity to use and initiate experience for present and future adjustment. However, infant behavior is so integrated and generalized that this adaptivity must always be considered in relation to the motor, language and personal–social aspects of behavior. Unlike the IQ, the DQ is not limited to a single inclusive formula. It is an adaptable device which registers changes in the growing complex of behavior. Significant fluctuations in a general DQ or in specific DQs denote intrinsic and extraneous factors which require interpretation. In clinical hands, the DQ is an analytic tool, a diagnostic indicator of both neuromotor and intellectual functions. Fluctuations in DQ over a range of 10–15 points may be benign, due in part to the imperfection of the measuring device, in part to the normal variability of behavior. In a word, the DQ must be taken with the proverbial grain of salt. But it is infinitely more useful in the problems of diagnosis than salt alone. It takes the estimate of developmental status out of the realm of subjective impressionism.

The developmental quotient has an additional merit. It reminds the examiner that, contrary to popular view, the younger the child, the more serious the prognostic significance of every degree of true retardation. Other things being equal, retardation, like a shadow, lengthens with the lapse of time. This makes the determination of even short shadows significant for the developmental diagnosis of infants. A month counts heavily in the calendar of development in infancy. Although 1 or 2 weeks may give rise to a spuriously large arithmetic error at 3 months, retardation of only 1 month at that chronologic age may well signify mental deficiency. Two months is to 3 months as 2 years is to 3 years, and as 6 is to 9 years. In terms of DQ, 1 month of retardation in infancy may be the equivalent of a whole year and then of 3 years in later childhood.

A final warning must be emphasized: Each different area of behavior makes its own unique contribution to the judgment of neuropsychologic function. For adequate diagnosis and prognosis, these distinctions must be appreciated and maintained. Cavalier combinations, reassignments of items and relabeling of areas of behavior in the mistaken idea that such changes clarify or simplify conceptualization can lead only to grief.[3,11,23,28,33] Such changes distort the entire approach to differential diagnosis; in the difficult diagnostic problems, in those patients with selective handicaps, they may result in disaster. The single formula concept is inadmissible in the diagnosis of infant behavior; it cannot do justice to the complexity and variability of infant development. Any adaptation of our methods which, for psychometric convenience, would affix IQs to infants is undesirable, and is inadequate for the scientific study of growth processes.

§6. RELIABILITY OF INFANT EVALUATIONS

Before proceeding to the question of the validity and predictiveness of the infant examination, some comments on its reliability are required. One classical method of evaluating reliability, that of split halves, must be dismissed immediately. There was never an intent to develop an equal number of items at every age, each of which was assigned a numerical score. That some aspects of behavior are more important than others, and that any individual item can be assessed only in the context of the total behavior picture, is implicit in the conceptualization. Neither can reliability be studied by reexamining the infant a week later to compare his response on individual items. Change is expected with time, and growth is a gradual process; it does not occur in 4-week leaps comparable to the age intervals used in construction of the developmental schedules. Even in successive examinations on the same day, variation on individual items might be expected. How the individual behavior patterns contribute to the overall maturity level is the important factor.

The degree to which it is possible to transmit the perceptions of one clinician to another can be measured by another classical method—the correlation between the independent findings of one or more observers and the examiner on a single examination. Approximately 100 clinical examinations were performed by 18 different pediatric residents who had had 5 or 6 weeks of exposure to the methods of developmental diagnosis; the correlation between the general DQs they assigned and those of their instructor was 0.98.[45] The same process was carried out by four different qualified pediatricians near the start of their training periods. The correlations ranged from 0.98 to 0.995 when abnormal patients were included in the samples and were 0.96 in different series containing only normal infants; the numbers of patients in any sample varied from 12 to 44.[43] A more stringent test takes into account changes in the behavior of the infants themselves. Two independent examinations of the same infant were done; one usually followed immediately upon the other, but occasionally 2 or 3 days elapsed. The correlation between two examiners for these DQs was 0.82 for 65 patients.[40]

The first clinical impression of the infants stated by the residents prior to recording their observations may have been in considerable error, but close agreement for DQ was obtained by systematization, a knowledge of the precise meaning of the behavior patterns itemized, and constant referral to the developmental schedules. Even the specialist must be systematic if precision is to be achieved. However, interpretation of observations for diagnosis and estimation of prognosis requires more training and experience than for the assignment of a DQ, and there were greater disparities in residents' judgments in these areas. For the four experienced pediatricians, correlations for neurologic diagnosis and intellectual potential ranged from 0.83 to 0.995, depending on the nature of the sample and their own particular skill.[40,43] From these results it can be stated that the methods of developmental diagnosis are precise enough to be transmitted.

§7. VALIDITY OF INFANT ASSESSMENT

The predictive value of infant examinations for later development hinges on what the purpose of the evaluation is considered to be. A basic assumption must be reiterated. Behavior is rooted in the central nervous system. If a healthy cerebral cortex is demonstrated in infancy by a normal tempo, quality and integration of behavioral development, cortical integrity will continue to be normal provided there are no intercurrent noxious events. Performance can be depressed by biologic factors leading to organic disease of the brain or by social and psychologic factors resulting from adverse environmental circumstances. On the other hand, acceleration in developmental rate can only result from learning in an enriched and stimulating sociocultural milieu.

Clear delineation of what is expected from clinical diagnoses in infancy is essential. First is the identification of the subnormal infant with organic disease of the brain which precludes normal development, even under optimal circumstances. Next is the differentiation of primarily neuromotor and sensory from intellectual handicaps. In addition, there is the ascertainment of diseases and environmental factors which may depress developmental rates, particularly those factors amenable to treatment. On the basis of his infant performance, the individual without organic disease of the central nervous system, who later will be culturally retarded, cannot be detected. Neither is it clinically important, nor generally possible, to identify the infant who later will be superior because of exposure to increased opportunities for learning, except by using nonbehavioral indices such as parental status. In the *undamaged infant,* the parents' sociocultural level is a better index of later performance on a standard intelligence test than is the infant DQ.

Clinicians would be satisfied with the following statement: This infant has no central nervous system impairment, and his intellectual potential is within the normal range; depending on what his life experiences are between now and school age, at that time he will have a Stanford–Binet IQ that is average or above, unless qualitative changes in the central nervous system are caused by noxious agents, or gross changes in milieu alter major variables of function (Chapter 8).

Predictions are much more precise than this clinically acceptable statement. Longitudinal data from several studies of infants define the contributions made by infant intellectual potential and neuromotor status to later function, and identify several factors that modify the course of development and the direction in which they do so. The literature on the subject emphasizes numerical correlations; such correlations are not the most important aspects of development to examine. In children without organic impairment, school age tests of intelligence have limited usefulness as indices of the validity of infant developmental examination methods. Errors of clinical application will be avoided if we remember that the DQ and IQ refer only to the end products of development. In themselves, they do not take account of the etiologies of defects and deviations, the medical history of the child, the presence of specific disabilities and differences in environmental and experiential factors.

When the developmental evaluation is used as a clinical neurologic tool, the numerical correlations found between infant and later evaluations must be viewed against certain background information. Correlations from our infant evaluations are as high as those obtained when standard intelligence tests are administered at similar widely spaced intervals but at two older ages; however, they still do not indicate the closest possible relationship between infant and later behavior, i.e., a perfect correlation, or r value of 1.0. In a dynamically developing complex organism, it is not surprising that the values fall short of the ideal goal. We know that organic, psychologic and social factors may alter behavioral development. The correlations also must be contrasted to those reported previously by psychologists, which range from small positive values to negative values as low as −0.34.[56]

In a variety of groups composed of infants with a normal intellectual potential, the correlations we found between infant and later examinations are all about 0.50. These groups are as diverse as a population of black infants reexamined at 7 years of age, a group of noninstitutionalized infants recommended for adoption placement and seen at 5 years, 300 infants reevaluated at 3 years of age, and 200 followed up in the early school period at about 7 years of age.[42] When a sample is composed only of infants with neuromotor and intellectual defects, or when those with mental deficiency are included in the sample, as in the last two groups mentioned above, the correlations between early and later examinations rise to 0.70. When the correlations are weighted for parental socioeconomic status and seizures after the infant examination, they rise to 0.75 for infants with DQs above 80, and to 0.85 for the total group.[46] Some psychologists have reported that 60% of infants change more than 20 points in DQ on subsequent examinations.[4] In contrast, 75% of the 300 seen at 3 years and 60% of the 200 reexamined at school age had changed their quotients less than 15 points between the two examinations. Other physicians working in the United Kingdom have obtained results similar to ours.[19,34]

When such results are obtained, the burden of proof that infant evaluations are invalid rests on those who do not find such correlations. The most logical conclusions to draw from their failure are either that they are using inadequate examinations or that they are interpreting those which they are using mechanically and incorrectly. It would seem unwarranted to translate the inadequacy or misinterpretation of an evaluative tool into vagaries in the process of development, or to state that infant and later examinations measure completely disparate aspects of behavior.

The wide variation in acceptance and comprehension of the validity of the developmental method and quotient, too complex and lengthy to discuss here, is illustrated by two contradictory statements: "The findings of these early studies of mental growth of infants have been repeated sufficiently often so that it is now well established that test scores earned in the first year or two have relatively little predictive validity (in contrast to tests at school age or later), although they may have high validity as measures of the children's cognitive ability at the time." The same investigator made a statement regarding "results which strongly suggest that developmental psychologists need to rethink their previous conclusion that infant developmental test scores are unrelated to later measures of intelligence."[55a]

Some of the interrelationships between infant adaptive DQ, other aspects of infant central nervous system integrity, and some subsequent experiential factors were demonstrated during a study in Columbus in the followup evaluations of 199 infants at early school age, who were given a 4–5 hour test battery. Thirty-three of the infants had been diagnosed clinically as functioning at a level of mental deficiency, and all had DQs of 75 or less. At followup only eight had IQs between 76 and 85; for six of the eight, improvement had been predicted because of modifying factors at the infant examination—seizures, marked growth failure, normal language development or good quality of the behavior. With the objective of detecting what constellation of infant characteristics were most likely to aid in the prediction of the future course, the remaining 166 infants were divided into impaired (63) and unimpaired (103) groups. Impaired infants were defined as those having a DQ of 96 or more associated with *both* abnormal neuromotor signs and seizures, or a DQ between 76 and 95; almost all of the latter also had one or both of the associated abnormal findings. Unimpaired infants had DQs of 96 or more with either abnormal neuromotor status *or* prior seizures but not both; 75% had

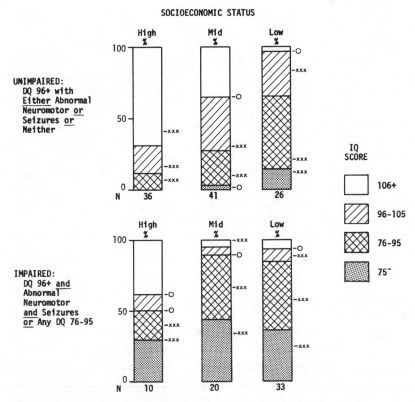

SOCIOECONOMIC STATUS

UNIMPAIRED:
DQ 96+ with
Either Abnormal
Neuromotor or
Seizures or
Neither

IMPAIRED:
DQ 96+ and
Abnormal
Neuromotor
and Seizures
or Any DQ 76-95

IQ
SCORE

106+
96-105
76-95
75⁻

DQ = Infant Adaptive Developmental Quotient
Neuromotor = Infant Neuromotor Status
Seizures = Before or During the Infant Examination
   -xxx = % of IQ Group with Seizures After the Infant Examination

Fig. 5-2. Percent of children with indicated school-age IQ according to infant central nervous system integrity and socioeconomic status. Children mentally defective in infancy are excluded. Unimpaired: DQ 96+ with either abnormal neuromotor or seizures or neither. Impaired: DQ 96+ and abnormal neuromotor and seizures or any DQ 76-95. DQ=infant adaptive developmental quotient; neuromotor=infant neuromotor status; seizures=before or during the infant examination. -xxx = % of IQ group with seizures after the infant examination.

neither. Figure 5-2 shows the relationships between infant DQ and school age IQ, taking into account socioeconomic status and subsequent seizures. In broad terms, it indicates that the outlook for the unimpaired infant in all socioeconomic groups is significantly better. If the infant is in the lowest socioeconomic group, his IQ is lower than his infant DQ, even if he was unimpaired and had no subsequent seizures. On the other hand, IQs of those in the high socioeconomic group rise, some in spite of impairment in infancy or subsequent seizures.

Thirty of the 166 infants had IQs of 75 or less at school age; 25 of these were in the impaired group in infancy. For only one of the 30, the fall in IQ could not be explained by subsequent seizures and/or low socioeconomic status, or the presence of another condition such as trisomy 21 or congenital hypothyroidism. In contrast, 60% of the 48 with IQs of 106 or more were from the high socioeconomic group; only three were from the low socioeconomic group. On the basis of their infant behavior alone, an IQ of 106 or more would not have been expected for five children. No child with an infant DQ of 116 or more fell to 75 or less, and 60% had IQs of 106 or more. In contrast, 7% of infants with DQs between 96 and 115 but 45% of those with DQs between 76 and 95 had a school-age IQ of 75 or less.

These predictions were based on only two factors: on DQs derived from the clinical estimate of general (adaptive) maturity and on the clinical diagnosis of neuromotor status in infancy; they took into account only two of the subsequent events, seizures and socioeconomic status. These four factors appear to be the major ones determining later school functioning. The IQ at school age correlates highly with all other tests in the battery and has definite value as a predictor of school performance. Chapter 11 discusses aspects of ability other than IQ test scores in more detail.

§8. OTHER DIAGNOSTIC PROCEDURES

The objective of differential developmental diagnosis is the prevention, cure or amelioration of the adverse consequences of developmental deviations. The history and basic methods of developmental and neurologic assessment have been discussed in detail in preceding chapters. Certain other information must be obtained for all patients, but diagnostic procedures should not be routine, done to satisfy the academic curiosity of the clinician or performed to impress the parents by extensive but nonproductive investigations. Special procedures which may carry a risk should be employed only when there are specific indications.

Often the physical examination will reveal features pointing to associated conditions that sometimes have prognostic importance, but it may be more valuable for purposes of genetic counseling. Special attention should be directed to the skin and eyes for clues to hereditary disorders or treatable conditions. Physical growth charts, particularly when longitudinal data are available, more often have general medical import, but direct attention to the need for studies of endocrine function, particularly of the thyroid and pituitary glands. A decreasing rate of growth in height often is the only clue to hypothalamic dysfunction from a third ventricle tumor; in their early stages such tumors produce virtually no symptoms except for occasional visual abnormalities, which often cannot be detected in younger children. A large or an increasing head size might denote a need for neurosurgical investigation. Transillumination of the head is a useful adjunct in infants less than a year of age, when the skull still is relatively thin.

Laboratory investigations to detect potentially treatable conditions should include urine analysis for reducing substances, phenylpyruvic acid and amino acids.

Blood studies for sugars and amino acids supplement the urine examinations and should include lead levels when indicated. In specific circumstances enzymes, antibodies, immunoglobulins, inclusion bodies and metachromasia should be investigated. Chromosome analysis is a helpful but less routine procedure. Lumbar puncture, muscle biopsy and even brain biopsy have restricted indications.

The frequency with which routine skull X-rays will produce useful information is low but definite. The presence of calcifications or anomalies have diagnostic but not necessarily prognostic importance, except in special circumstances. If premature closure of the sutures is complete, surgical intervention must be carried out in the first 2 or 3 months to prevent interference with brain growth and to achieve cosmetic benefit. If synostosis is not complete, brain function is not modified by operative procedures which improve skull configuration.

The electroencephalogram has limited usefulness as a routine procedure. It correlates positively with most paroxysmal disorders and is specific for a diagnosis of petit mal and hypsarhythmia. A single or several normal tracings do not exclude a diagnosis of convulsive seizures when there is a positive clinical history; neither is an EEG abnormality without a history an indication for treatment. The EEG provides evidence of abnormal neuronal discharges but no information about other functions of the brain. It is not likely to detect hemispheric space-occupying lesions in the absence of other clinical findings pointing to their presence. However, nonspecific slowing may suggest further study for the presence of deep midline lesions associated with increased intracranial pressure, even without other signs. The electromyogram and nerve conduction studies have their own specific indications in the differentiation of neurogenic from myogenic disease.

Air contrast studies and angiography are not without risk of morbidity and even mortality. They should be reserved for the detection of conditions where surgical intervention is a possibility. Air contrast studies should not be performed to make a diagnosis of "cortical atrophy"; there is no correlation between the thickness of the cerebral cortex, or the ventricular size, and the intellectual potential of the infant. On the other hand, an echoencephalogram is another noninvasive procedure like the EEG or brain scan which can be done without inconvenience, and it often may detect situations in which more definitive procedures would be productive.

§9. SUMMARY

In the final analysis, the history and behavior of the child are the most sensitive indices of the function of his central nervous system. The hazards of development are so numerous one may wonder that normality is ever achieved. It is possible that we all may have suffered some degree of insult. Fortunately, there is a tendency toward the normal inherent in all developmental processes, and there is an unexplained process called compensation, perhaps through the assumption of function by remaining healthy brain tissue. Moreover, these factors may be fostered by the child's environment or by planned rehabilitative care. Nevertheless, in almost all instances when damage has occurred, some dysfunction can be found by sensitive measures throughout later life.

The remainder of Part II is directed toward differential diagnosis by considering various organic and environmental factors which may depress or deflect the course of development. In certain instances, trends of development can be elevated by improved environmental conditions; in other selected instances, recourse may be had to therapeutic tests, endocrine therapy, anticonvulsants, stimulating or inhibiting drugs and other rehabilitative programs. The DQ then becomes a valuable aid in determining the efficacy of therapeutic measures.

The more complicated problems of differential diagnosis cannot always be solved on the basis of a single examination. Several examinations at spaced intervals may be necessary to offer a critical judgment of the rate and course of development. Differential diagnosis then becomes a program of orderly investigation combined with supervision. It entails identification, exclusion and progressive evaluation.

6

Mental Subnormality

An understanding of mental subnormality is fundamental to differential clinical diagnosis of behavioral disorder.[44] In all cases of defective and deviant development, the first inquiry is whether the consequent retardations and deformations of behavior are deep-seated or transient, generalized or delimited, ameliorable or irreducible. Mental deficiency must be recognized and ruled out.

Mental subnormality includes a protean group of conditions as varied in their clinical manifestations as other forms of neuropsychiatric disorder. Classic types occur, but individual variation is the rule. Many cases escape recognition in infancy because the undiscriminating eye fails to make critical distinctions between different degrees of immaturity. On the other hand, partial disabilities often simulate mental deficiency; it then becomes important to detect the normal potentials which are masked by misleading visible defects.

Mental subnormality is defined as subnormal general intellectual functioning which originates during the developmental period and is associated with impairment of either learning and social adjustment, or maturation, or both. It is extremely important to recognize that subnormal intelligence is composed of two distinct categories, which may overlap. In one instance, the subnormality is a result of some pathologic condition of the brain which precludes normal development, and properly is referred to as *mental deficiency. Mental retardation* is a term which should be reserved for individuals who function below their potential level of ability; it is usually the result of suboptimum environmental situations, and not due to organic central nervous system disease. However, many workers still feel that individuals so affected represent the lower end of the normal curve on a hereditary rather than an environmental basis (Chapter 8). Today the term mental retardation has replaced all previously applied terms such as amentia, oligophrenia, feeble-mindedness, moronity, imbecility and idiocy; it is well that this is so. However, in the ensuing chapters we propose to maintain a distinction between the terms *deficiency* and *retardation*.

In mental deficiency the physician's responsibility is a direct one of diagnosis and some aspects of patient care; in mental retardation it is frequently indirect, as a consultant to schools and child-caring agencies when he is not involved with direct medical care. He also acts as a concerned citizen. In general, the physician will be called upon for help most frequently during the infant or early preschool period and will be dealing almost entirely with mental deficiency; it is his main responsibility to make a diagnosis, as it is in other pathologic states. Nevertheless, he should be cognizant of the overwhelming numerical importance of the disadvantaged retarded group in the totality of subnormality. Moreover, he must recognize that a child with organic pathology also may function below his capacity because of adverse environmental conditions.

In discussion, some intermingling of the various facets of impaired central nervous system function is inevitable; however, we will attempt to keep these aspects distinct by devoting separate chapters to each of the major neuropsychiatric disorders. The focus in Chapters 7 and 8 on mental subnormality will be on differential diagnosis, particularly in infancy. We will not attempt exhaustive descriptions of the numerous clinical syndromes which may be associated with intellectual impairment. The clinician should become familiar with the constellations of physical abnormalities outside the central nervous system which comprise specific entities; useful references are listed in Appendix E. Two specific syndromes will be discussed, primarily to indicate where our experience has led us to conclusions different from those commonly reported.

§1. BIOLOGIC CRITERIA OF MENTAL DEFICIENCY

Mental deficiency *is evidence* of organic disease of the brain, and impairs that aspect of function most uniquely human. It is manifested by an impairment of developmental potentials. As a consequence, the rate of maturation is retarded, and the ultimate maturity level of behavior is lowered.

Infants vary with respect to their developmental capacities, which depend first of all upon biologic integrity. More precisely, human RNA and DNA are so programmed that unless something intervenes, the template will produce the expected result in development. The normal individual has an inborn power to adjust to or change his environment and to profit by experience. He is able to meet the normal expectations of development as embryo, fetus, infant, child and adolescent—he is able to mature. As an adult, he also meets the normal range of requirements of family and community life. He manages himself and his affairs with some efficiency. The normal individual "gets along," because he has the requisite biologic equipment and experience, prenatally and postnatally.

If the individual's original equipment is impaired, if it becomes damaged *in utero,* if it is blemished during birth or if it is impared by accident or disease after birth, he cannot meet adequately the demands of his environment, even in infancy. His development may be completely arrested or seriously diminished, to such a degree that as an adult he will continue to require extraordinary assistance and support. This lack of potential usually displays itself early, and nowhere more strikingly than in the field of behavior.

A curious anomaly exists in regard to early development in pediatric texts and in articles on the detection of mental deficiency. Such materials rightly emphasize the importance of a developmental history, and state that a child of school age who has mental deficiency did not pass his developmental milestones at a normal age. These statements merely indicate that a child usually does not become defective suddenly, but has been so all along. If a history of early delay in behavioral maturation is accepted later in childhood as evidence of mental deficiency, surely attention should be paid to the *observation* of abnormal behavior in the first year of life. The purpose of developmental evaluation is to systematize and facilitate the detection and interpretation of maturational delay *as it is occurring.* Mild as well as gross deviations can be recognized in infancy.

§2. TRENDS OF DEVELOPMENT

Table 6-1 charts the broad trends of normal and defective development. It is quantitative only, and does not consider those qualitative changes which so frequently accompany deviant development. The table covers the first 3 years of life, the period in which timely diagnosis of developmental defects and deviations still is most neglected. Four major clinical types are illustrated: normal, mild, moderate to severe, and profound mental deficiency.

The *normal* infant of 28 weeks has normal behavioral equipment and performance. At 3 years he remains normal; he has progressed enormously; his development as measured by DQ still approximates 100. The term "normal" is used as synonymous with "healthy."

The *mildly defective* infant at 28 weeks is functioning at about a 16-week level; this represents an absolute retardation of only 12 or 14 weeks, but denotes a reduced developmental rate of 50–60%. At 3 years this same child usually will be functioning between an 18- and a 21-month level, with a DQ of 50–60.

When the defect is *moderate to severe,* the infant of 28 weeks is functioning at a lower level, represented by the maturity zone of 8–12 weeks, with a DQ or developmental rate of 30–40%. Deceleration is a frequent phenomenon, and a DQ of 30 at 28 weeks may signify *either* moderate *or* severe deficiency for the age of 3 years. Consequently, at 3 years he may prove to be functioning at about the 1-year level, with the same DQ, or he may function near the 16-week level. Even the mildly defective infant may decelerate and be more severely impaired when he attains the age of 3 years. Lastly, the *profoundly defective* infant functions at a neonatal level at the age of 28 weeks, and makes scarcely any advance over 3 years of time.

All forms of mental deficiency may be interpreted in terms of greater or lesser degrees of general behavioral impairment. Certain adverse conditions produce selective impairments which result in restricted disabilities and uneven trends of development. Consideration of such conditions, both inborn and acquired, their influence on the subsequent developmental course and the ways in which they

Table 6-1. COMPARATIVE DEVELOPMENT AT 28 WEEKS AND 3 YEARS OF AGE: NORMAL, MILD, MODERATE TO SEVERE AND PROFOUND MENTAL DEFICIENCY

28 Weeks	Maturity Level	3 Years	Maturity Level
ADAPTIVE BEHAVIOR		**ADAPTIVE BEHAVIOR**	
Normal: reaches, grasps, transfers...........	28 wk	*Normal:* builds 3-cube bridge.............	3 years
Mild: regards object in hand.............	16 wk	*Mild:* builds tower of 3-5 cubes.........	18-21 mo
Moderate to Severe: disregards or only glances at object in hand.............	8-12 wk	*Moderate to Severe:* dangles ring by string......	52-65 wk
Profound: stares vacantly; may hold object reflexly without regard.............	0-4 wk	*Profound:* grasps object near hand or on contact; or stares vacantly; or drops object in hand...	4-16 wk
GROSS MOTOR BEHAVIOR		**GROSS MOTOR BEHAVIOR**	
Normal: sits leaning on hands for support, head erect.............	28 wk	*Normal:* climbs stairs with alternating steps....	3 years
Mild: sits supported, head steady but set forward.............	16 wk	*Mild:* walks well.............	18-20 mo
Moderate to Severe: sits supported, head unsteady.............	8-12 wk	*Moderate to Severe:* stands or toddles.............	52-65 wk
Profound: head droops.............	0-4 wk	*Profound:* sits supported, head steady or wobbly; or lifts head in prone.............	4-16 wk
LANGUAGE BEHAVIOR		**LANGUAGE BEHAVIOR**	
Normal: vocalizes m-m-m.............	28 wk	*Normal:* speaks in sentences, using plurals........	3 years
Mild: laughs aloud.............	16 wk	*Mild:* names 1-2 pictures.............	18-21 mo
Moderate to Severe: smiles; coos.............	8-12 wk	*Moderate to Severe:* says 2-6 words.............	52-65 wk
Profound: vague throaty sounds.............	0-4 wk	*Profound:* laughs; or crying and vague ejaculation.............	4-16 wk
PERSONAL-SOCIAL BEHAVIOR		**PERSONAL-SOCIAL BEHAVIOR**	
Normal: takes feet to mouth.............	28 wk	*Normal:* feeds self, little spilling.............	3 years
Mild: anticipates feeding.............	16 wk	*Mild:* carries and hugs doll.............	18-21 mo
Moderate to Severe: watches moving person......	8 wk	*Moderate to Severe:* gives toy on request.......	52-65 wk
Profound: stares blankly at persons.............	0-4 wk	*Profound:* anticipates feeding; smiles on social approach; or stares blankly at persons.......	4-16 wk

modify prediction are discussed in subsequent chapters. However, familiarity with the characteristics of mental deficiency is one of the first essentials in diagnostic orientation.

§3. SOCIAL CRITERIA OF MENTAL DEFICIENCY

From the standpoint of the law, a mentally deficient person is one who will *always* require special care and help for his own, his family's and others' social welfare. Developmental diagnosis cannot ignore these social and medicolegal criteria. Every diagnosis of mental deficiency in a child carries the prognostic implication that when he becomes an adult he will have some limitation in managing himself and his affairs with ordinary prudence. He will always show some lack of intelligence and independence.

Impairment in social functioning in itself is not synonymous with mental subnormality, but it is generally a concomitant; the manifestations depend on the age of the individual and the degree of impairment. The terms educable, trainable and custodial have been applied in the past, and correspond roughly to the three degrees of deficiency discussed; they are mentioned here only to be disparaged.

In broad terms, since the rate of development will be relatively consistent, the *profoundly defective* infant at maturity will have behavioral capacities less than those of the average 3-year-old, in some cases less than those of an infant. Presumably he will be incapable of guarding against ordinary physical dangers, will be totally incapable of self-maintenance and will require complete care and supervision. The *moderately to severely defective* infant will have the behavioral capacities of a 3- to 7-year child. He is conceived of as capable of guarding against simple physical danger in a controlled environment, but as unable to learn functional academic skills and in need of complete supervision in order to contribute partially to self-support. The behavioral capacities of the *mildly defective* child range from the 7- to 12-year level at maturity. With special education, his academic achievement will range from fourth to seventh grade. With proper training and under mild conditions of social and economic stress, he may be capable of self-maintenance in unskilled or semiskilled occupations; he will require assistance under more serious socioeconomic stress.

Some of the most important functions of a social worker involved in the care of the mentally subnormal are to find appropriate jobs and living arrangements, to obtain adequate financial support and to locate leisure time activities in which the handicapped individuals can participate.

Rigid predictions of what these children will be able to accomplish during their life span have been based on many misconceptions: underestimating the abilities of 3-, 7- or 12-year-olds; failure to distinguish between pathologic conditions of the brain and environmental retardation; assumptions that routine and repetitive rather than challenging and difficult tasks are the proper educational approach; and tendencies to herd the mentally subnormal out of sight in large stultifying institutions. Recent new approaches with behavior modification techniques have shown that we grossly underestimate what can be accomplished with simple conditioning; previously helpless and totally disorganized adults have been helped to live in acceptable social relationships, take care of all their own physical needs and engage in simple productive work under supervision. Such techniques can be employed with young children with equally promising results; marked modification of their later functioning might be expected. The increasing provision of community facilities for education and training and the wider use of hostels and sheltered workshops permit the greater stimulation of family living. We will be able to raise our sights considerably in the future.

It is impossible to establish sharp distinctions between the various categories of mental deficiency. One category merges into another, and theoretically, the milder grades of mental deficiency shade into the dull normal zone. However, it is necessary to make a clear-cut distinction between mental deficiency and normality. Mere lowering of measured intelligence does not constitute mental deficiency if the individual shows no marked social incapacity. Integrative and organizational capacities also must be taken into account; often they are of more importance than intellectual ability. The diagnosis of mental deficiency should be reserved for those individuals who always will need external support and supervision because of their inadequate behavioral capacity.

7

Mental Subnormality: Mental Deficiency due to Brain Disease

Mental deficiency is not a single disease entity. It represents subnormal intellectual ability due to a pathologic condition of the brain, and results from a variety of disease processes which may arise at any time during the developmental period. It may be accompanied by any of the other manifestations of chronic organic brain disease, or may be the only expression. Except in the case of postnatal insults or degenerative processes, mental deficiency shows itself in the infant's behavior from the very beginning of postnatal life. Behavior is the most sensitive index of the integrity of the central nervous system. Evaluation of intellectual potential must be based on evaluation of adaptive behavior, the forerunner of later cognitive behavior. Reflexes and motor activity have important implications for neuromotor integrity, but they are not the basis for judging intellectual adequacy. These principles underlie the following discussion of mental deficiency.

§1. MILD MENTAL DEFICIENCY

Brain pathology most often results in mild rather than gross impairment of intelligence. Lacking pronounced physical abnormalities, the mildly defective child may present a superficially healthy developmental picture. Even as an adult he may pass for normal, in the absence of an adequate diagnosis or demands for adult performance. In infancy the parents often report."He is no trouble at all; he is a good baby." Perhaps too good; there may be some disquietude because of the lack of vigor in his behavior, but it is optimistically assumed that as he grows older he will be different. The optimism is not warranted. A series of examinations will fail to show any trend toward improvement. Even mild mental deficiency can be detected with considerable confidence by the fourth month of life, using the techniques of developmental diagnosis.

The Case of P.B.

Typical is the case of P.B., whom we examined at 8, 32 and 60 weeks, 54 months, and $8\frac{1}{2}$ years. An outline of the biography of his development serves as a frame of reference for an understanding of the milder grades of mental deficiency.

Age: 8 Weeks

The first examination was made when P.B. was 8 weeks old. He was the third child of parents in their late twenties who had two normal children. The mother had elevated blood pressure and slight edema of the hands and face in the last 2 months of pregnancy. The infant was born at term with a birth weight of 7 lbs, 14 oz, and was delivered by emergency cesarean section because of complete separation of the placenta, which necessitated transfusion of 1000 cc of blood. P.B. required incubator care for 8 days because of intermittent cyanosis and had some sucking difficulty in his first few weeks of life.

In the 8-week examination, *adaptive behavior* fell below expectation. P.B.'s facial expression showed no attentional responses, and no visual fixation could be elicited. He did not regard the dangling ring in his field of vision, but there were slight eye movements as the rattle was shaken and moved. There was no response to the bell; whether this was due to deafness was not yet clear. *Motor symptoms* were not immediately reassuring. The infant's supine posture was a normal t-n-r attitude, but his head lagged completely on tentative elevation, sagged when he was held in the sitting position, and drooped in ventral suspension. In the prone position he cleared the bed, lifting his head momentarily to Zone I. *Language behavior* was very meager; no throaty sounds were heard. His facial expression was quite bland and impassive. In the *personal–social* field he showed no regard for the examiner's face on social approach. He stared indefinitely at surroundings. By the mother's report he was said to follow a moving person (this response ruled out blindness) and to stare at a window. The mother did not report either social smiling or facial brightening.

The average 8-week infant gives delayed regard to a dangling ring in the midline, follows the ring past the midline and shows some facial animation on hearing a bell. In early infancy the head is a very important area for observation, because development moves in a cephalocaudad direction. In an 8-week baby we wish to see evidence of organizing head control. The normal infant holds his head bobbingly erect. Lowered to prone, he erects his head while in ventral suspension; having been placed prone, he turns it to midposition and lifts it to Zone II at 45° recurrently. In addition, he regards the examiner's face, shows an alert expression from time to time, and smiles socially. He is also capable of making vowel sounds like "ah" and "eh."

On all these counts, it was clear that P.B. was retarded, not only in the motor field but in all fields of behavior. The motor retardation evidenced in defective head control had ominous import. He was chronologically 8 weeks old; his maturity level was in the neighborhood of 4 weeks. This represents only four weeks of retardation—a negligible amount, unless it signifies a permanent lag. At 8 weeks, a lag of 4 weeks creates a ratio of 4 to 8, a DQ of approximately 50. A provisional diagnosis of mental deficiency was made. His developmental status was summed up as follows:

Maturity Level

Approximate DQ   Weeks
    50 .... 4 or less .... General Developmental Level
    50 .... 4 or less .... Gross Motor Behavior
    50 .... 4 or less .... Fine Motor Behavior
    50 .... 4 or less .... Adaptive Behavior
    50 .... 4 or less .... Language Behavior
    50 .... 4–5 .... Personal–Social Behavior

Diagnostic Summary

Intellectual: Probable Mental Deficiency
Neuromotor: Motor Retardation without Abnormal Signs for Level of Function
Seizures: None
Special Sensory: Hearing Defect?
Qualitative: None
Specific Diseases or Syndromes: None

Age: 32 Weeks

P.B. was 32 weeks of age on the second examination. We were pleased to note on first glance that the facial expression was somewhat more alert and the regard more direct. Since the mother reported that he was able to sit up in a propped position for over an hour, we were warranted in beginning the examination by placing the child in the examining chair. This represented a postural gain, but its significance would not become apparent until we had made a careful survey of the behavior patterns in the five major fields.

Adaptive behavior tended to gravitate toward the 16- to 20-week level. The baby looked down at his hands and grasped one of the massed cubes on contact. In supine he gave immediate regard to the ring and grasped it when it was near his hand. He also regarded the rattle in hand, and he brought the free hand up to it. These were considerable gains when compared with the profound ineffectuality of his behavior at the age of 8 weeks.

Motor gains were registered in increased head control. The baby no longer showed marked head lag, and in the supine position kept the head predominantly in the midposition. This indicated a 16- to 20-week level of maturity in head control.

His head was steady but set forward, and he propped on extended forearms in prone. The arms and hands likewise showed an advance in patterned behavior. In supine the hands now engaged at the midline. Prehensory grasp was sufficiently advanced to result in retention of the dangling ring. The cube also was held precariously—another indication that the prehensory patterns were undergoing development and now approximated a 20-week level of maturity. The general postural behaviors, supine and prone, were near the 18-week level. Nevertheless, there was mild hypotonicity of all extremities, with all deep tendon reflexes increased, and sustained ankle clonus was present on one side.

P.B. laughed aloud, gurgled and cooed in his vocal play. He smiled spontaneously in social situations; he vocalized as a social response. He turned to the sound of a bell, a 24-week behavior pattern. With this single exception, his *language* and *social behavior* approximated a 16-week level.

His behavior gains had been notable and consistent. Evidence of hearing was now definitely established. However, there had been no acceleration of developmental rate, his attention was poorly sustained, and there were some neuromotor abnormalities. The DQs in the various fields of behavior were again in the neighborhood of 50. He had advanced from a 4- to an 18-week level of maturity, but the relative retardation remained constant. The diagnosis of mental deficiency made provisionally at the age of 8 weeks was confirmed. His mother's toxemia with abruptio placentae was the most likely etiology—a prenatally determined impairment.

Maturity Level

Developmental Quotient	Weeks	
56	18	General Developmental Level
56	18	Gross Motor Behavior
53	17	Fine Motor Behavior
56	18	Adaptive Behavior
50	16	Language Behavior
50	16	Personal–Social Behavior

Diagnostic Summary

Intellectual: Mental Deficiency, Mild
Neuromotor: Motor Retardation with Abnormal Signs of Minor Degree
Seizures: None
Special Sensory: None
Qualitative: Mild Disorganization
Specific Diseases or Syndromes: None

Age: 60 Weeks

The third examination of P.B. fell just past his first birthday at 60 weeks. How had he used this first year of chronologic time when growth normally proceeds at its maximum pace? Had he made up the lag of 3—4 weeks which was noted when he was 8 weeks old?

The lag had lengthened. His attention was difficult to elicit, his interest fleeting and variable. A normal child of 14 months dominates the examination with eager, restless attention, seizing each new test object avidly. P.B. in *adaptive behavior* had coordinated looking, approach and grasp into a single movement, grasped the second cube when presented, freed himself from the limitations of postural symmetry, engaged in vertical banging and shaking and even occasionally transferred from hand to hand, a universal propensity ·in normal infants at 28 weeks. We were obliged to consider his adaptive behavior as no more than 30 weeks in maturity.

He had an atypical combination of *gross motor* abilities which suggest that his postural and locomotor patterns were undergoing very slow and imperfect organization. He sat alone—a 40-week pattern—pivoted in the prone position and managed to support his weight briefly when his hands were held, but he was still unable to roll from supine to prone. Some hypotonia persisted, and his gross motor behavior approximated 32 weeks. Likewise there were problems in *fine motor* control. Well before 14 months he should have been plucking a pellet with precise finger prehension, but he merely raked at it with 28-week crudity. He had some difficulty retaining objects, and a fair proportion of the time he tended to keep his hands fisted with the thumbs adducted into the palms—the so-called cortical thumb.

Language behavior was similar in level. He vocalized "m-m-m-m" when crying and occasionally made single consonant sounds. He clearly localized sounds and turned to the radio in listening. *Personal–social behavior* was also between 28 and 32 weeks. The care and stimulation he had from his mother did not perceptibly raise his level. His play interests were limited; he played repetitively with familiar toys and was "afraid" of new toys. He put his feet in his mouth, biting and chewing them, but he still looked occasionally at his own hands, a pattern more appropriate to 12 weeks, and usually fully outgrown by 28 weeks. He often engaged in repetitive and stereotyped scratching of the tabletop, regardless of the presence of toys thereon.

P.B. cried at attempts to teach him patacake. Patacake games require 40 weeks of maturity; he could not learn because he scarcely had the motor, adaptive and personal–social equipment of a 32-week infant.

The diagnosis now was established firmly. At 14 months he had not mastered some of the elementary problems of earlier infancy. Uncritical optimism might have suggested that this child made a good showing in postural control (sitting alone); yet it would have been fatuous to think that he would make up his deficits in later childhood. He would in a sense outgrow some of them, but new deficits would come into evidence. He would not make up lost time.

Maturity Levels

Developmental
Quotient   Weeks

50 .... 30 .... General Developmental Level
53 .... 32 .... Gross Motor Behavior
47 .... 28 .... Fine Motor Behavior
50 .... 30 .... Adaptive Behavior
53 .... ..32 .... Language Behavior
50 .... 30 .... Personal–Social Behavior

Diagnostic Summary

Intellectual: Mental Deficiency, Mild
Neuromotor: Motor Retardation with Abnormal Signs of Minor Degree
Seizures: None
Special Sensory: None
Qualitative: Moderate Disorganization
Specific Diseases or Syndromes: None

Age: 4½ Years

An examination of P.B. at the age of $4\frac{1}{2}$ years, when the normal child is beginning to turn his face toward kindergarten, made our developmental story more complete. It took him 2 years to learn to walk, and still longer before he began to put blocks and words together and learned not to touch "mother's toys." If we forgot his chronologic age he made an encouraging impression; but for diagnostic purposes we had to be mindful of his $4\frac{1}{2}$ years. At $4\frac{1}{2}$ years P.B. was a cooperative, friendly boy, attractive and rosy-cheeked, with occasional flashes of alertness and attention. He walked alone and ran well, seated himself in a chair, kicked a ball and attempted to stand on one foot. He built a tower of seven cubes, and imitated the four-cube train but not the three-cube bridge. He scribbled vigorously, and imitated the vertical stroke and the circle. He placed two color forms correctly. He named ten pictures; his articulation was poor, but he used short sentences and knew parts of one or two songs. He did not feed or dress himself, but he asked for the toilet during the day.

His general maturity level was approximately $2\frac{1}{2}$ years. Development was defective but of relatively high grade. He had been well managed, had thus far presented no difficult problems at home, and was enrolled in a preschool community class for the retarded. In our treatment of the boy and our guidance of his parents, almost exclusive stress was placed on his truest and most fundamental age—his developmental age.

Maturity Levels

Developmental
Quotient   Months
57 .... 31 .... General Developmental Level
57 .... 31 .... Gross Motor Behavior
55 .... 30 .... Fine Motor Behavior
57 .... 31 .... Adaptive Behavior
59 .... 32 .... Language Behavior
57 .... 31 .... Personal–Social Behavior

Diagnostic Summary

Intellectual: Mental Deficiency, Mild
Neuromotor: Motor Retardation without Abnormal Signs for Level
Seizures: None
Special Sensory: None
Qualitative: None
Specific Diseases or Syndromes: None

Age: 8½ Years

P.B.'s last examination was at 8 years, 5 months. On a Stanford–Binet test his mental age was 4 years, 11 months, IQ 56, with a fairly even performance. He was able to participate in a variety of motor, language and perceptual–motor tests, but in all of these his performance was little more than that of a 5-year old. He could not perform on school achievement tests in reading, spelling and arithmetic. He was continuing on a regular basis in the community classes and was making a good adjustment.

P.B.: Past, Present and Future

The course of mental growth in P.B. was more or less typical of many cases of mild mental deficiency. We could see that the behavioral patterning, which is in fact mental growth, had been proceeding at a slowed rate throughout infancy, preschool and the early school period of childhood. Looking back, we could be certain that the retardation probably was present even during the late fetal period. This child was born with a developmental potential definitely below normal.

Looking forward, we could project a similar course of growth. This boy looked attractive, was obedient, and now and then alert, but this was no reason for believing that he would outgrow his present retardation. His nervous system would not develop any new growth potentials with the eruption of his second teeth, or with the onset of puberty. He would continue to develop at his present rate for a dozen years or more until he reached chronologic "maturity" as all adults do. To that extent he would improve; however, his mental abilities would still be at a defective level when he reached adulthood.

His parents had accepted the fact that at $8\frac{1}{2}$ he was not yet ready for formal academic education in the special classes in a public school system; in a few years he would be ready to acquire simple academic skills that he would need for participation in community life. He was relatively stable and organized and was not a management problem.

If adequate hostels or sheltered workshops are available, a child like P.B. will not require institutionalization and should be able to become at least partially self-supporting, provided that adequate assistance is available. His final position will depend not so much on his own capacities as on what society can offer.

As P.B.'s case shows, mental deficiency proves to be a medical, a social and an educational problem. All three aspects are interrelated. First, however, it is a medical problem; the doctor must make the early diagnosis and use his strategic position to give constructive oversight and guidance during the growing years. In this instance, the need of oversight began as early as the age of 8 weeks.

§2. BORDERLINE DEVELOPMENT

There are infants who, without being definitely defective, are nevertheless well below average with respect to developmental status and outlook. Emphasis has been placed on the importance of making a distinction between dullness and mental deficiency. For practical clinical reasons, the diagnosis of mental deficiency is reserved for the child who will need special help in adult years. Dullness is not a mild form of mental deficiency in this medicolegal sense; it is a form of normality, albeit of low degree and of poor quality.

The clinician must recognize this marginal group of cases in infancy which borders on mental deficiency. This is a highly diversified category, which should not, however, be made into a catch-all. Two types of cases may be distinguished: borderline dull and borderline defective.

Borderline dull denotes a mild general reduction of performance in adaptive behavior. The reactions are slow, limited and very mediocre without, however, being seriously inadequate. In quality the behavior is relatively normal. *Borderline defective* denotes a degree and form of impairment which approximates mild mental deficiency. The behavior may be relatively well organized and balanced, but more often it is erratic and unstable. In quality and caliber it is defective, but not sufficiently so to warrant a diagnosis of outright deficiency.

The foregoing distinctions must rest on clinical impressions rather than on precise objective criteria, on the quality and organization of the behavior rather than on the numerical value of a developmental quotient. They are useful as descriptive diagnoses. A borderline classification is far better than a poorly supported diagnosis of mental deficiency, but the per cent of expected maturity achieved cannot be ignored in the diagnosis.

A diagnosis of borderline function in infancy is always indicative of some degree of impaired central nervous system integration. Such infants will have some handicap in later life, and are at risk of deteriorating. The ultimate prognosis can be determined only by serial examinations, taking into account the environment and subsequent events. In favorable circumstances the child may be able to function in a regular school situation, although not as well as his schoolmates and siblings. Under adverse conditions he will not be able to keep up with a regular academic program and will require special educational facilities, although he will be capable of making an adult adjustment.

Case 1 made a poor showing on the developmental schedules, but was diagnosed as *borderline dull* rather than mentally defective. He was referred to the clinic at the age of *24 months* because he was slow in talking. He did not respond to simple questions; his sole vocalization was "uh" when the picture card was presented. He did not scribble imitatively, but simply turned the crayon end over end, and tapped it on the paper. He built a tower of four cubes, but not a train. He dumped the pellet from the bottle and piled the three blocks on the formboard. In sum, his adaptive performance was at 18 rather than 24 months, with a DQ of approximately 75.

This degree of retardation was serious enough to suggest mental deficiency, but there were mitigating factors. In spite of the slowness of the boy's reactions and his unprepossessing appearance, the general tenor of his responses was normal. His word comprehension was in advance of his speech. He adjusted fairly promptly to the rotation of the formboard. He was cooperative and well organized during the examination. Therefore, a diagnosis of mental deficiency was not warranted.

Case 2 presented an interesting contrast, by virtue of her attractive personality. She was classified as *borderline defective;* from infancy her mental growth consistently had been retarded at a subnormal or borderline level. Her development was followed over a period of 15 years.

She first came to our attention at the age of *40 weeks* as an orphan who was considered for adoption. She had every appearance of being a normal infant—in countenance, responsiveness and general reactiveness. Her amiable personality cast a spell which tended to conceal the fundamental limitations revealed by the developmental examination. She rated coherently at a 28-week level, with DQ approximately 70.

Her intelligence quotient during 10 years at school showed a similar retardation. At $9\frac{1}{2}$ *years,* her reading and spelling were below the second-grade level of performance. At *15 years,* her reading and spelling were near the fifth-grade level; her other capacities also approximated 10–11 years.

Her personality picture had changed scarcely at all during the long period of developmental observation. The mental growth trend and temperamental traits had remained remarkably constant in spite of checkered environmental changes, in institutions and a succession of foster homes. As an infant she was amiable and amenable; as an adolescent she revealed the same traits. The somewhat lowered quality of her intelligence and judgment made it necessary to provide good supervision and training through adolescence. If she were adequately protected from being exploited there was an excellent prospect of her making a satisfactory social and vocational adjustment in adult life.

§3. MODERATE, SEVERE AND PROFOUND MENTAL DEFICIENCY

We turn now to the graver degrees of mental deficiency—which also declare themselves in infancy. The ultimate limits of development are reflected in the progress which is made in the early years of life; however, it is not possible to base a precise prognosis on developmental quotients derived in the first 2 or 3 months after birth.

Even when more severe degrees of mental deficiency are present, the early picture, while abnormal, may engender overoptimism about the eventual level of function that will be attained. Subcortical mechanisms may produce oculomotor and other postural behavior patterns which simulate more mature patterns, or degenerative processes may be cumulative and exceed the rate of aging.

In the neonatal period, looking and listening are the only two aspects of behavior indicative of cerebral cortical activity. If the infant pursues an object dangled in his field of vision and quiets his activity in response to sound, one can expect the normal progressive elaboration of these patterns to continue. If he does not, but merely shows reflex responses to light and noise, one may be suspicious. But his state of arousal and of hunger may modify his responsiveness at the time of the examination, even though he is not abnormal. The normal infant will continue to show his normality in following months by the steady organization of his behavior repertoire. Not until 16 weeks, with the expected release from the domination of the tonic-neck-reflex, is adaptive behavior sufficiently defined that one can be fully confident about the integrity of the cerebral cortex.

In profound deficiency, mental development is almost completely wanting. The autonomic system is least disturbed: the vegetative functions of respiration, digestion and excretion are preserved, but the capacity to eat solid foods and even sucking may be deficient. In his behavior patterns the profoundly deficient infant scarcely rises above a fetal level, and may even maintain a huddled prenatal posture. He is capable of stereotyped movements but does not acquire powers of prehension or locomotion. His needs and wants are extremely limited and are readily satisfied by food and warmth. His developmental potential is virtually absent.

When the defect is generalized, the child may undergo an extremely slow yet progressive course of development in the motor field. However, he is not likely to rise to a 1-year level of maturity, even in 3 or 4 years. For example, he may learn to stand with support by the end of 3 years, but it may be another 3 years before he walks independently. His postural stances, his prehensory attitudes and his locomotor gait show crudities or even discoordination. His vocalizations are sparse, exaggerated and inarticulate. His emotional life is shallow and unmodulated. His neuromotor equipment is so faulty that he eats solids with difficulty, and usually does not learn to manage a spoon by the age of 3. Lacking the requisite cortical development, he does not acquire sphincter control. Within narrow limits, he is conditionable in childhood. He may learn a few nursery tricks; he establishes associations between bib and bottle; he enjoys simple infantile pleasures like bouncing and cuddling.

So extremely slow is the pace of development in the profoundly defective child that even in adult years he may continue to function at an infantile level, always lacking the dynamic vividness and vitality of a normally developing infant. Only in a limited descriptive sense is he comparable to the normal infant, and he seldom attains as much as one-fourth of expected development. The intervening levels between profound and mild mental deficiency differ only in the rate at which developmental progress is made, and require no separate description. The ultimate function for these degrees of defect ranges between 20 and 50% of normal.

Like normal infants, defective infants show differences in "temperament" and organization of behavior which have diagnostic significance. Some may be quite mild and placid. In the early months they may be regarded as "very good babies." They eat and sleep with docile regularity; they gain weight so steadily that parents are satisfied with the progress made. The eyes are wide open and give a false impression of attention. The coordinate eye movements impart a suggestion of normality.

If the infant is excitable rather than apathetic, he is likely to be troublesome and given to excessive crying and irritability. In later years such an infant may be destructive and impulsively violent. He may acquire pronounced stereotyped movements—body swaying, head rolling, tongue chewing, scratching, brushing, head banging, grunting, snorting, bizarre variations of breathing, fetichistic attachments and other idiosyncrasies. These stereotyped movements are not perversions. They are fixations of pattern. A normal infant does not ordinarily establish permanent fixations because he is constantly changing and expanding the frontiers of a growing reaction system; he progresses from scratching to grasping. However, the most defective infant has such low-grade potentials that his reaction system is relatively static. It does not yield to the ferment of development; instead it settles here and there into rigid patterns of response which are so unvarying that they seem to possess the child.

The disorganization may be so severe that a diagnosis of infantile psychosis, or "autism," is made. In our experience, this symptom represents but one aspect of chronic organic brain disease; it is usually associated with mental deficiency, but is present in only a small proportion of defective children. The subject, which will be considered in detail in Chapter 16, has given rise to an inordinate amount of confusion in the literature. Through application of the techniques of developmental diagnosis, precise delineation of potentials and deficits is possible, and much of the mystique of the problem may be dispelled.

The defective child is most comparable to a normal child when the deficiency is due to a generalized deficit which impoverishes overall development in a symmetric manner. Such classical reductions are extremely rare. More commonly, the physiology of development is so disturbed that the resultant structures of behavior are not only weak and unformed, but distorted and malformed. When the impairment is due to intrinsic pathologic changes within the central nervous system, as in progressive degenerative diseases, the organization of behavior is not only retarded, but also undergoes disintegration. A series of behavioral examinations in the course of the first 3 years shows actual decline and diminution. Such infants are at their best in the very first months of life.

The largest group of defective children come by their defect through a variety of prenatal, natal and postnatal exogenous factors. This group naturally presents a vast array of clinical features, because the cerebral insults have a selective and unevenly destructive effect. Some specific developmental capacities may remain more or less intact. Accordingly, even a profoundly defective child may walk at a relatively early age. Children suffering from such selective deficiencies may even display an impressive perfection of physique and countenance. Curious residuals of normality crop out incongruously in their behavior traits. These children are entitled to discriminative interpretation. If they are profoundly involved, their defect has a different cast.

Physical appearance, however, is an untrustworthy criterion. Some children look normal but are profoundly defective. Because of their motor disabilities, other children give the impression of severe deficiency, but their intelligence is not impaired at all. While poor integration and scattered spotty responses are more common with the severe degress of mental deficiency, they may occur at any ratio of function. The organization of the child's behavior is as important as the maturity of the child in determining his ability to function in society.

Illustrative Cases

The following cases illustrate severe mental deficiency resulting from the continuum of reproductive casualty and various postnatal factors.

Primary Mental Deficiency of Unknown Etiology

Case 3 had been placed with a view to ultimate adoption with a young couple who became concerned over his slow progress. At *45 weeks* his head circumference was 40.9 cm (9-week level); his general maturity level was about 16 weeks (rolls from prone, arms activate and contact toy, laughs, automatic social smile). The behavior patterns were defective in quality (DQ about 35).

At *20 months* his head circumference was 42.6 cm (15-week level). Attention was very poor, and he crawled about aimlessly. His general maturity level was about 20 weeks (grasps toy on contact, obtrusive hand regard, no regard for pellet). Gross motor behavior was slightly more advanced (DQ about 25).

This case illustrates slow, decelerating development. The small head size is associated with lack of cerebral development but not causative.

Case 4 had always been a very "good baby," content to be left alone for hours; development had always been slow. He was first examined at $3\frac{1}{2}$ *years* of age. Left to his own devices, he wandered about the room aimlessly, climbing, screaming, whistling and fingering objects idly. He did respond in some measure to loud, stern, insistent commands and could thus be induced to conform to the requirements of the examination. His general maturity level was approximately 18–21 months, DQ 45–50. He built a tower of cubes, dumped the pellet from the bottle, turned the pages of a book, and placed all the forms in the formboard; he had no words.

At $5\frac{1}{2}$ *years,* after 2 years in a special school, he was controlled, obedient and "trustworthy," having stabilized his activities and advanced in social adaptability. Developmentally, however, he had made essentially no progress (DQ 25–30).

In a suitable environment and with skillful training, much of this child's disturbing erratic behavior had disappeared. Nevertheless, his developmental rate had decelerated.

Aplasias and Malformations

Case 5 was born 4 weeks prematurely; he required resuscitation at birth and respiratory stimulants for 3 days. The head was peculiarly shaped (oxycephaly), the eyes very prominent and vision was doubtful; the infant was very irritable.

At *15 weeks* the anterior fontanelle was closed; the infant was considered probably blind. Irritability was extreme. His general maturity level was approximately 4–6 weeks (DQ about 25).

At *28 weeks* there was no evidence of progress. He was quieter, but still irritable, though receiving phenobarbital. General maturity level was 4–6 weeks (lifts head 1 inch in prone, vocalizes "ah," responds to bib under chin). DQ was about 15.

Death overtook this child at 11 months of age, the cause of death being given as croup. The outstanding features of his brief life were congenital abnormalities, irritability and almost complete lack of developmental progress. Many defective infants react poorly to the birth process.

Case 6 had an older defective sister of similar appearance; there were five normal siblings. At birth the facies was large and flat, and the cranium excessively small and flat, giving him a froglike appearance. At 19 weeks the anterior fontanelle was closed, the head circumference 36.5 cm (2-week level).

At *24 weeks* he showed a very defective picture of 12-week development (t-n-r and symmetry, coos, laughs softly, regards a cube, hand regard). DQ was about 50.

At *25 months* his behavior was disorganized and had deteriorated, though fragments of his earlier behavior patterns were still evident. Head circumference 40.8 cm (8-week level). DQ was about 15.

Congenital anomalies are common among this group of defectives; in this case the malformation and maldevelopment of the cranium and the malformation and maldevelopment of the brain were closely related. The presence of the same condition in a sibling points to a specific hereditary factor.

Degenerative Processes

Case 7, a large well-formed Jewish infant, presented no unusual symptoms during the neonatal period. The first developmental examination at *56 weeks* revealed an atypical behavior picture, with neuromotor signs. Neck, back, shoulders and arms were hypotonic; legs were variably hypotonic and rigid; reflexes were hyperactive; feet were everted. Unable to sit alone, she was supported in her mother's lap; her head sagged forward, and her back was markedly rounded. She grasped a cube with a weak radial palmar grasp, regarded a third cube and also a pellet. Eyes were half-closed and showed alternating strabismus. Motor signs were much more prominent than visual signs. Exploitive drive was very low. Behavior patterns were meager, and did not rise above the 24-week level, but they were not in themselves distorted.

On reexamination at the age of *18 months,* a full blown picture of amaurotic family idiocy unfolded: progressive retardation, heightened reactiveness to sound, increased rigidity, blindness, a conspicuous alternating tonic-neck-reflex, easily induced by passive head rotation. All social responses had vanished; she no longer recognized her mother; she was unable to grasp a cube. Ophthalmoscopic examination revealed a white patch with a central cherry-red spot in the macular region of each eye.

Hemorrhage

Case 8 was resuscitated with difficulty after birth. Spinal fluid was grossly bloody, a diagnosis of cerebral hemorrhage was made and he remained in the hospital for 15 weeks with symptoms of twitching and vomiting.

At *35 weeks* he was a large irritable baby with a small head and closed fontanelles. He had a left unilateral strabismus, hyperactive reflexes and hypertonic extensor muscles. His general level was not above 4 weeks (lifts head 1 inch in prone, attends bell, follows ring briefly, no social responses). DQ was about 10.

At *52 weeks* his level was in the 8–12-week zone (regards cube, coos responsively and smiles, engages in hand play). Neurologic signs persisted. DQ was 15–20.

This boy was making slow but consistent progress at the level of profound mental deficiency, probably secondary to damage suffered at birth.

Case 9 was born at home and developed hemorrhagic disease of the newborn. He was hospitalized on the sixth day, but by that time he was very ill, had numerous ecchymoses, the fontanelle was tense and he had a hemorrhage of the optic disk. With heroic treatment he survived.

At *29 weeks* he was totally blind, and his behavioral responses were very meager. With respect to sleep and activity rhythms he was near the 4-week level. DQ was about 15.

At *18 months* he was limp and hypotonic and subject to minor convulsive seizures. His general level was below 4 weeks (quiets to sound, pursues bottle with mouth, quiets in bath). DQ was 0–5.

This mental deficiency is due to devastating destruction from hemorrhage in the neonatal period.

Infection

Case 10 was born with some difficulty; the left femur was fractured. He had congenital syphilis with osteitis, periostitis, ephiphysitis, white patches on the tongue, rhagades about the mouth, snuffles and general lymphadenopathy. Antiluetic treatment was instituted. At 4 months he had pneumonia, at 6 months pneumonia again.

At *30 weeks* vision was obviously defective, and his behavior was retarded to the 12–16-week level (lifts head to Zone III in prone, coos and smiles as he regards his hand; follows the ring 135° and regards it briefly in hand). DQ was about 45.

At *48 weeks* vision seemed slightly improved, but his responses showed very little alteration. General level was 12–16 weeks; DQ was 25–30.

This is mental deficiency of severe degree due to congenital syphilis.

Case 11 was circumcized on the ninth day after birth. He promptly developed a fever and by the 14th day had convulsions, signs of meningitis and frank pus in the spinal fluid (*E. coli*). After strenuous treatment he recovered from the meningitis but slowly developed a hydrocephalus.

At *28 weeks* the head circumference was 47.3 cm (52-week level), he had a hydrocephalic squint, and he could not support his head. The arms were rigidly semiextended, prehensory approach was incomplete, and grasp was defective. No response to sound was elicited; there was no evidence of social interest. His general maturity level was approximately 14 weeks (regards rattle in hand, hand regard, regards cube). DQ was about 50.

At *56 weeks* the head was still slowly increasing in size, but at a normal rate. He was a happy playful infant, oblivious to sounds and to social approaches. He played with a rattle, regarding it in hand, and he played with his fingers. His general maturity level was approximately 16 weeks. DQ was about 30.

This is another example of mental deficiency of infectious origin: *E. coli* meningitis followed by hydrocephalus and deafness.

Case 12 developed normally to the age of *25 months,* when she had measles with severe convulsions; a diagnosis of measles encephalitis was made. After that time, definite character and personality changes took place. The child became overactive, violent, destructive, stubborn and generally incorrigible.

At *33 months* she was a disorganized deteriorated child, controllable only for brief intervals. Her general maturity level was approximately 15 months (fills cup with cubes, imitates scribble, throws ball, 2–3 words). DQ was about 45.

At *44 months,* after 10 months of institution life, she was quieter and more manageable, though she had frequent attacks of excitement. Although her behavior was socially more acceptable she had made essentially no developmental progress; DQ was about 35.

In this instance, measles encephalitis resulted in mental deficiency.

Anoxia

Case 13 was born prematurely, weighing 3 lb 2 oz (fetal age 29 weeks). He gained well and was considered a normal infant. At 6 months of age he smothered in his blankets in bed. He was lifeless and black when found; on resuscitation he was pallid, had a fixed expression and increased respirations. The parents dated his retardation from this episode.

At *55 weeks* (corrected age about 44 weeks) his behavior was retarded and deformed. His movements were distinctly athetotic. His general maturity level was approximately 20–24 weeks (approaches objects, grasps on contact, no regard for pellet, coos and laughs). DQ was about 45.

At *18 months* (corrected age about 15 months) his greatest gains were in the motor field, in spite of his motor handicaps. He could sit alone, creep and cruise, but in all other fields of behavior his general level was not above 28 weeks (transfers toy, holds two cubes, stereotyped hand regard, no "da-da"). DQ was about 45.

The deficiency in this case is a sequel to a serious postnatal asphyxial episode.

Prenatal Rubella Virus

Case 14 was born with a birth weight of 2 lb 12 oz, but was adjudged to be at full term on the basis of menstrual history. The mother had contracted rubella 65 days after her last menstruation. There was placenta previa with excessive bleeding. The infant gained to a weight of 5 lb after 7 weeks, was active and of normal facies. At the age of 10 months an overoptimistic estimate by one physician attributed the retardation to a dense cataract of the microphthalmic right eye which had been needled at the age of 12 weeks. Other physical anomalies included a markedly asymmetric cranium, overlapping middle toes, undescended testicles, poorly defined junction of upper lip and nasal philtrum and a cardiac lesion.

At *52 weeks* developmental examination revealed extreme and irregular behavioral retardation. The infant stared vaguely at overhead lights. He gave no social regard to persons. His preferred activity was mouthing of one or both hands. From time to time he removed his hands from his mouth, extended one arm in a salute-like pose and fixated on it in a manner suggesting hand inspection. He needed support in sitting. Head station was unsteady. He looked down recurrently at the table top and vaguely regarded his hand. There was no voluntary grasp or reaching, and no reaction to sounds. The behavior picture was irregular, with maturity level 4–8 weeks. The diagnosis was mental deficiency of profound degree following maternal rubella.

Summary

These case reports could be multiplied almost endlessly. Each story differs in detail, each child presents a unique behavior picture, and each has his own individual growth career. Some are quiet and inert; others plod laboriously and slowly through the early phases of development; others are bizarre and disorganized in behavior; still others are excitable and violent; there is a wide variety of neuromotor signs and patterns. The common feature in the more severe degrees of mental deficiency is an extreme failure of normal development.

Development is an all-consuming task for the infant and child; if he fails at this task, it is a very serious matter. There is no second chance; he cannot do it later and make up for lost time. There can be no lighthearted, offhand extenuation; failure of normal development in infancy due to mental deficiency usually is insuperable because of the indivisible unity of life, growth and age. Behavior may be improved but the situations in which treatment can restore developmental potentials to normal are rare.

§4. TRISOMY 21

Until recently, trisomy 21 was referred to as *mongolian idiocy,* the designation applied to the condition in 1866 by Langdon-Down[52] ; the first clinical description by Seguin was published in 1846.[67] The term mongolism has been discarded because of its pejorative implications of an atavistic reversion to an ancient racial stock. The eponym of Down's syndrome also is being replaced gradually. The major purpose of this section is to dispel other misconceptions arising from the designation of mongolian idiocy.

Trisomy 21 is one of the most distinctive forms of mental deficiency; this very distinctiveness has led to a certain overemphasis on the subject in medical writings. Tredgold states that between 40 and 50% of all children diagnosed as mentally defective during the first year of life have this condition.[76] However, they constitute only 5–10% of the total population of defectives. This only can mean that other forms of infant defect should have more attention, because practically all forms can be recognized in the first year. Trisomy 21 nevertheless presents problems of medical and social importance which justify special consideration.

The relationship of trisomy 21 to maternal age long has been recognized, as has its association with complications of pregnancy, especially bleeding; the latter disturbed maternal physiology clearly is not causative but more probably is secondary to the presence of a defective fetus. While the overall incidence of trisomy 21 is reported as 1 in 300–600 births, there is a sharp increase at maternal age 35, with 1 in 30–40 births over the age of 45, compared to 1 in 2000–2500 in mothers under 25. However, younger mothers contribute a significant proportion of the cases, because they bear the greater number of children.

Trisomy 21 is the most common of the chromosomal abnormalities; in 1959 the presence of an extra small acrocentric chromosome, resulting in 47 chromosomes, was demonstrated.[53] In the vast majority of instances this is due to nondisjunction of the chromosome pairs during meiotic formation of ovum or sperm. In a portion of the patients the total chromosome count is the normal 46, the extra Number 21 chromosome being carried as a translocation attached to one Number 15 chromosome, or sometimes to another Number 21 or 22 acrocentric chromosome. Mitotic nondisjunction also occurs, as evidenced by mosaicism, or the existence of both normal and abnormal cell types; skin as well as blood culture is sometimes necessary to demonstrate its presence. Rarely have other tissues been studied, but at least one instance has been found of an abnormal clone of cells in a testicular biopsy of the normal father of two children with trisomy 21. The translocation type is found most often, but not exclusively, in younger mothers and sometimes in the fathers. This factor has importance in genetics counseling, since when a parent carries the translocation chromosome the risk of subsequently affected children is markedly increased. Newer cytogenetic techniques will permit more precise determinations of translocation types than has been possible before.

While the clinical picture of trisomy 21 is due to the extra chromosome, this knowledge brings us no closer to the reasons for the nondisjunction. We are still left with the concept of what can be termed reproductive inefficiency, because of the syndrome's appearance most often in older mothers of any parity or in the firstborn at other maternal ages.

In practical terms, a diagnosis on the basis of anatomic characteristics, amply detailed in numerous texts and articles, can almost always be made at birth—even in an infant born prematurely. None of the characteristics is peculiar to the syndrome; some may be absent in any given case, and all of them may be found in other types of mental deficiency. However, in trisomy 21 the characteristics present a distinctive composite, one so striking that the experienced eye may make a diagnosis by a mere glance at the profile or posture of the infant. There are occasions when a differential diagnosis on the basis of physical characteristics is more difficult; a premature infant sometimes bears a mild though wholly fictitious resemblance to the syndrome, and errors of diagnosis are made if too much weight is placed on obliquity of the eyeslits. The infant with trisomy 21 is under no constraint of fulfilling the specifications of the fullblown textbook model; he may remain unidentified if the physician expects to find all of the grosser features in the period of infancy. Additional aids in diagnosis are the presence of a constellation of atypical dermatoglyphic patterns and of certain bony abnormalities (absent nasal bone and widened acetabular angle) in young infants. Whenever the diagnosis is in doubt, definitive chromosomal studies should be done; they also should be done in younger mothers to detect the translocation carriers.

The term mongolian idiocy has led to a misunderstanding of the infant's developmental course and often affected the advice given to parents. There is a wide range of abilities in these infants. Even though the diagnosis can be made at birth with the certain knowledge that there will be some impairment in function, the extent of the disability cannot be determined at that age. It is certain, however, that trisomy 21 differs from most forms of mental deficiency in that the developmental course is one of premature aging and progressive deceleration in developmental rate. New behavior is added with the passage of time, but it is not steady progress, and the pace at which it is acquired declines.

The typical trisomy 21 child is at his best in his first year of life; an increasing proportion have normal or near-normal development until about 9 months of age. Some infants even lack the supposed *sine qua non* of the syndrome, hypotonia, and can be distinguished only by physical abnormalities and/or chromosomal findings. Almost all children have associated neuromotor disabilities of varying degrees, in addition to the hypotonia, as well as variable amounts of qualitative disorganization of their behavior.

Those patients who are clearly impaired from the beginning will decelerate further and eventually will fit the former classification of "idiocy." Others maintain developmental quotients of 75 or 80 at 3 or 4 years of age or even longer, and their ultimate function will be more advanced. However, the deceleration continues; for how long has not been established definitely. The level at which the IQ stabilizes depends on a variety of factors, e.g., occurrence of seizures and subsequent life experiences.

Equally misleading as the old view of the child's intellectual capacities is the stereotype of his emotional characteristics. Temperament varies quite widely; not all patients are placid, affectionate, cheerful, imitative and have a fondness for music, rhythm and social attention. It is an affront to the human dignity of any individual, however handicapped, to suggest that his love of praise and attention and his amiability make him a pet, or that his mimetic capacity enables him to learn tricks which will amuse the family.

Because diagnosis can be made at birth, it was usually—and unfortunately still often is—recommended that the infant be placed away from home directly from the newborn nursery; in most instances this means in an institution. The evidence is abundantly clear that what usually happens in large regimented institutions is a decline in the child's functional ability. All children benefit from the individual care and stimulation to learning that is provided in a good family setting. The decision must be made by the parents; it is the responsibility of the physician not to impose his own value judgments, but to provide them with the information on which they can reach a rational decision. This must include the fact that a reliable estimate of eventual function cannot be made until a much later age in trisomy 21 than in most instances of mental deficiency, as well as what the community has to offer in terms of foster care, nursery schools, educational facilities and sheltered workshops for the care of the mentally subnormal. At older ages the child's distinctive physical appearance may necessitate more sheltered supervision than would be required by other defectives of comparable mental abilities. Fortunately, attitudes are changing, and the community is more accepting than in the past. In those cases where the parental attitudes are such that they cannot accept the child into their own home under any circumstances, every effort should be made to arrange for foster home care—at least until it is determined whether or not such severe deficiency already is present in the early months that the child's developmental potential always will be profoundly restricted.

It has been a prevalent belief that intellectual function is related to the amount of abnormal chromosomal material present in the child, and parents of mosaic children sometimes have been encouraged unduly, without reference to the behavior of the child. Not all mosaic trisomy 21 patients are "high level," while some patients who are straight trisomy 21 by blood and skin culture are. It is likely that there is the same degree of variability in both types, when due account is taken of the age at which the behavioral evaluation is conducted.

A final word about specific treatment is necessary: there was some evidence that administration of 5-hydroxytryptophan ameliorated the hyptonia, which normally disappears spontaneously with increasing age. Completion of the investigation demonstrated that whatever beneficial effects there were did not persist for more than 3 months.[14] More important, there was no improvement in intellectual function. Consequently, there is no indication for undertaking treatment with this medication. No other specific therapy has been demonstrated to be effective in improving the mental deficiency. However, hypothyroidism appears to be associated with trisomy 21 in 5–6% of the children. When there are clinical signs suggestive of this disorder, appropriate laboratory study and treatment should be instituted. Life expectancy of trisomy 21 children has been prolonged by advances in other fields of medicine, and associated congenital anomalies should be corrected surgically, on the basis of the usual criteria for such procedures.

§5. INBORN ERRORS OF METABOLISM

Phenylketonuria (PKU) is the prototype disease used most often in any discussion of inborn errors of metabolism associated with mental deficiency. It is the most common of these disorders, yet the incidence is only about 1 in 10,000 births. In all, metabolic disorders do not account for more than 4–5% of cases of mental defect. PKU is a recessively transmitted hereditary disorder with a deficiency of a single enzyme, phenylalanine hydroxylase. Its inheritance and biochemistry are well understood, but the mechanism by which it produces the mental deficiency is not. As with all gene-borne disorders, there is a wide phenotypic expression. The condition can be detected in the newborn by blood phenylalanine levels; identification of the heterozygous carrier is possible by phenylalanine loading tests; and there is supposedly a definitive treatment available, a diet low in phenylalanine. Consequently, PKU has received wide publicity, and legislation for mandatory newborn screening and treatment exists in most states. Controlled studies of the efficacy of dietary treatment are no longer possible in the current climate.

Detailed descriptions of the clinical picture and biochemical features of PKU are available in texts and articles. It should be emphasized that seizures—when all types of episodes are considered—and "autistic" behavior are present in 75–85% of

PKU patients who are diagnosed because they already present abnormal development. We are concerned here with some of the unanswered questions and their relevance for diagnosis, prognosis and treatment. Almost all articles and texts state that untreated patients are severely mentally defective, that all are normal at the time of birth and that each week treatment is delayed results in some loss of intellectual function, because damage occurs progressively in the postnatal period. Each of these assumptions must be examined in turn.

First, the initial surveys were done on patients in institutions for the mentally defective; it is therefore not surprising that they demonstrated subnormal intelligence. No systematic screening of a preschool or school-age population has been reported; indeed, it might scarcely be worthwhile in view of the low incidence of the disease. However, reports began to appear of older children with biochemically classical PKU who were functioning normally in school, had normal measured IQs, and were diagnosed accidentally or only when another PKU sibling was identified.

Second, as already stated, a developmental quotient cannot be determined in the first month of life. There is little significant difference in the behavioral accomplishments of normal 1-week and 4-week infants. A variety of developmental quotients could be assigned, but they are usually spuriously advanced rather than retarded. Thus, normality at age 2 or 3 weeks only can be assumed. Case reports of early development reveal documentation of normality only by lists of motor items; characteristically, the vast majority of PKU children have gross motor behavior much closer to their chronologic age than is their language and adaptive behavior.

Third, a pitfall of earlier evaluations of response to treatment was failure to recognize the existence of a group of atypical cases, with elevated blood phenylalanine usually at lower levels than in classical disease, and transitory in nature in many instances; this condition appears to be unassociated with intellectual impairment. More important is the failure to distinguish among the cases on the basis of the means of ascertainment; there are three separate groups. The first comes to attention because of the presence of developmental retardation; these children are older and already clinically abnormal. The second group is detected because they are siblings of known cases; they may be diagnosed in the newborn period, or if at later ages, they are often not functionally impaired. The third group are those found on routine newborn screening. In both these latter categories, there are children who in prior years would not have been diagnosed, in the absence of any abnormality in function; what proportion of the total cases they represent is unknown and will remain so because of the current legislative mandates. Reports in the literature seldom provide adequate data on individual cases; if they do differentiate on the basis of the ascertainment method, the data give indications which do not support the conclusions that early treatment and good subsequent dietary control are responsible for normal intellectual progress. In all of the reports one can find instances of children treated from the neonatal period with excellent dietary control who are defective, and some treated not at all or well after a year of age, with poor dietary control, but with a normal IQ. In fact, one recent report contains the following statement: "Twenty-two children were not treated due to late diagnosis associated with profound mental retardation. This group presented at a mean age of $11\frac{8}{12}$ years. The mean IQ was 36 (range nonmeasurable to 96)."[50]

Finally, dietary treatment clearly results in control of seizures, including often unrecognized prolonged staring episodes, and in earlier disappearance of "autistic" behavior (Chapters 13 and 16). However, little attention is paid to the role of these factors in the improvement in the child's function; putting him back in contact with his environment and organizing his behavior may be the factors that result in improvement in measured intellectual function. Furthermore, data on the socio-economic level of the family is not provided, nor is its effect on later function considered. The efficacy of the diet still is in question.

Thus, there are at least two important considerations to be borne in mind in the approach to metabolic disorders. The first is that the diet necessary for treatment is very restricted in an essential amino acid and is not without inherent hazards. Irritability, lethargy, anemia and growth failure may result, and the consequent malnutrition in early months may contribute more to abnormal central nervous system function than does the disease itself. The second consideration is the danger of assuring parents that if treatment is carried out from a very early age, normal development invariably will result. In all instances, the behavioral development of the child must be monitored closely and adequately, and the observed function must be the basis on which recommendations are made.

An ethical consideration which confronts the involved professional is the fact that the total gene pool of PKU carriers will increase slowly, if dietary treatment improves behavior and permits reproduction. Further, there still are no clear data defining the risk of abnormal outcome of pregnancy in PKU patients, treated or not. These are crucial social problems. At the very least, the statistical probabilities should be discussed with the patients involved so that they might consider abortion or sterilization.

8

Mental Subnormality: Environmental Mental Retardation

Throughout this volume we have stressed the close relationship of intrinsic and environmental factors in the development of behavior. Growth and development are processes of anatomic and functional integrative organization which bring "heredity" and "environment" into productive union. Development constantly creates its own conditions as it proceeds; the products of present development influence later development. The manner in which an organism functions today has an effect on how it will function tomorrow. Surely, in the prognostication of development much depends upon what happens to a child!

How much? That is a clinical question which always demands an estimate of developmental potentials in relationship to a given environment. Sometimes the environmental factors seem so significant that a new environment must be provided to put the question to a therapeutic test. The problem is one of differential diagnosis, requiring a discriminating estimate of the responsiveness of the organism to its environment. These general principles become very pointed in clinical situations; they then lose their abstractness.

In appraising developmental potentials, we cannot ignore any environmental influences: cultural milieu, siblings, parents, illness, trauma, education. But these must always be considered in relation to the organizational integrity of the child's central nervous system, which ultimately determines the degree and mode of reaction to the environment. Environmental impoverishment leads to behavioral impoverishment. It produces palpable reductions of behavior. It does not produce mental deficiency, but it does produce syndromes which may be severe enough to make diagnosis difficult and to call for therapeutic intervention.

§1. MENTAL RETARDATION DUE
TO ENVIRONMENTAL DISADVANTAGE

We turn now to that larger group of children without organic disease of the brain who function at a subnormal level of intellectual ability as measured by IQ and school performance. Such children are found almost exclusively in the lowest sociocultural groups, in this country particularly in minority groups. The term *mental retardation* should be reserved for this type of subnormal mental ability often referred to as "physiologic," "familial" or endogenous retardation. Many professionals contend that this behavior is a gene-determined characteristic—that because of the lack of demonstrable neurologic or other physical abnormalities, such individuals represent the "lower end of the normal curve" of intelligence. The evidence cited for this is the inter- and intra-generational familial aggregation, and the fact that the closer the blood relationships, the higher the correlations in measured IQ scores. Cited also is the higher correlation between IQ scores of adopted children and IQ or education of their natural mothers than between scores of these children and education of their adoptive parents, as reported by Skodak and Skeels.[69] Three facts are ignored in such citations: there was a 20-point difference in mean measured IQ between the children and their true mothers; the infants of mothers with higher educational and IQ levels generally were placed in more academically oriented homes, on the assumption that this would result in better "matching"; and there was a substantial correlation between the educational levels of the natural mothers and the adoptive parents.

Cotwin control studies also have their problems. Twin pairs differ in several considerations other than the fact that dizygous twins are comparable to any pair of siblings, while monozygous twins are presumably identical. Monozygosity is a fetal abnormality, a fact often overlooked. It is associated with increased mortality rates, lower birth weights and a greater incidence of neuropsychiatric disabilities. As with dizygous twins, there often is a significant disparity in birth weight between members of the twin pair, the lighter one evidencing more impairment. Differences in the intrauterine environment could account for such discrepancies. An alternative explanation could be that the genetic material is not identical, depending on the time at which the embryo split. However, upbringing tends to be more comparable for twins of the same sex, particularly if they are thought to be identical.

In the lower socioeconomic strata of society there is an increased incidence of organic mental deficiency, due to the increased incidence of many interrelated antecedent etiologic factors. Disadvantaged children are not only born *into* poverty, they are conceived *of* poverty. As a group, their mothers give evidence of malnutrition throughout their own life cycle. Maternal and infant mortality rates are increased, and there is a higher incidence of complications of pregnancy, other diseases associated with pregnancy, low birth weight as well as premature birth, and subsequent illness, malnutrition and lack of medical care. A comprehensive review of relevant data has been written by Birch and Gussow.[7] These biologic factors contribute to a depressed performance, and all the adverse conditions have a higher incidence in minority groups.

But what of those who escape any significant injury to the central nervous system? The largest proportion do so, in spite of the accumulation of adverse factors. What is their developmental progress?

The generally depressed function on school-age tests in the lowest socio-economic strata and the vigor of most infants seen in well-baby clinics has led professionals to say it is not possible to detect mild mental subnormality in infancy. The majority thus affected cannot be identified for a very simple reason: Those children with so-called familial or physiologic retardation are *normal* in infancy. Those with organic disease of the brain impairing intellectual potential, regardless of the degree of impairment or of their social status, *can* be identified in infancy.

Abundant data indicate there is an increased incidence of subnormality and increasing socioeconomic disparity in function with increasing age, at least during the school years. Two different epidemiologic surveys of individuals considered to be mentally subnormal illustrate the first point. An Onondaga County, New York, survey revealed subnormal labeling at less than 1% in the preschool years, 3–4% at 5–10 years, a peak of 8% in the 10–15-year range (greater for boys than girls), and a drop back to 4% in the 15–20-year group.[59] A survey in the Eastern Health District of Baltimore, Maryland, obtained similar results with somewhat lower rates, since more objective measures were used for identification of subnormality: less than 1% before 5 years, 1% at 5 years, 4% at 10 years, 3% at 15 years, 1–2% at 20 and 25 years, and again less than 1% over 60 years of age.[54]

A clearer picture emerges from the variety of studies in which individuals were evaluated by detailed examinations at various times in their life cycle. Data from the Baltimore Study of Prematures* indicate that in an infant population of 1000, adjusted for population distributions by birth weight and race, 1.4% of infants had adaptive developmental quotients of less than 75, and 1.8% less than 85.[41] The comparable rates were 4.5% and 14% for the white school-age population on which the 1937 Revision of the Stanford–Binet Test was standardized.[70] The curve for the distribution of DQs in infants rose abruptly at DQ of 90, and over 85% had developmental quotients between 95 and 125.

Nearly 800 of these 1000 Baltimore infants were diagnosed as having normal intellectual potential and neuromotor status; there were no significant differences in developmental quotients between white and black infants or between infants whose mothers had different levels of education. For whatever criteria used at 40 weeks of age—mean DQs, distributions of DQs, or item analysis of all the individual

*This study was initiated in 1952 under the auspices of the Maternal and Child Health Division of the Johns Hopkins University School of Hygiene and Public Health. Information was gathered about the subjects at five different age periods between their 1st and 12th years; a series of reports have been published and are cited at various points. The coeditors examined all of the infants in the first year and one-third of them at 3 years of age. The present volume contains some previously unpublished data derived from the study.

Table 8-1. Percent of Population with Adaptive Developmental Quotients Below 75, by Age and Socioeconomic Status (Adjusted for Proportion of Premature Infants in Each Group)

Socioeconomic Status	AGE	
	40 Wk	3 Yr
White upper half	0.2	0.3
Black upper half	1.5	0.6
White lower half	2.5	2.3
Black lower half	2.0	8.1

Data from Study of Prematures, Baltimore, Maryland
Knobloch, H, Pasamanick, B: Predicting intellectual potential in infancy. Am J Dis Child 106: 43-51, 1963

behavior patterns—inspection of the developmental examination protocol gave no clue to the race or socioeconomic level of the infant.

Table 8-1 indicates that disparity in the incidence of organic abnormality does exist in infancy, when each racial group in the study was divided in half by an index of socioeconomic status.[45]   After adjusting for differences in birth weight distributions, the incidence of DQs of less than 75 was 0.2% in the white upper-half, and ranged from 1.5 to 2.5% in the remaining three groups. Marked divergence already was apparent in 300 of the original infants examined at 3 years. Three-tenths percent of the white upper-half children had quotients of less than 75; the rates for the remainder were 0.6% for the black upper-half, 2.3% for the white lower-half, and 8.1% for the black lower-half. Table 8-2 shows the divergence for the smaller number of 3-year-olds with birth weights above 2500 g, using education of the mother as the only index of socioeconomic status.[45]   At 40 weeks of age there was essentially no difference in either race in the average general (adaptive) quotients. However, at 3 years, the mean DQ for the white children whose mothers had a high school education or better was 115; in contrast, the black children whose mothers had less than a ninth grade education fell to 90.

Table 8-3 shows Drillien's data on the effect of the standard of maternal care at ages 2–5 for fullterm control infants.[18,19] For the children with the best grade of

Table 8-2. Adaptive Developmental Quotients by Age in Fullterm Infants, According to Race and Education of the Mother

Mother's Education	AGE			
	40 Wk		3 Yr	
	White	Black	White	Black
Less than 9th	103	100	109	90
9-11 Grade	104	104	108	102
High School +	102	104	115	105

Data from Study of Prematures, Baltimore, Maryland

Knobloch, H, Pasamanick, B: Predicting intellectual

potential in infancy. Am J Dis Child 106: 43-51, 1963

Table 8-3. Developmental Quotients by Age and Grade of
Maternal Care in Mature Control Infants

Grade of Maternal Care	AGE			
	2 Yr	3 Yr	4 Yr	5 Yr
1. Best	107	108	110	118
2. Middle	103	103	103	106
3. Poorest	98	97	98	95

Data from Drillien [18,19]

Knobloch, H, Pasamanick, B: Predicting intellectual

potential in infancy. Am J Dis Child 106: 43-51, 1963

maternal care, from middle-class and superior working-class homes, the mean
quotient rose from 107 at 2 years of age, to 118 at 5 years. In average working-class
homes, there was essentially no change with age. In the poor working-class homes
with the poorest maternal care there was a downward trend, which was not
statistically significant. However, the comparison between the best and the poorest
maternal care indicates the effects of learning, a difference of 9 points at 2 years of
age and of 23 points at 5 years of age.

Another study by Nelson and Deutschberger was directed towards correlating
head size at 1 year with 4-year IQ.[58] Fortuitously, it provides data regarding the
effect of the mother's education upon the child's test score. The sample size was
very large, but no exclusions were made for birth weight, gestational length or
neurologic damage, factors which would tend to confound the observations. Table
8-4 shows differences between boys and girls; it also demonstrates that the mother's
educational achievement did not have the same absolute effect in each racial group.
However, a systematic relationship was present in all four race and sex groups: the
higher the mother's education, the higher the child's IQ score.

The 6–7-year Stanford–Binet IQ results for almost 700 of the 800 infants in
the Baltimore Study of Prematures who had normal infant neuromotor status and
intellectual potential extend these findings further. Again there were no significant
differences in infancy, when the infant was an *undamaged* black or white baby,
premature or fullterm. For these normal infants, Table 8-5 shows clearly the

Table 8-4. Mean IQ at Four Years by Sex,
Race and Mother's Education

	No.	MOTHER'S EDUCATION			
		0-8	9-11	12	13+
White Males	2154	96	100	104	113
Black Males	2585	85	89	93	98
White Females	1982	99	102	108	118
Black Females	2658	88	91	95	101

Adapted from Nelson and Deutschberger [58]

Table 8-5. Comparison of Infant DQ and 6-7 Year IQ by Birth
Weight, Race and Education of Mother

	EDUCATION OF MOTHER								
	9th Grade			9-11 Grade			High School +		
	N	DQ	IQ	N	DQ	IQ	N	DQ	IQ
White Prematures	47	105	93	34	106	100	44	106	105
Black Prematures	80	103	87	72	104	90	32	106	95
White Controls	45	105	96	47	105	101	54	107	108
Black Controls	82	104	89	85	105	92	38	107	97

Data from Study of Prematures, Baltimore, Maryland
    Includes children with normal neuromotor and intellectual status
in infancy and testable with the Stanford-Binet at school age.

systematic relationship to the mother's education in the early school years. Further, whites did better at all educational levels than blacks, again indicating that a comparable level of education does not denote equivalence, in the quality of the mother's education or that of her child. Finally, Table 8-6 demonstrates that the children who were abnormal in infancy had a greater risk of poor performance at school age, for all levels of maternal education.

These racial and socioeconomic phenomena have their roots in the total milieu in which children grow and develop: in medical and nutritional problems; in the noisy crowded conditions of slum living; in the lack of academic orientation in the home; in the accompanying suppression of verbal communication and curiosity; in feelings of hopelessness; and in the inferior educational facilities which are usually provided for the ghetto culture. Hurley presents eloquent and graphic descriptions of the brutal conditions of poverty.[32]

Improvements in measured test performance and academic achievement with improved environments have been demonstrated in a variety of situations and at different ages. A recent experimental study by Heber has highlighted this dramatically.[29] Pointing out that children living in very poor circumstances whose mothers have IQ scores below 75 show a progressive decline in test performance, from 100 at 2 years to 70 at 18, he instituted an intensive program of stimulation for 20 infants with 20 control patients. All were black. The intervention measures

Table 8-6. Children Untestable or With Stanford-Binet IQ
Below 80 at 6-7 Years of Age, by Mother's Education and
Infant Central Nervous System Integrity

	INFANT STATUS			
	Normal		Abnormal	
Mother's Education	#	Per Cent Untestable or IQ <80	#	Per Cent Untestable or IQ <80
<9th Grade	259	16	67	41
9-11th Grade	243	10	59	23
High School or +	168	2	33	16

Data from the Study of Prematures, Baltimore, Maryland

were begun at 3 months of age and were carried out in a study center and at home. Stimulated and control infant groups both had mean DQs of 115 at 12 months. The stimulated infants did better than the controls in the early preschool years, and their Stanford–Binet scores remained high at $4\frac{1}{2}$ years. The mean IQ level was 120, while the control group already had started their downward drift, to 95. Heber provides no information on whether there was associated improvement in the performance of the mothers and the older siblings, an indication that a total family reorientation might have been the major influence on the infant's subsequent development. Nevertheless, he does show that a radical impact can be made in a population where the familial aggregation of low test scores generally is attributed to inherited differences in intellectual ability.

A word of caution is indicated in the interpretation of all this data. The tests used in evaluating "intelligence" are not culture-fair. They almost always are biased in favor of the white academically-oriented middle-class and make their own contribution to the differences which are found.

A final word must be devoted to the adult functioning of children identified in school as mentally subnormal, by virtue of their placement in special classes. The findings of various followup studies fit with the results of the epidemiologic surveys on the differential age distribution of mental subnormality. One typical study, in which the children did not come from poverty-stricken families, showed that as adults about 80% were married, had a lower than average divorce rate, raised families and were gainfully employed with a stable occupational pattern.[12] Their children did not exhibit more mental deficiency than is found in the general population. Their own IQ scores increased by about 25 points over what they were in school. Thus, the greater proportion labeled as subnormal were self-sufficient members of the community.

These data emphasize the importance of the sociocultural milieu and its effect on the intimate interrelationship of biologic and psychologic factors affecting development. They have definite implications for the controversy which is raging anew about the relative contributions of genetic and environmental factors to intellectual performance, not only between races, but also within each racial group. There is a contemporary preoccupation with the heritability of IQ test scores, and a tacit assumption by many that such a score reflects innate ability. A recent review of present knowledge of such heritability data supports, but does not prove, the hypothesis that there are different environmental factors determining IQ between blacks and whites, but that the genotypes are similar.[24] Hirsch has stated, "The plain facts are that in the study of man a heritability estimate turns out to be a piece of 'knowledge' that is both deceptive and trivial."[30]

Until optimum conditions for conception and subsequent development are provided for the entire population, it is not possible to study or define the relative contributions of "heredity" and "environment" to intellectual function. Under present circumstances, it is a disservice to humanity to attempt to do so. Important educational, social and political decisions must be directed toward maximizing opportunities for each individual to develop to his fullest potential. In the present state of society, few individuals can achieve this ideal goal.

Man has apparently reached the stage where, because of his tremendous plasticity in psychologic functioning, significant upward intellectual change does not take place on a structural level. Scientific parsimony seems to lead to the most useful theory: while man's fundamental structure—and consequently his basic functioning—is genetically determined, it is chiefly the sociocultural milieu affecting biologic and psychologic variables which modifies his behavior and, in the absence of congenital organic brain dysfunction, makes one individual function significantly differently from the next.

§2. INFANT CARE PROGRAMS

For a long time it had been fashionable to assume that "one intimate and continuous relationship with his mother (or permanent mother substitute)" is essential for the mental health of the child. The growing interest in maternal deprivation was thus summed up by Bowlby.[8] Such deprivation supposedly can lead not only to a variety of psychologic disturbances, but to mental deficiency. Little attention has been paid to the retraction of the statement made by Bowlby himself some years later: "Meanwhile it is clear that some of the former group of workers, including the present senior author, in their desire to call attention to dangers which can often be avoided, have on occasion overstated their case. In particular, statements implying that children who are brought up in institutions or who suffer other forms of serious privation and deprivation in early life *commonly* develop psychopathic or affectionless character (e.g., Bowlby, 1944), are seen to be mistaken."[9]

In orphan asylums where there is little or no care, or even when the standards are high and humane, infant development can be depressed. However, no definitive evidence exists that early institutional experience for an otherwise intact individual results in *permanent* damage, particularly if the child is removed from the institution. In one orphanage in which we had experience, infants who demonstrated retardation in behavioral development after they were 16 weeks old functioned normally after later placement in adoptive homes. Whether their ultimate function would have been better had their institutional experience never occurred remains unanswered.

The growth career of C.B. illustrates the point in less abstract terms. An illegitimate child, she was placed in institution A where she remained to the age of 17 months; she was then placed in foster home B, and at 29 months in adoptive home C. Three examinations were made during her long institutional period—17 months is a very long time for an infant. At each of these examinations she was judged clinically as dull normal. With more superficial diagnosis she might well have been considered defective, because she was definitely retarded on the developmental schedules. At the age of 35 weeks she still regarded her hands in the manner of a 12-week infant. This and other behavior characteristics were attributed to the unfavorable institutional environment.

Her subsequent career can be told briefly: As she progressed from less favorable to more favorable environments, she improved in her showing on examinations in almost exact proportions, and so promptly as to make the relationship convincing. After 6 months of foster home experience, she earned a dull normal to low average rating. Four months later, a low average status was indicated. Placement in adoption with a full year of probation was recommended. Seven months after she had entered her adoptive home, her development had risen to a full average level. Six months later it was slightly above average. The examiner's comment was, "C.B.'s adoptive placement seems ideal."

Why did it seem ideal?—because at last there was compatibility between her capacities and her opportunities, between her surroundings and her behavioral assets. If in her institutional days, at the age of 35 weeks, she looked at her hands, it must have been because she had nothing better to do. Later she had constant chance and occasion to exercise her growing powers; this made for her happiness. It also was a safeguard against developmental deviation.

Recently, reports have stated that maternal deprivation leads directly, by psychologic mechanisms, to growth failure as well as to retardation. However, these reports have not included documentation of caloric intake.[62] One study emphasized atypical hand posturing, seen so frequently in infants with abnormal neuromotor function, as an index of "sensory deprivation"; but it failed to pay due attention to the fact that the infants and young children who exhibited this posture had evidence of significant mental deficiency as well.[51] Little attention has been directed to a study by Whitten which demonstrated that the caloric intake of presumably deprived infants with growth failure was, in fact, inadequate.[77] He showed further that provision in the hospital of "tender loving care" in the face of continuing undernutrition did not induce weight gain, while adequate calories under conditions of continuing social deprivation did.

The philosophic approach regarding social group experience for infants and young children has a great deal to do with its outcome, as does the question of whether such experience results from economic necessity or from a deliberate approach to a form of child-rearing considered beneficial. In this country there are many current efforts to provide daycare centers for infants from disadvantaged homes as early as 2–6 months of age. The data cited in the first section of this chapter indicate that this is not necessary at so early an age. Differential experience for young infants may accelerate the emergence of more mature patterns which are in their nascent stages, but differences disappear once the infants reach the age when the particular behavior normally appears in the behavioral repertoire. At the proper age, infants not specifically "trained" or "stimulated" acquire a particular behavior pattern spontaneously and rapidly. Infant care programs have more virtue if there is concurrent reorientation of the mothers toward interaction with their children. This interaction will come to fruition in the toddler and preschool ages, when positive reinforcement of the child's curiosity and communication is so important. Daycare projects undoubtedly have been influenced by models such as the Soviet Union nursery schools and the Israeli Kibbutz settlements, were practices have arisen from a combination of the needs of working mothers and a communal orientation. Isolation from a family unit is not complete in these models, and a definite educational program is part of the daily activity.

There are mothers who must work from economic necessity and others who do so because they have professions or wish to engage in productive activity outside the home. The number of good quality day care centers is inadequate to meet the needs of these women, and should be expanded. Well-staffed and well-organized day care centers are not harmful for the developing infant and child.

§3. INSTITUTIONAL SYNDROMES

However, many infants and young children are obliged to spend much of their lives in institutions, hospitals and congregate nurseries. Of course, the level of personnel and organization of any institution, even of a family home, determines its benefits and its hazards. Therefore, we shall discuss the subject from a functional standpoint and show how the typical patterns of institutional arrangements enter into processes of infant development. It is not our purpose to discuss abuses or substandard and unsanitary institutions; the effects of institutional life can be examined even in presumably well-conducted, humane institutions designed for normal children, which seem to be doing all or even more than should be expected of them. We can analyze objectively the dynamics of their equipment and methods.

The following discussion describes in concrete clinical terms the impression which prolonged institutionalization makes upon the behavioral characteristics of infants and young children. We depict an XYZ institution, fortunately becoming less common, of near average size, moderately well staffed and equipped, and under medical supervision. The children range from a few weeks to a few years in age. The population is ever changing. Some children come on a brief emergency basis, but there is a strong tendency for all to remain longer than was intended. The institution has a good local reputation for the care which it bestows on its charges. Some of them have come from miserable homes. The general level of the education and intelligence of their parents is low rather than high, but there are always some exceptions in both directions.

Psychologically speaking, the children who fare best in this institution are the very youngest babies. They are on a schedule; they are getting regular and frequent physical care. This physical care coincides well with their current psychologic needs. The bath, the cleansing, the rubbing, the changing, the dressing, the undressing, the weighing—all add up to a fairly busy and slightly exciting behavior day, particularly when so much time normally is expended in sleep, in staring and in sensory experiences possible to a baby in almost any crib or bassinet anywhere. The very young infant doesn't need much more than he is getting. An institution provides at least a major portion of his most basic needs, both physical and mental.

A hospital provides even more; diagnostic procedures afford the necessary sensory input, even though they may be painful and contrary to our concept of appropriate "tender loving care."

As the baby grows older, his basic physical needs remain much the same, but his psychologic needs increase with every day. In a busy institution the physical care continues, but the progressive new psychologic needs are met only partially. There are too many babies and not enough attention to go around. The baby belongs, but to what and to whom?—to the institution. Sometimes the very vastness of the rooms and the repetitive multiplicity of furniture prevents the building up of natural associations with a settled and comprehended *place*.

By 4 months the young infant is straining to sit up; he is developing new powers of ocular fixation and pursuit; he is picking up moving objects with his eyes; he is ready for increasingly varied visual expeditions. He has a need for perceptual experience, for elementary knowledge of the physical world. Is this need satisfied? Only partially, because of the inevitable limitations of an XYZ institution. He is propped up, possibly at regular intervals, and for predetermined periods—but not always at the psychologic moments which are most favorable, and not with the endless variations and surprises which naturally enter into the flexible living of a domestic circle. The caretaker, having propped him for the sitting-up period, even places a toy at his disposal. However, the propping is of necessity somewhat hurried and impersonal, because the very same attention must be repeated for many babies. There can be no waiting for or adaptation to psychologic moments; neither is there much time for improvisational play with the baby. There is too much to be done. In a well-organized family which considers children an accepted aspect of its orientation, there are innumerable psychologic moments during the day. The mother and other people help to create them and are on the alert to detect and to exploit them. That is the supreme advantage of the home over the institution in the matter of psychologic care.

Superficially, the difference in the two environments may seem small, but over a course of months this difference proves to be far-reaching. A home builds up the psychology of the baby by countless opportunistic impacts varied to meet the fortuities of each day. An institution tends to channel the psychology of the baby by restricted and standardized impacts. It delimits the scope of the infant's behavior by paucity of impacts. This paucity has nothing less than an impoverishing effect.

We can see this effect in behavioral syndromes elicited by developmental examinations of institutionalized infants, even by the time they are 16—28 weeks of age. These infants often react better in supine situations than they do while seated at the test table. They are accustomed to lie on their backs—overaccustomed, because they have acquired exaggerated, circular forms of hand play, hand and mouth play, head nodding and head rolling. Such activity becomes congealed into stereotypy, into blind-alley behavior patterns which are not sloughed off sufficiently or displaced by normal developmental elaborations. Even hand inspection, which should disappear between 16 and 20 weeks, may usurp other forms of activity and assume an unnatural dominance at 24 weeks. Why not? The child has spent an unnatural preponderance of time on his back and has become an overexpert hand inspector—hyperplasia rather than morphogenetic differentiation.

In the seated position, such an infant begins to show his limitations. He may not even look at the cube on the test table; he looks at his hand instead, or he fastens a transfixed gaze on the examiner, smiling blandly in an overfascinated manner. He seems overfascinated because the examiner is a new sight. An XYZ baby has very narrow experience with persons; this tends to produce a certain ineptness, and has narrowed the scope and adaptability of his social behavior. The end-result is a species of environmental retardation, revealed by the developmental examination: a 24-week baby scarcely giving heed to the tabletop or the cube on it, not bending his head to the task in hand, instead gazing inordinately at the examiner or looking recurrently at his own hand, with semiautomatic jerks of attention. Even a normal 20-week baby will concentrate his ocular, manual and postural powers avidly upon the focal object on the tabletop in an effort to corral it.

The retardation of the 24-week institutional baby may be only slight, but it is significant. It becomes increasingly serious if that same baby stays in an institution for 6 months, or perhaps a whole year, more. Environmental retardation works by attrition as well as by impoverishment; effects tend to be cumulative in susceptible infants. Unfortunately, there is an increased proportion of susceptible infants in such institutions because of the increased likelihood of adverse antecedent conditions in the mother, with subsequent central nervous system dysfunction. Increased maturity does not bring increased power to overcome these effects, because it is only a partial maturity which comes, and because the behavior patterns are incessantly organized to accept the institution. The most susceptible infant is the infant who most completely accepts.

The very acceptance may reach an abnormal degree of intensity. The baby becomes overweeningly attached to the institution, not so much from sheer love of the place as from ignorance of other places. By the age of 1 year he may be terrified when taken somewhere else; he resists strangeness, he clings to the attendant, he cries. A new situation is altogether too much for his limited experience and for his atrophied adaptability. The social ineptness noted at the age of 24 weeks comes to its developmental issue.

Such resistances should not be interpreted as abnormal fears; they are perfectly natural emotional manifestations of restricted and restrictive personal—social behavior patterns. They are the products of meager, overchanneled social experiences. The XYZ type of institution, in spite of its high standards, is not arranged physically or personally to supply a well-balanced social diet. The "vitamins" are left out.

Contrast the typical behavior of an average 1-year child who has been brought up in ordinary home surroundings or a good day nursery. He may show shyness in a new situation, and we rather like to see him show it, but he thaws out, sizes up and adjusts emotionally. Confidence mobilized, he bends to the tasks of the developmental examination with eagerness. There may even be a burst of protest as he is about to leave. He enjoys new experiences, he profits by them and he gets them in abundance.

In the development of the child, one of the most critical transition periods is that between 1 and 2–3 years. Woe befalls the child who does not get discriminating individual attention during that difficult period—when, more or less simultaneously, he is learning to walk, talk, acquire a sense of personal identity, a reciprocal sense of other persons and an adaptation to strange social mores, including bladder and bowel control! The demanded controls are so multifarious that the institutional child, being subjected to less insistent cultural pressure, may seem to have some advantage over the household child. But the institutional child pays too heavy a price for this apparent leniency; he lacks the stimulus that comes from the changing, albeit sometimes excessive, demands of family living.

First and foremost, the child in an XYZ institution lacks the normal stimulus of language—the excitement of intercommunication by facial expression, gesture, pantomimic action, social laughter, interjections, words and sentences, and other forms of expressional behavior, both on the give and take sides—which occurs in the intimacy of home life. No matter how noisy the institution sometimes is, with wails and crying, no matter how footsteps and activities of the caretakers break the quiet, a veritable pall of meaningless sound tends to hang over the nursery where the runabouts and the creepabouts are congregated. At first blush they seem to be having a fine time. It is a smooth expansive floor, and they are excellent creepers; indeed, some are creeping who under other auspices would be walking. Just as the institution puts an unconscious premium on supine behavior for young infants, it overweights prone behavior in older infants. This arena of quadrupedal and bipedal locomotion is relatively devoid of speech. There is little social laughter. Even crying has lost much of its language value; it is only a primitive form of emotional release. There is no jargon among the children, and very little conversation between adult and child.

Picture a scene: a dozen or a score of infants on the floor, getting in each others' way, or occupying islands of isolation; play objects are promiscuously exploited in a fragmentary manner; there are no cohesive, continuing small groups with an adult and a baby as a focal center of the group. There are no stable focal centers; the centers are ever shifting, the activities scrambled and more aimless than they would be in a home. This is a kind of ordered chaos so far as patterned personal—social behavior is concerned. The major activity is motor activity, and vacuums are constantly being filled with stereotyped, circular, repeated reactions. Here is one infant, tired of hitching about, who sits in the middle of the floor with a rubber toy and sways back and forth for minutes at a time as though doing some incantation. Two or three children are standing, but not still; they are weaving back and forth with incessant rhythm, reminiscent of the head rolling of their supine days. This too is environmental stereotypy. Another child is transfixed in a bent-over stance, similar to that of a football center about to pass the ball. But the child is poised for inaction; he peers through his legs for minutes at a time—another postural perseveration. Other children are indulging in unwonted, persisting, chewing movements—a stereotypy of mandibular action.

To a discriminating observer there is only one child in the entire group who seems to be behaving normally. He is a newcomer just arrived, for emergency reasons, from his natural family home, where he learned to speak. He is talking to one of his creeping colleagues, and offering him a toy, but there is no language response. In time the prattling visitor also will adopt the institutional silence.

There can be no doubt that institutional children are retarded in language development. Our portrayal has not been overdrawn, if it reveals the mechanisms and the circumstances which choke the growth of speech and muffle social interchange, with all its give and take of humor, echoing back, repeating over and over again, laughter, praise, mock surprise, dramatic play and expressed affection which are part and parcel of a baby-centered home or good day nursery. Lacking all these repercussions, the institutional child often acquires an impassive face, because his facial muscles have not been adequately animated by social behavior. He is not so much oversensitive to strangers as he is socially stupid with respect to their advances. He has not had much training in the subtleties of social advance and retreat, nor can he meet halfway the overtures of speech and gesture when they come from another child. He has learned to be indifferent to many of the activities of an institution, because most of them are not personally directed toward him. He overgeneralizes his indifference and withdrawal. He may "act strange" with men, because he has seen so few of them. He has had both too much and too little privacy. So many of his spontaneous initiatives have been unobserved and unheeded that they were virtually stillborn. Many activities will not be born at all—why should they? Likewise, he has often cried or tried to speak without being heeded. This has dampened his speech development. He has been denied the conversations of bedtime, mealtime and toilet time. His toilet training has been more or less futile because of its regimentation—ten tots on as many toilets at the same time! His caretakers often are clothed in uniforms; the uniformity of their clothes, the uniformity of his own and the lack of opportunity to build up a sense of place and individuality all have conspired to blunt the edge of his self, and to confine the margins of his growing personality.

It is not our desire to exaggerate this portrayal of institutional life, but to indicate how the environmental mechanisms operate to bring about the syndromes of retardation. We call them syndromes because they are constituted of more or less characteristic behavioral symptoms. Again, some of the effects may be permanent, but an institutional environment does not create mental deficiency, even when it seriously depresses the DQ. It produces lags, and bogs down both initiative and expressiveness, but fortunately it does not necessarily impair latent maturation. The behavior improves with improvement of environment.

A final qualification serves to prove the rule. If a child has an abundance of initiative and vigor, if he is not too sensitive, if he has energy and sufficient vitality of temperament, he may not show environmental retardation. He may indeed become the pet of the institution, but even then he will not escape altogether unscathed—if he stays too long.

A list of cumulative signs of environmental retardation and deflection follows. They are illustrated further by a few brief case sketches in Chapter 19 on adoption. The symptoms are exaggerated in children with impaired nervous systems and in those with passive and acquiescent personalities. The approximate ages at which the symptoms become defined are listed; they tend to persist and summate. The syndrome consequently becomes more complex and intensified as the child grows older.

Signs	Approximate Age of Appearance
Diminished interest and reactivity	12–16 weeks
Reduced integration of total behavior	12–16 weeks
Beginning retardation evidenced by *greater* disparity between exploitation in supine and sitting situations	12–16 weeks
Excessive preoccupation with strange persons	12–16 weeks
General retardation (prone motor behavior relatively unaffected)	24–28 weeks
Blandness of facial expression	24–28 weeks
Impoverished initiative	24–28 weeks
Channelization and stereotypies of behavior	24–28 weeks
Ineptness in new social situations	44–48 weeks
Exaggerated resistance to new situations	48–52 weeks
Relative retardation in language behavior	12–15 months

The term *institution* is used for descriptive convenience. Similar conditions are present in many socially disadvantaged homes where there are too many children, too little room and too little money, and where the neighbors are too close. It also is clear that a well-meaning but uninformed middle-class mother, a faultily managed, oversanitary home or a misguided, domineering babysitter or governess may create a similar set of environmental circumstances and produce the counterpart of an institutional syndrome. Fortunately, in the ordinary home, the amount of stimulation provided in infancy appears sufficient, no matter what the socioeconomic status, and development proceeds in a healthy fashion. Special programs which drive the mother of a normal child to drive her child in turn may even prove harmful. Older children who receive adequate stimulation and education attain average or above-average achievement, provided an optimum environment continues.

9

The Developmental and Behavioral Approach to the Diagnosis of Neuromotor Function

An examination of infant behavior is an examination of the central nervous system. In the preceding chapters we have shown how to use this examination to determine the maturity status of the infant. We turn now to the use of this same examination to discover the presence of lesions and disease in the neuromotor system. The developmental examination thus includes a neuromotor survey which is vitally important during infancy.

Maturational status and neuromotor status are intimately interrelated. A maturity appraisal is an essential part of a neurologic diagnosis for an infant or young child. However, a clinical distinction must be drawn between signs of chronologic immaturity in motor behavior and signs of neuromotor dysfunction. This distinction rests upon an appraisal of the child's behavior patterns; his spontaneous reactions to the demands of the test situations are the most sensitive indicators of underlying neural structure and of neuronal activity. Functional tests of behavior define the *maturity* and *integrity* of the central nervous system. The developmental approach, systematic in scope and procedure, insures a complete survey of behavioral equipment and behavioral efficiency.

A knowledge of normal neuromotor development is the basis on which detection and elucidation of abnormality rests; this chapter outlines the growth trends in normal neuromotor development. Chapters 10 and 11 discuss differential diagnosis of neuromotor dysfunction.

§1. POSTURE

Postural behavior is the most fundamental concept for interpreting the integrity of the neuromotor system and the efficiency of its operation. All coordinations, both gross and fine, imply postural adjustments, adjustments of the organism as a whole to its environs. Locomotion is a dynamic, repetitive projection of posture. Prehension and manipulation consist of closely knit series of postural adjustments. Even eyes and fingers assume postural sets.

Postural sets are neuromotor fixations by means of which the child achieves station, balance, stance, steadiness and preparatory poise. Postural set may issue in overt movement, and is itself a form of action because it requires active counterbalancing inhibitions. With complete muscular relaxation, postural set dissolves. Postural set and movement patterns are so closely related that most perceptuointegrative motor reactions should be envisaged clinically in terms of posture.

Motor behavior develops from the beginning by expansion of a total reaction system. For example, thumb opposition is a pattern of this kind. As it emerges, it also becomes incorporated into the basic postural sets which make up the total reaction system. Early in the infant's life, thumb opposition is altogether lacking. In its incipient stage it is manifested in an imperfect, sporadic manner; its execution is dependent upon a few favorable and accessory postural attitudes. Later it becomes independent of these limitations and responsive to a wide variety of postural sets. Such relative emancipation (individuation), combined with obedience to the total reaction system, marks the maturity of a growing function.

All the movement patterns of the infant are constantly undergoing developmental organization similar to that just outlined. Clinical appraisal of any motor function must take into account the developmental status of that function in relation to age and maturity. The genetic steps in the normal development of a function can be summed up as follows:

0. Prenascent stage: Complete absence of function.
1. Nascent stage: Imperfect, inadequate sporadic manifestation of the function in loose and variable associations with several postural sets.
2. Assimilative stage: More positive performance of function, which is dependent upon particular postural sets and accessory reinforcing postural attitudes.
3. Coordinating stage: Perfected performance limited to these particular postural sets, but with sloughing off of the previously necessary accessory postural attitudes.
4. Stage of synergic individuation: Independence from restricted postural sets; versatile performance smoothly synergized with numerous and varied postural sets.

These categories enable us, to differentiate normal physiologic awkwardness from neuropathologic awkwardness. The normal infant, *qua* infant, is not to be regarded as awkward. He is awkward only with respect to a very new function while it is in a nascent or assimilative stage. He has an extensive array of established functions which are executed with grace and facility. Indeed, in numerous motor skills the year-old infant already approximates the adeptness of an adult. He may be crude in digital coordination, but expert in manual manipulation; he may be crude in manual movements, but expert in eye movements. Normally he is skillful in the functions which are part and parcel of his established maturity.

Neuromotor dysfunction is not always based on sheer absence or even impairment of specific structures; it may be due to a lack of functional correlation and of synergy between structures which are relatively intact. The facile operation of the nervous system depends upon balance and counteraction between antagonistic components. For example, the function of the sympathetic division is generally antagonistic to that of the parasympathetic. Extensors are antagonistic to flexors; excessive dominance of one disturbs their normal counterpoised relationship and produces neuromotor symptoms. Bilateral, unilateral, ipsilateral and contralateral members must be brought into parallel and diagonal coordination. This is accomplished through a kind of cross-stitching or reciprocal interweaving in the structural growth of the networks of the nervous system. Disturbance of the regulative growth factors or damage to the normal lines of communication in these networks produces asynergies and disharmonies which constitute an important group of neuromotor symptoms. Excessive individuation of behavior patterns accounts for yet another group of symptoms, some of which are not neuromotor abnormalities but rather stereotypies that may reach a psychiatric level in compulsive action.

The organization of an infant's perceptuointegrative motor behavior—that is, his integrated total pattern—proceeds from head to foot. He does not develop on an installment plan, but always by expansion of a unitary reaction system. It is neither a homogeneous balloonlike expansion nor a hierarchical stratification, but rather a process of reincorporation and consolidation with progressive corticalization. The neurologic result is an interwoven structured texture which expresses itself in progressive patterns of behavior.

§2. THE DEVELOPMENTAL ORGANIZATION OF NORMAL NEUROMOTOR PATTERNS

The following outline of the progressive organization of neuromotor functions is concerned with functional mechanisms and relationships, and with the neurodevelopmental significance of perceptuointegrative motor patterns. This survey of normal neuromotor organization serves to explain the nature of abnormal neuromotor signs and symptoms.

Head

The newborn infant may display considerable rotary head activity in the supine position. However, the predominating spontaneously assumed position of the head is rotation to one side. This position evokes the tonic-neck-reflex (t-n-r) posture of the arms. At about 16 weeks, spontaneous midpositions of the head predominate, with related symmetric arm postures and activities. Even at earlier ages, the hands come together, or the arms abduct symmetrically, if the head is placed in the midline. In the supported sitting position, hand engagement tends to be more prominent. Similarly, the t-n-r position disappears earlier in sitting than in supine, because shift to symmetrotonic postures is imposed by the midposition of the head when the trunk is erect. By 24 weeks head and arm postures have become relatively dissociated. The infant can turn his head without altering arm attitudes, and he can use his arms asymmetrically with his head in midposition.

Erection of the head against the forces of gravity requires coordinations, tonal distributions and sustaining powers that the newborn lacks. The first head liftings are fleeting and wobbly and require bracing of the back—as when the infant is held at the shoulder—or a favorable prone position for employing the extensors of both back and neck. The wobbling and plunging of the head, with only momentary erection, is superseded by more sustained erection with fine rhythmic nodding or bobbing (12 weeks). At 16 weeks accessory neck muscles are brought into play to assist the extensors, and a steady, erect but slightly forward position can be maintained. Rotation of the head in this position may disturb the newly acquired equilibrium, so that the head may plunge. By 20 weeks the head can be maintained freely erect, and can be rotated freely. Maintenance of head station is fully established; it has become more or less effortless and automatic. (Head control in prone is discussed under Creeping, later in this chapter.)

Although the head moves, the behavior described so far is essentially static. Body movement, such as pull-to-sitting, upsets the still precarious balance. The complete head lag evident in the newborn period gradually disappears, concomitant with the achievement of head station, but slight lag is still present at 16 weeks. Not until 20 weeks, at the time the head is held in line with the body in sitting, does the infant maintain this alignment when he is translocated to a sitting position. At 24 weeks he starts to lift his head and assists, simultaneously flexing his elbows, as soon as the pull on his arms begins. By 28 weeks the muscles of the neck have reached their adult capacity to erect and steady the head; the infant lifts his head independently from a supine position, foreshadowing attainment of the sitting position.

Persistence of head sagging is easy to recognize, but one must appreciate that the normal progression of control is from forward sagging to erect and steady. An infant who holds his head erect, in line with his body but still unsteadily, or one who retracts and pushes backwards, is abnormal. Increased extensor tone of the neck muscles is responsible.

Eyes

Ocular fixation, perception and pursuit are readily observed in the dangling ring situation and in all situations which bring the eyes into requisition. Fixation and perception are at best vague in the newborn, and ocular pursuit is fleeting. As a rule, objects are unperceived unless directly in the infant's line of vision; then they must be moving, massive or must offer a distinct contrast to the surroundings. When left alone, the newborn infant is particularly prone to stare vaguely at lights and light masses such as windows.

Looking, as distinct from reflex pupillary responses to light, is one of the earliest evidences of cortical activity. It can also be elicited by moving a series of lines of different widths and spacing across the infant's visual field, observing eye following or the opticokinetic nystagmus which accompanies following; a gross measure of visual acuity is obtained in this fashion. Failure to elicit looking does not necessarily denote abnormality, but its consistent absence raises high the suspicion of blindness, mental deficiency or other neurologic deficit. The presence of looking generally is an indication that intellectual potential is intact; the progressions of visual organization expected to follow at succceeding ages are definable.

Definite fixation, with convergence, focus and shifting of focus, begins to appear at about 8 weeks of age. Overconvergence (strabismus) is frequent at this age, because the ocular muscles are still used discoordinately. Visual following of a moving object is jerky; the eyes move too slowly to keep up, or move faster than the object, so frequently the object is lost. However, the infant is extremely alert to moving objects. By 12–16 weeks convergence and focusing are fairly accurately performed, and following is smooth and well coordinated. Macular acuity is well enough developed so that an object as small as a pellet is perceived and may be inspected with absorbed interest. By 24 weeks the child has sufficient voluntary command of eye muscles to maintain fixation on a stationary object, even in the presence of a competing moving stimulus such as the examiner's withdrawing hand.

After this mastery of the basic ocular movements, eye behavior is closely bound up with the development of visual perception. By progressive stages the infant learns to identify forms, and to associate the visual experience of objects with the visual experience of representations of objects (15–18 months). It usually takes 5 more years of maturation and experience before he is ready to discriminate word symbols for objects and to follow, with comprehension, a whole procession of such symbols across the printed page. These achievements are based on postural adjustments involving eyes, head and hands.

Mouth

In the normal newborn, sucking and swallowing usually are well developed; however, without reinforcement, when spoon or cup feeding is instituted from the start, sucking ability is lost. Even swallowing needs to be relearned if a gastrostomy is indicated for medical reasons and there is no practice. Early awkwardness in feeding shows itself in precipitate sucking, before the nipple is in the mouth, so that the tongue cleaves to the palate; drawing the lower lip in with the nipple; imperfect approximation of the lips with leaking from the corners of the mouth; inability to release a deflated rubber nipple; occasional choking; and considerable air swallowing during feeding.

By 16 weeks the infant opens his mouth adaptively and awaits insertion of the nipple; he closes his lips securely about it and permits a collapsed rubber nipple to reinflate.

When semisolid foods are first offered, sucking movements of the tongue are initiated with elevation of the posterior part of the tongue; the food is ejected with the tongue in pursuit. The infant may choke on food that reaches the pharynx. By 28 weeks coordination of tongue and pharynx has advanced so that these retrussive movements disappear, and there is no further difficulty in handling pureed food. At this same age the infant begins to coordinate his feeding performance with his nascent capacity to sit and to grasp.

By 32 weeks, biting begins to replace mouthing in the child's exploitive play as well as in feeding situations. By 36 weeks he can bite off a piece of cracker, munch and swallow it in a sophisticated manner. Air swallowing has ceased to cause any difficulties. Control of salivary overflow begins to improve at 40 weeks, with increased tonicity and command of lips, tongue and jaws, so that drooling practically disappears by the end of the first year. By 40–44 weeks the infant begins to drink milk from a cup.

The mouth also functions as a prehensory organ, a third hand, in the first year of life. Mouth-reaching is used as a substitutive pattern in the presence of motor handicap of the arms; otherwise, oral patterns become restricted to the feeding situation at about one year: toys and hands, except when thumb sucking is a persistent pattern, go less frequently to the mouth.

By 18 months, with the acquisition of well-defined chewing, oral patterns are fairly well differentiated and coordinated. The child needs only to integrate these patterns with his manual–adaptive behavior, self-feeding, and with social requirements—that is, table manners.

Arms and Hands

Prehensory approach is observed readily in numerous situations in which objects are offered within the child's reach, in both supine and sitting positions. Reaching responses make their first appearance in the normal infant at about the age of 16 weeks. They are then poorly differentiated, poorly coordinated and poorly directed. Both arms become active, but are as likely to be withdrawn or to extend laterally as to approach the midline; if the midline is approached, flexion is apt to be so predominant that the hands come to the mouth and lack the necessary extension to reach out toward the object. The sitting position reveals the tendency of the whole body to be involved in the response, so that forward leaning of head and trunk, projection of lips and tongue, eye widening and flexion of the legs accompany the arm activity. Sitting at this age may place the child in such an unaccustomed position in relation to the forces of gravity that he may be unable to release the approach mechanisms which he displays in the supine position.

With increasing age and perfection of central control, approach becomes prompter, better differentiated, more smoothly performed and directed. At 20 weeks both arms approach objects in the midline. At 24 weeks this bilateral approach and prehensory appropriation (grasp) are synthesized with visual perception in a coordinated movement. By 28 weeks one arm leads in approach, the movements of the other being partly or completely suppressed. Handedness as such does not appear until much later, and clear preference for one hand in the first 18 months of life frequently indicates overt or subtle impairment in the peripheral or central control of the other hand. As many as 30% of infants without neuromotor impairment still show ambidexterity at 3 years of age, and there is some evidence that completely integrated dominance does not occur until 8 or 9 years of age.

The reasons for the clear preponderance of right-handedness, the close association of the speech and language centers with hand dominance and the time when the association occurs in the developmental cycle are not clear. Man probably is the animal with clearest hand preference relatively early in life, in the absence of neurologic impairment. Persistent ambidexterity, failure to develop timely hand dominance and left-handedness have been associated with low birth weight and complications of pregnancy; all may be the result of brain dysfunction. However, an open mind must be maintained about the influence of cultural pressures and environmental influences; as any left-handed person will tell you, it is functionally a right-handed world.

Grasping also goes through numerous well-defined stages. The neonatal hand is closed. The first requisite for grasp is an open hand (12 weeks); the hand then must close around the object and maintain that closure. This act requires coordinated interaction between flexors and extensors. Active grasp of an object placed in the hand at 12 weeks is evidenced either by the infant's lifting it off the supporting crib surface or by whitening of his knuckles as the hand closes. Automatic opening and closing of the fingers is present until the appropriate inhibition of one muscle group is achieved, at 24 weeks, so that top-heavy objects such as a rattle fall from the hand, even in supine. In sitting, a placed object is retained precariously and often at the ulnar side of the palm; grasp may occur as the hand contacts the object (20 weeks). From this age on, the term grasp denotes prehension—the integration of visual perception, approach and seizure with retention into a single coordinated movement. The first specialization of the radial digits which occurs is demonstrated best with an object such as a cube. Early grasping at 24 weeks is whole-handed or palmar, and even includes flexion of the wrist. Grasp then shifts to the radial side of the hand (radial palmar at 28 weeks), and later becomes a function of fingers rather than hand, as an adult pattern appears—a free space between the object and the palm (radial digital at 36 weeks).

Initially, digital differentiation occurs with larger objects; special development of thumb and index finger for fine prehension of smaller objects then parallels and overlaps this earlier progression. At 28 weeks the infant contacts a pellet with his whole hand or rakes at it with fingers outstretched, with concomitant movement of the entire arm. At 32 weeks radial specialization for smaller objects has begun. The hand is used less as a paw as the infant attempts to grasp the pellet by raking with the thumb and two radial digits. The fingers are still relatively extended; the thumb shows rudimentary opposition as it is adducted against the curling four digits in an inferior scissors grasp, which occasionally is successful; arm movement has almost disappeared. At 36 weeks the ulnar digits become completely suppressed in pellet prehension, but the infant still does not use the ends of his fingers. He has a scissors grasp of the pellet—acquisition between the side of the curled index finger and the thumb. At 40 weeks the pellet is plucked promptly between the *ventral* surfaces of thumb and index finger, but not perfectly. The grasp is an *inferior* pincer grasp because the infant must rest his arm on the table for stability. Not until 48 weeks does he have enough facility to use a *neat* pincer grasp. Accessory arm support no longer is needed; the pellet is approached from above and is prehended promptly and precisely between the fingertips. Adult man is not capable of a more refined grasp on an object of this size.

Release is more mature than grasping. When release first appears, it is inextricably bound to simultaneous grasp by the other hand, evidenced by transfer, and by the dropping of a cube held in one hand as the other goes out to pick up a second cube. When transfer begins, the second hand approaches the held cube and pulls it jerkily out of the first, or else transfer is two-stage, the mouth or table top being used as an intermediate way-station. Maturation occurs rapidly; at 28 weeks there is simultaneous release by one hand as the other grasps the cube, and the cube is shuttled back and forth adeptly. By 32 weeks there is the first inhibition of the simultaneous grasp and release pattern: the infant picks up and holds the first and then the second cube, but the inhibitory aspects are so strong that he is unable to drop one of these cubes to pick up a third. At 36 weeks, the first volitional dropping occurs; however, dropping cannot be called release until control is achieved. Release normally appears in the last quarter of the first year, when at 40 weeks the infant puts the cube down and then removes his hand from it.

In succeeding months, release becomes more precise, better timed, and combined with grasp, exploitation and placement; the child releases at the correct moment in the correct place. At 44 weeks the confines of a cup inhibit release; at 52 weeks he releases a cube inside the cup. At 52 weeks, when he tries to build a tower of two cubes, he pushes too hard or releases too soon, and his tower falls. Similarly, the smaller pellet usually falls outside the narrow confines of the bottle neck. By 15 months all the complexities are sufficiently integrated so that both these tasks are accomplished: the tower of two stands; the pellet goes into the bottle. At 18 months he can release a cube in fair alignment on top of a tower of two or three cubes he has built, without knocking down the tower; however, it is another 18 months before he can stack ten 1-inch cubes. When manual release is well coordinated with arm movements, projected placement and throwing with some accuracy of aim is possible. Release also must be integrated with stance and postural attitude. A 15-month child cannot throw a ball without falling down; he sits to throw. Not until 18 months can he throw a ball from a standing position.

Finesse and diversity in manipulation depend on maturational factors, and on the integrity of neuromotor equipment. Early manipulatory patterns are simple and somewhat clumsily executed. Manual exploitation goes through rapid, successive cumulative stages of development: simple regard for an object in hand, mouthing, shaking, banging, transfer from hand to hand, matching of two objects, putting one object into another, putting one object on another, aligning objects, fitting objects together and other more elaborate combinations. All these acts have an adaptive significance, but the neuromotor elements are of equal importance. Precise manipulations of increasing complexity require coordinations of increasing precision and complexity. With each new function the child shows the newness by awkwardness in execution; with the integration of each new function into the action pattern system, the child shows facility and expertness.

Trunk, Legs and Feet

We have traced the organization of arm and hand activities in the development of their specialized functions of prehension and manipulation. Trunk, legs and feet also have specialized functions—those of body posture and locomotion. The ultimate goal of their development is independent bipedal walking in an upright position. This is the framework on which all more complex gross motor skills such as running, climbing, skipping, skating, bicycle riding and dancing depend.

Development in the human infant is orderly; however, it is not necessarily so orderly that he achieves one function in its perfection and then develops another which he appends to the first. Two functions which are to be integrated tend to develop almost simultaneously, at first apparently unrelated to each other, first one and then the other taking lead or precedence. They seem to weave in and about each other as they develop, until they finally merge, synergize and coordinate; it is a reciprocal interweaving. So it is with the development of upright posture and locomotion.

Achievement of erect head station is the first step in the assumption of upright posture. In broad outline, the succeeding steps are sitting, crawling, creeping, standing and finally walking, first with support of decreasing degrees and then independently.

Sitting. At the earliest ages, the trunk and legs are passive in the supported sitting position: the back is bowed, and the legs flexed. By 16 weeks the infant holds his head erect, though not perfectly so, and he begins to evince some pleasure in propped sitting. At this same time both thoracic and cervical spines participate actively in the erect posture; only the lumbar region is bowed passively. By 28 weeks the infant lifts his head spontaneously from the supine position as though straining to sit. Also by 28 weeks he maintains the passive sitting position on a hard surface for a brief period, without outside support. He sits on an ample diamond-shaped base with his legs widely abducted, knees flexed and resting on the surface for lateral support, leaning forward to insure anteroposterior balance and using his hands as accessory forward props. This is not sitting alone; he cannot use his arms for manipulation at the same time, although he may sit erect momentarily. He increases the amount of time that he can sit alone and, lifting his arms, begins to master forward balance. Sitting erect but unsteady, with a straight back, he maintains the posture for about 1 minute at 32 weeks and ventures into the problem of backward balance. Before he has mastered the art, he may fall backwards, but at 36 weeks he sits steadily for approximately 10 minutes, leans forward and reerects without having to push himself back up stepwise with his arms. With the acquisition of anteroposterior balance, he begins to narrow his sitting base. At 40 weeks, when he has achieved lateral balance relatively independent of leg posture, he is a free and able sitter, and both hands can be used in play. This is *sitting alone.* He leans forward and turns to the side within his sitting posture; he hitches or moves about within that posture. The hands and arms have been freed for manipulatory duty, and eyes have been elevated to a commanding position. By 48 weeks he can pivot, using only his legs.

Creeping. The progressive patterns of postural attitude and activity which the infant displays in the prone position may be regarded properly as stages in the development of locomotion. Over a score of such stages have been identified for the entire ontogenetic sequence, and they illustrate clearly the principle of reciprocal interweaving. There are stages in which flexor components predominate, and others in which extensor components are more prominent.

The cephalocaudad and integrative trends in the development of prone posture merit notice. In the earliest weeks the infant is helpless, peculiarly so in the prone position. Because head and arm responses are so poorly developed, with the head barely clearing the crib, the arms flexed under the chest and the hips high, he tends to pitch forward on his head. The legs are comparatively free and engage in reflexive, alternating crawling movements. As the hips begin to lower, head lifting in prone becomes possible, at first recurrently to 45° at 8 weeks, and then sustainedly at 12 weeks; by 12 weeks there also is control of its return to the crib surface, and the arms no longer are tucked under the chest. As long as the hips are high, head lifting in prone is difficult or impossible, but by 16 weeks the legs are fully extended, if still relatively passive; elevation of the head and upper chest is well developed and the infant looks straight ahead at a 90° angle. As one arm extends fully at the elbow, it throws him off balance, rolling him passively to the supine position. By 20 weeks he props up on his fully extended arms, rearing his head and chest well above the supporting surface. At 24 weeks he can roll from the supine into the prone position with considerable agility, getting both arms out from under himself. This is the child's first successful voluntary change of positional orientation. When his body is fully supported in the supine position, the legs are active as he lifts them high enough in extension to see or grasp his feet; by 28 weeks he puts his feet into his mouth.

The first attempts at coordination of both arms and legs in the prone position to produce movement appear at 28 weeks; they are symmetric and simultaneously executed, producing swimming movements which are ineffectual for translocation. By 32 weeks, alternating coordinated flexions and extensions of the arms as they cross each other, with the legs essentially passive, result in effective circular pivoting. This is the first successful voluntary change of position that requires alternating coordinations. *Crawling,* i.e., dragging the body along the supporting surface by coordinated action of arms and legs, develops directly from pivoting.

Finally the trunk is elevated, and the infant assumes the *creeping* position, at 36 weeks. At first he must maintain a static posture of all four extremities simply to hold this position; any movement results in ignominious collapse. By 40 weeks he has combined his alternating coordinations with mastery of balance, and he creeps on hands and knees. He progresses so long as trunk and extremities give each other mutual support in the quadrupedal position. At the same time, he integrates his prone and sitting abilities; he can go directly forward into prone from the sitting position, creep expertly and then sit up again. He can now move about under his own power, take himself where he wishes to go, pursue and secure remote objects. He also shows a tendency by 52 weeks to creep on hands and soles, instead of hands and knees. This plantigrade stance is the final transition to upright posture. It puts him in a position to stand erect and to walk on two feet. A small proportion of infants never creep, or walk on palms and soles. Some hitch along in a sitting position; others fail to develop the alternating coordinations and progress by "frogging," using all four extremities simultaneously. Whether these patterns represent abnormalities in motor control or normal variations depends on the presence or absence of associated disturbances in coordination, particularly in fine motor control. A few infants omit quadrupedal progression entirely and go directly to the upright posture.

Standing and walking. Neonatal stepping and placing responses are reflex acts mediated by the spinal cord and lower centers, and have little relationship to cortical control. The earliest voluntary response to a supported standing position is seen at 12 weeks, when there is some active leg extension, with brief partial assumption of weight, and repeated lifting of one foot. An infant's shoulder girdle muscles· are generally strong enough by 16 weeks to prevent him from slipping through the examiner's hands placed in the armpits, but the legs tend to be passive in the upright position. The base is wide, the hips are more or less flexed and the knees hyperextended. Not until 28 weeks does an infant assume any large fraction of his weight when he is held firmly around the chest. He delights in this new ability and exercises it by active bouncing; when his hips and knees relax, he extends his legs with an active thrust against the supporting surface. The hips are now in the normal extended position, the knees no longer need to be locked in hyperextension and are held slightly flexed, and the base has narrowed considerably. By 32 weeks he tends to maintain active extension of the legs, hips and trunk; posture is sufficiently stabilized so that he can stand briefly, supported only by the hands, held at shoulder height for balance. In another 4 weeks he uses his own hands to maintain this posture, and can stand holding onto the railing of his crib or playpen without leaning his chest against it. This is the assimilative stage—a rigid fixed posture can be held, but not assumed, with accessory use of the arms. Movement is incompatible with maintenance of posture, but the child is experimenting with and developing balance.

The shift to a dynamic erect posture is made at 40 weeks. Balance and control have been sufficiently incorporated into standing so that the infant can coordinate it with his newly acquired ability to sit. By combined alternating integrated coordinations of arms and legs, he both pushes and pulls himself to a standing position, still holding on, and he can lower himself again.

Independent, coordinate action of the legs, combined with maintenance of the upright posture and balance, is yet to be achieved. At 44 weeks he begins to lift and replace one foot. By 48 weeks he can walk when both hands are held just to provide balance, with coordinated, alternating leg action and some forward drive. He can also cruise, walking sideways, abducting one leg, bringing the other to it, shifting first one and then the other hand at the same time. In this manner the infant walks about his crib, playpen, and furniture in the room. By 52 weeks he is so versed that he prefers to have only one hand supported when he walks, leaving the other free to carry, reach and touch. At 56 weeks he "forgets" to hold on as he stands in his playpen, and he stands alone briefly.

The infant now is ready to walk. His first independent steps are propulsive; he lunges forward a few steps into his mother's arms. By 15 months he can rise to his feet independently, assume his wide stance, toddle about, stop and start again. Only this is truly *independent walking*. Posture and gait are somewhat rigid and easily upset; and he falls by sitting down suddenly rather than falling headlong. Further progressive stages entail acquisition of smoothness, speed and versatility. Rigidity, propulsiveness, awkwardness, falling and wide stance gradually disappear as function is perfected. Running first appears at 2 years; at this same age the child can kick a ball by swinging his foot against it without capsizing. He is 3 years old before he can stand on one foot even momentarily.

Walking can be retarded by bad falls or by sickness, and it can be accelerated a little by practice and training; however, the normal child does not need to be taught to walk. We provide him opportunity and he learns. The problem with a normal infant is not how to get him to move about, but how to stop him from combining his mobility with his curiosity about his environment in ways that are physically dangerous for him.

Sphincters

Excretory functions are controlled by a complex combination of voluntary and involuntary mechanisms. Action of the sympathetic nervous system involuntarily maintains the urethral and anal sphincters in tonic contraction when bladder and bowel are empty or only partially filled. When a certain threshold in bowel or bladder content is reached—varying greatly from individual to individual and in a given individual under different conditions—the sphincter relaxes and the smooth muscle of the wall of the bladder or bowel contracts, expelling the contents. Expulsion may be complete or partial, again depending on stimulus thresholds. This is the basic excretory mechanism upon which voluntary action under cerebrospinal control is superimposed. In the early weeks and months of life, it is essentially the only mechanism in operation, although even in this stage accessory voluntary muscles may be called into play to assist in the act of expulsion.

In order to be completely "toilet trained," the child must: consciously associate the excretory act with certain internal sensations, with a particular and appropriate place, and with certain words; voluntarily inhibit relaxation of the sphincters, and terminate that inhibition (release) voluntarily; verbalize or otherwise indicate the need; differentiate between stimuli from bladder and bowel and inhibit or release the appropriate sphincter; and foresee sufficiently the urge to urinate or defecate—a formidable series of tasks, the complexities of which are not always appreciated.

The successful early toilet training about which some mothers boast depends upon a conditioning process in which the child makes a very simple association between toilet seat and toilet need. The association is of such a nature that an impending excretion is released more or less promptly by the stimulus of the toilet seat; if excretion is impending and no toilet seat is provided, events take their natural course; if excretion is not impending, no results ensue from the stimulus of the toilet seat. The "success" is highly dependent on the mother's timing of the toilet seat stimulus, and on a large preponderance of positive associations (full organ plus toilet seat) as opposed to negative associations (full organ minus toilet seat, or empty organ plus toilet seat). Such associations may break down easily under slight alterations in conditions: an illness, a different bathroom, conflicting activities—the development of walking, a new baby sitter or a cold day—may disrupt the conditioned association. Also, so many negative reactions may be built up by overzealous training as to establish a negative association: the toilet seat inhibits.

If a positive association is established at a favorable period in development (around 15 months of age, the same time that precise release of cube and pellet has been achieved), the child may himself take the next step, which involves inhibiting release until the proper conditions are established for release—i.e., waiting with a full organ a reasonable length of time until the toilet seat is provided. At the same time, he may begin to form new associations between excretion and a general word (18—21 months). The word is first applied to the products after excretion, then to the process as it occurs; only after a long developmental process can it be applied to the internal sensations which precede the act. As this is accomplished, the child "tells" (24 months). First he tells after he has acted, then as he acts, then before he acts (but not soon enough) and finally he tells in good time.

Reciprocal interweaving is occurring all the time in the development of these functions as it always does when antagonistic components are involved. At times *inhibition* takes the upper hand; then the child withholds valiantly as long as he can, and is unable to release at will. Then *release* mechanisms are dominant, and the ability to inhibit is overpowered. This is another example of physiologic awkwardness due to immature coordinations.

When positive associations between excretory need, toilet and word have been well established, time relations have been worked out and mastered, and differentiations have been made between bowel and bladder urgencies, the child still must coordinate these abilities with a mastery of impeding clothes. At 3 years he begins to free himself from dependence on adult help and reminders, and from ideal and specific conditions. At about the same time he acquires an ability to maintain inhibition of release during sleep, and to respond to the stimulus of a full bladder during sleep by awakening rather than by releasing; however, as many as one-third of normal children still are not dry at night at age 3.

All these aspects of sphincter control are slowly acquired; lapses may occur at any time before coordinations are completely and permanently established, by 6–7 years. In fact, check and countercheck—progress, lapse, progress again with breaks in the mechanism reinforced and strengthened, lapse in a new direction, progress with new reinforcements, etc.—is the way in which a strong, durable pattern is developed. The final pattern is fairly proof against mishap.

Ears and Larynx

In the neonatal period an infant responds with startling or crying to loud sudden noises such as the ringing of the telephone, the slamming of a door or the backfiring of a car. Listening, as distinct from startling or an eyelid blink, is the only evidence of cortical intactness other than looking which can be evaluated in the neonatal period. It is perhaps less definitively elicited than visual pursuit, but can be recognized by immobilization or diminution of activity in response to a bell rung or a rattle shaken close to the ear. By 6 or 7 weeks of age the infant accepts, more or less, the cacophony of the civilized world, or at least noise no longer violently disturbs his tonal or emotional equilibrium. He listens to sounds about him and displays transient auditory attention by immobilization. By 24 weeks of age he locates sound with considerable accuracy, turning his head appropriately. He may respond at first only if a toy with which he is playing is removed, or only to the relatively loud sound (60 db) of a bell, but he learns to divide his attention. By 32 weeks clear responses to high and low pitched, and soft and loud sounds can be obtained, even when his attention is directed elsewhere.

The vocal apparatus develops slowly but progressively. The earliest sounds an infant makes are no more than squeaks or mews. By 8 weeks some of the middle vowel sounds like "ah-eh-uh" are enunciated, and by 16 weeks expressive laughter is well differentiated. Pitch is modified first as squeals and crows of high tones at 20 weeks of age; grunts and growls of guttural quality follow (24 weeks). By 28 weeks control of the lips modifies the air stream, and the consonant "m-m" is heard, chiefly in association with crying. As larynx and vocal cords are controlled, clear single syllables, combining consonant and vowel, are heard by 32 weeks, and the doubling of syllables ("da-da") emerges by 36 weeks. The first evidences of verbal comprehension usually appear at the same time, when the infant responds correctly to his name, to "no-no," and to "come" accompanied by a gesture. Deliberate imitation of sounds—cough, click, razz—also appears first at 36 weeks, a critical age in the development of speech.

Emergence of speech depends on reinforcement of the infant's spontaneous vocalizations by others. "Da-Da" acquires meaning when his parents exclaim "Look, he said daddy." The infant acquires his first word, the association of a definite articulated sound with a particular object, person or action, at 40 weeks. It is not surprising that this first word may not sound much like an adult word, or that its associations may be loose and variable. "Baa-baa" perhaps may mean bottle, food, eating and even kitchen. Many more months are required to develop the necessary association between the sound of the thing and the thing itself, and to make both associations and differentiations.

The jargon stage (13—24 months) is the period when a matrix for connected speech is laid down. Fluency and variety of sound combinations are developed into an incomprehensible language, more or less free floating and nonutilitarian, because adults do not understand it. Out of that matrix, words (15—18 months) and phrases (21 months) crystallize. Words become tools: language burgeons rapidly; vocabulary increases apace; utilization expands to include past and future, the absent and finally the abstract. Even so, not until $4\frac{1}{2}$ years do most infantile pronunciations disappear. Many more years are required to develop the necessary neuromotor skill to articulate correctly and accurately, with ease and diversity.

Attentional Sets

Attention is the integrated expression of psychomotor set. Patterns of attention depend on: age and maturity; absent acute or chronic illness; special individual interests; and visual, auditory and experiential factors—the novel experience commanding attention by virtue of its very novelty. Attention shows great individual variation, in terms of the ease or difficulty with which it is elicited, its incisiveness or vagueness, and its sustained character or its brevity. However, many of these qualities are dependent on *temperament*—a confusing term to describe the organization of the central nervous system characteristic for a particular individual. To describe an attentional pattern as "long" or "vague" tells little of its quality or maturity.

Even in the neonatal period, an infant is attentive at times. At this age he shows his attention by brief immobilizations, assuming a listening postural set. His own internal sensations interest him when they are pleasant, and there is little doubt about them when they are unpleasant. Sights and sounds that impinge upon him, if not immoderate, interest him and he quiets to attend them.

By 6–8 weeks, nearby moving objects begin to catch his eye and evoke his attention. He follows moving persons and every now and then catches sight of his own hand. He begins to inspect objects that are within his near range of vision: an animated face, a toy hung on his carriage. His attentions are brief but unmistakable. By virtue of his beginning head and eye control, he seeks new visual experience.

The acquisition of the erect head station at 12–16 weeks and the beginning of propped sitting provide new postural sensations and orientations, and attention at this time tends to be more definite. In the examination situation, however, attention to the examination materials may be somewhat difficult to elicit, partly because of immature head and eye coordinations, and partly because his attention is directed more readily to larger and moving objects, and hence to people.

As head–eye control advances, the infant's visual range increases and his interests widen. Simultaneously, prehensory powers dawn. He spies things promptly and expertly as they are presented on the table, and they become things to encompass, hold and feel. By 28 weeks his hands are so obedient that they grasp and hold objects and bring them to his mouth. Everything within reach excites his interest and invites grasping, feeling and mouthing. He is accustomed to the sitting position. In the examining situation his attention is prompt and tenacious; it is highly channelized and limited to the object immediately in front of him.

His first attentions are chiefly internal; then they become more external, but diffuse, relatively undifferentiated and lacking versatility. By the end of the 1st half-year they become selective, though they are still very restricted. He gives sustained attention to one object; if a second object is presented, he attends one to the exclusion of the other, or he may attend the two objects alternately. By 40 weeks, three or more objects can be "kept in mind" simultaneously; the infant can attend a large and a small object at the same time, with special interest in the small. The scope of his attention widens to include the whole tabletop, instead of just the circumscribed area immediately before him.

In the last quarter of the 1st year, the infant can attend to the examiner or to his mother without losing track of his play objects; he also traces objects from their source and to their destination. He exploits the undersurface of the table, the inside of the cup, the crib rails, and the shade over the mirror behind him. He seems aware of the whole room and everything in it, and he can choose what he will attend to. Throughout the whole latter half of the 1st year, the infant's attentions are consistent, durable and related to immediate objects and events, but the scope of attention continually expands in space.

With the acquisition of walking, attention shifts become more rapid and diversified. Attention, as well as posture, no longer is sedentary. It shifts from one interest to another; it is deflected by almost every intervening object or occurrence. In fact, diversion seems to be the most outstanding quality of the attention of the 18-month child. He appears to be led here and there by the immediacy of his shifting interests and by his impacts against the world about him. His whole attentional complex is in a transitional but constructive stage of unstable equilibrium. The ability to maintain an objective, while surmounting an intervening obstacle to that objective, begins to appear shortly after 18 months. This projection of attention into the immediate future is the first real conquest of time—space barriers. Further conquests are made possible by elaboration of his language powers.

In summary, recognition of the relationships between chronologic age and functional integration is the key to differential diagnosis of neuromotor dysfunction.

10

Neuromotor Dysfunction

The development of the different functional areas has been traced because an understanding of normal developmental processes is essential to the diagnosis of sensory and motor deviations. As a function develops, it goes through various stages, and is correlated with other functions. Normal development is dependent upon an intact organism; disease, defects or damage that impair the integrity of the organism deflect the normal currents of development.

In this chapter, it is not our purpose to describe all the neuromotor diseases, defects and insults that may befall an infant, but to show how the developmental examination establishes integrity or exposes dysfunctions and faults. Abnormal behavior patterns are interpreted in terms of functional developmental stage, integration with other functions and equipment with which to perform that function.

§1. DIAGNOSIS OF NEUROMOTOR DYSFUNCTION

Normal equipment includes normal developmental potentials, receptors and effectors. Loss or impairment of vision, hearing, touch or proprioception, the most important receptors, may interfere seriously with acquisition and integration of experience, and with development of appropriate responsive behavior. An infant cannot develop normal responses to things he cannot see, hear or feel. Loss or impairment of movement or speech, the two most important effectors, precludes normal responsive behavior and thus may interfere with the acquisition of adequate experience. This does not mean that responsive, age-appropriate behavior is never developed by handicapped individuals, for it is. However, it is not developed with normal ease, or through normal channels, and it is not fully normal behavior in its organization.

It is axiomatic that it is easier to exercise a skill than to acquire it. An adult has acquired his motor functions; he exercises his skills. A superimposed motor disability impairs motor function, but it does not necessarily abolish previously acquired skills. A man may still walk without much difficulty after losing the proper use of several muscle groups normally used in walking. In infancy the problem is a little different. In this period, motor functions are in the process of development, and functions are being integrated into skills. Motor disability not only impairs motor function, as it does in the adult, but it also impairs the infant's ability to develop motor functions. The infant is under a double handicap: the handicap to function imposed by the disability, and the handicap which the disability imposes on learning the function. A disability which merely affects an adult's gait may delay the acquisition of walking in a young child for years.

Thus, motor handicaps in infancy greatly increase the difficulty of acquiring a skill; they greatly increase the length of time needed to acquire a skill; and they exaggerate the awkwardness displayed in the nascent and assimilative stages of the development of a skill. These facts make motor handicaps readily apparent in infancy; their recognition is the first step in diagnosis.

In essence, the developmental examination is a series of functional tests. Fortunately, the infant is so constituted that, although he cannot respond to verbal commands, motor performance can be elicited easily. Positional change, lures and toys, and his own visible spontaneous activity induce him to resist the forces of gravity. He does this if he can—reflexly at an early age, voluntarily later. We induce him to reach, lift and hold, by offering him a plaything. The examination tests the infant's power to turn his head, lift his head, open and close his mouth, move his eyes, brace his shoulders, move his arms in various planes, grasp objects, sit erect, move his legs freely and assume weight support. We expect him to perform in all positions—supine, prone, sitting, standing—that we would evaluate appropriately for his age. We also investigate his ability to swallow, chew, articulate and control his sphincters. Finally, we compare the ability of the child with the normal motor behavior appropriate for his level of maturity.

In infants and young children the signs and symptoms of nervous system disease tend to be diffuse rather than localized. Classic neurologic syndromes may be approximated, but because the lesion or defect occurs in a developing organ—in the germinal, embryonic, circumnatal or postnatal period—the pathology tends to be widespread, even when visible damage is not gross. As a rule, lesions are not limited to the internal capsule, or neatly located in the sphenoidal fissure. Few hemiplegias in children are true hemiplegias; usually both sides of the body are involved, one more seriously than the other. It is perhaps more important to recognize the diffuseness of the lesion than its limits. This diffuseness accounts for the injuries to intellect and personality that so often accompany impairment of the neuromotor system. Intelligence and personality are not localized in any single gyrus or lobe; they both are mediated by the entire cerebrum.

Neuromotor impairments, whether mild or severe, local or general, transient or permanent, express themselves by *reduction* or *disorder* of motor performance. On the other hand, simple motor *retardation* implies a performance normal in quality, and abnormal only in terms of age. A careful distinction must be made between reduction and disorder in function and retardation in function, even when, as is usually the case, they appear in combination. This distinction is discussed in detail in the two following sections and in Chapter 11.

The examination of a child with motor disabilities always presents practical problems, and requires infinite patience. It demands ingenuity in adapting the situations to fit the child, and alertness to his use of substitutive patterns of behavior. It involves the provision of accessory postural aids for successful performance—holding his head firmly supported, lifting his arm to place his hands in a favorable position for prehension, providing adequate sitting support and even presenting the tabletop situations on the crib platform while he is in a reclining position—in order to differentiate as precisely as possible motor disability from intellectual defect. Rest periods during which the child is permitted to lie back often permit him to renew his attack on the examination with revived zeal and interest.

Often it is difficult to distinguish between a performance which fails for mechanical reasons and one which fails from lack of insight and maturity. Is the child with "cerebral palsy" who fails to build a tower of six cubes too handicapped to place his cubes accurately, or does he lack the fundamental maturity to make such a structure? Is his inability to imitate a stroke due to manual incoordination or to mental deficiency? We can hardly expect a severely hemiplegic infant to transfer a toy from hand to hand. The interpretation of each performance must rest upon its own merits. Evidences of insight or of effort should not be overlooked; some children will not even attempt a task when it is clearly beyond their capacities. The examiner should offer as much assistance as the child will accept, encourage effort and even reward effort deliberately by simulating success, if these measures will help in eliciting concealed abilities. On the other hand, errors probably are made as frequently in excusing failure on grounds of motor incapacity as in penalizing a child because of motor incapacity. Errors in either direction are unfair to the child. Situations that are clearly impossible in the face of the specific handicap should be omitted. "Snap" diagnosis on the basis of a single examination is to be avoided; repeated observations over a period of many months often are necessary to establish the diagnosis.

§2. DEGREES OF NEUROMOTOR DYSFUNCTION

The continuum of neuropsychiatric disabilities has its parallel in a continuum of neuromotor impairments. When there is a qualitative change in movement control, it is generally accepted that the abnormality is due to some lesion of the central nervous system, usually demonstrable on pathologic examination. Lesser degrees of neuromotor impairment are characterized by the presence of the other abnormalities in neuromotor integration, such as cortical thumbs or fisted hands, which accompany qualitative changes in movement control. There is a decreasing gradient in the frequency and pervasiveness of the signs. These less severely involved infants do not die from their central nervous system disease, so there have been few pathologic studies. The minor deviations from normal neuromotor integration are demonstrable, however, when the intimate relationship between neuromotor integrity and maturational level is understood. For any infant, his adaptive maturity level is crucial, because the diagnostic interpretation of any observed neuromotor pattern depends on the stage of his development. It is not possible to list abnormal neuromotor patterns and apply this list to infants of all ages. The neuromotor abnormalities, the ages at which they assume diagnostic significance and a further discussion of their recording and interpretation are found in Appendix A-5 and in Chapter 11.

The minor disorganizations are easiest to detect in infancy, when the rapidity of developmental changes causes lesser impairments to distort normal behavior definitively. Compensation for the disabilities occurs with increasing maturity. In the late preschool and early school period, neuromotor evaluation generally is not formulated in terms of developmental stages, although increasing recognition is being given by neurologists to so-called "soft" neurologic signs.

Distinctions must be drawn between normal neuromotor function and varying degrees of abnormality, as in the evaluation of intellectual potential. These distinctions, which derive from a necessarily complex terminology, carry prognostic as well as diagnostic import. A careful differentiation must be made between those infants who have abnormal neurologic integration with intellectual potential within the normal range, and those infants who have motor retardation—by definition, gross motor development significantly below their chronologic age *because of mental deficiency*. A very small number of infants and young children with mental deficiency have motor behavior which is appropriate for their chronologic age; a somewhat larger proportion have motor behavior which is retarded, but qualitatively normal for the adaptive maturity level at which they are functioning. In the vast majority, the motor retardation is accompanied by abnormal neuromotor signs; thus, there are parallel degrees of neuromotor dysfunction when the intellectual potential is normal and when mental deficiency is present. Management and subsequent education are different for those children with mental deficiency.

There are five diagnostic categories of neuromotor status. When mental deficiency is present, the phrase 'motor retardation with' precedes the appropriate category in the first four stages.

NO ABNORMAL NEUROMOTOR SIGNS. Both gross and fine motor behavior are qualitatively appropriate for the chronologic or functional age. The infant may show occasional or fleeting abnormal patterns, but the overall picture is well integrated. When intellectual potential is normal, there is no interference with his total performance in either motor or adaptive behavior. When mental deficiency is present, motor behavior is appropriate for the maturity level at which the infant is functioning.

ABNORMAL NEUROMOTOR SIGNS OF NO CLINICAL SIGNIFICANCE. These infants have some definite abnormal patterns, and cannot be given a clean bill of health. However, there is no interference with total performance, and the signs are insufficient to consider them significantly outside the normal range. When mental deficiency is present, the functional level is the criterion against which the motor behavior is judged. Technically, the patterns signify some aberration, but clinically they are of no *importance*.

ABNORMAL NEUROMOTOR SIGNS OF MINOR DEGREE. In these infants there is an increase in the frequency and severity of distortions in motor integration, which usually causes delay in the rate of motor development. Motor achievements may be at age in those instances in which the abnormalities are chiefly unilateral. While there are often accompanying disorders of attention, personality and integration, the term *minimal cerebral dysfunction* in infancy refers specifically to the *motor signs.* This diagnostic label can be used for these infants only when intellectual potential is normal; mental deficiency is evidence of major pathology of the central nervous system. Usually gross compensation occurs by 15—18 months; no abnormalities are detected when a standard neurologic examination is used, but persistence of deviations can be demonstrated by developmental evaluation. Minimal cerebral dysfunction is discussed in detail in Chapter 11.

ABNORMAL NEUROMOTOR SIGNS OF MARKED DEGREE. The abnormal patterns are more frequent and more severe than in the previous categories, but there is no significant qualitative change in movement control. Regardless of the intellectual potential, there is greater disparity between motor and adaptive maturity levels. If the findings were present in an older child, a diagnosis of "cerebral palsy" would be made, but clinical experience indicates that almost all of these infants have gross compensation before 2 years of age; a standard neurologic examination then shows no residua. Even at school age, abnormalities are evident by developmental assessment if motor behavior is compared with that appropriate for chronologic age; at school age such children also are diagnosed as having minimal brain dysfunction if they have normal intelligence. In a few instances, the abnormal signs of marked degree, and sometimes those of minor degree, are precursors of various degenerative diseases of the central nervous system.

ABNORMAL NEUROMOTOR SIGNS OF SEVERE DEGREE. In these infants there are qualitative changes in movement control—a reduction or distortion of motor performance. The smaller proportion have space-occupying lesions, relatively clearly defined disease processes in the spinal cord, nerve roots, or muscles, or hereditary or nonhereditary degenerative diseases. The majority suffer from a static nonprogressive insult to the brain acquired in the developmental period, prior to 8—9 years. The term "cerebral palsy" is applied to the heterogeneous group of conditions resulting from such insults; this diagnosis is made independently of the intellectual potential of the infant, although it is highly associated with mental deficiency. A diagnosis of "cerebral palsy" often is made erroneously when mental deficiency is present because of failure to take into account the level at which the child is functioning. The rate of motor development is almost always delayed. However, hemiplegics who have unquestionable unilateral disabilities may have motor achievements at age. A diagnosis of "cerebral palsy" implies that a standard neurologic examination at school age will show definite abnormality, even though it may be so mild no treatment is required. An exception to this rule exists when hypotonia is the only manifestation of disordered movement control, since gross compensation occurs.

A neuromotor diagnosis has prognostic implications for maintaining the normal intellectual function present in infancy. When infant neuromotor status is normal or when there are abnormal neuromotor signs of no clinical significance, fewer than 5% of the previously normal infants will have an IQ of 75 or less at school age. For those with abnormal signs of minor degree, the risk of failing to maintain an IQ above 75 at school age is 25%; for those with abnormal signs of marked or severe degree, there is a 45% risk. The two most important factors in the child's subsequent life experience in the interval appear to be the occurrence of seizures and the socioeconomic status of the family.

§3. DISORDERED MOVEMENT CONTROL ("CEREBRAL PALSY")

Table 10-1 is the most useful classification of the "cerebral palsies"; it separates the different types by the character of the movement disorder. The colloquial name should be discarded; it is better practice to designate the specific type of disorder and append a term indicating the number of extremities involved. Convention uses hemiplegia (one side), quadriplegia (all four extremities), etc., recognizing that the dictionary definition of -plegia is paralysis, but that dysfunction rather than absence of movement is the problem.

Hypotonia, the spectrum of dyskinesia and mixed types are more common than pure spasticity; ataxia and tremor are relatively rare. Hypotonia often is referred to as atonic diplegia, because it remains undiagnosed until the stage when some arm control already is achieved and the major involvement is still in the lower extremities.

Table 10-1. CLASSIFICATION OF "CEREBRAL PALSY"

REDUCTION IN MOTOR FUNCTION
    Hypotonia
DISTORTIONS OF MOTOR FUNCTION
    Spasticity
    Dyskinesia
        Chorea and choreoathetosis
        Athetosis
        Dystonia
        Rigidity
    Ataxia
    Tremor

Reduction in Motor Function

Infants with this problem often are referred to as having "the floppy infant" syndrome. Reduction in motor function is present when there is hypotonus, muscular weakness or flaccid paralysis; these three signs represent gradations in loss of power. Outright paralysis is recognized readily. The weaknesses and hypotonias often are overlooked unless functional ability is evaluated strictly in terms of age and maturity. Even if noticed, they are dismissed too frequently with a shrug: "He is such a fat, heavy baby," or "He's just lazy." They are misunderstood almost as often, because too many diagnoses of mental deficiency are made solely on the basis of motor performance: "Your child is retarded."

Since an infant is not mature enough to respond if told "Don't let me bend your knee," a diagnosis of hypotonia or weakness in the early years requires more than a decreased resistance to passive motion. This *must* be present, but there must be poor postural adjustments and decreased spontaneous activity in addition. A normal 9-month-old may enjoy the game when his extremities are manipulated, and he may go limp. However, he sits alone, creeps and pulls himself up at the crib rail; he is not hypotonic. Further, it must be determined that the hypotonia is real, not simply retardation compatible with the maturity level at which the infant is functioning; mental deficiency as a cause must be ruled out.

The causes of weakness and hypotonia are numerous and diverse. It is beyond the scope of this volume to consider in detail the differential diagnosis due to a host of general systemic conditions and other disorders. However, hypotonia in infancy is common enough that a differential diagnosis and prognosis are essential. The clinician will be aided in this task if he has a conceptual framework in relation to the site of origin of the disease process against which to view his observations. For the most frequently encountered disease conditions, Table 10-2 illustrates the anatomic origin of the disease process, the common clinical prototype and the various symptoms, signs and laboratory findings usually associated with each condition. Hypotonia is one condition in infancy in which the presence or absence of deep tendon reflexes is of prime importance for diagnosis and prognosis. The course of motor behavior, indicated in the table by asterisks, is of equal or greater importance.

Hypotonic quadriplegia is probably the most common cause of infantile hypotonia and constitutes perhaps one-third of the cases of "cerebral palsy" in this age group; it is the exception to the persistence of findings on standard neurologic examination at school age. Paradoxically, in hypotonia of cerebral origin, there is always some element of hypertonia and discoordination; the abnormal neuromotor patterns associated with hypotonia are the same as those observed in the other degrees of neuromotor disability discussed in the previous section.

In the absence of progressive disease, hypotonia *in infancy* has a good prognosis. The picture in the first year of life may seem gloomy to the unsophisticated observer, but when the hypotonia is of central origin there is

Table 10-2. Differential Diagnosis of Infantile Hypotonia

Site of Origin Prototype Disease	CP	WH	IN	MuD	MyD	BCH
Abnormal Pregnancy	+	-	-	-	-	-
Abnormal Neonatal Period	+	-	-	-	+	+
Early Motor Retardation	+	(±)	-	-	+	+
*Motor Regression	-	+	+	+	-	-
*Motor Recovery	+	-	+	-	(±)	(±)
Adaptive Retardation	+	-	-	(±)	(±)	-
Other Abnormal Neuromotor Patterns	+	-	-	-	-	-
Tendon Reflexes	2-4	0	0	0-1	2-4	0-1
Sensory Changes	(±)	-	+	-	-	-
Seizures	+	-	(±)	-	-	-
Electromyography	(±)N	+N	+N	+M	+M	-
Abnormal Nerve Conduction	-	-	+	-	-	-
Spinal Fluid Changes	-	-	+	-	-	-
Elevated Serum Enzymes (Creatine Phosphokinase)	-	-	-	+	+	-

CP:	Cerebral Palsy	+: Usually present
WH:	Werdnig-Hoffmann	±: Sometimes present
IN:	Infectious Neuronitis	-: Usually absent
MuD:	Muscular Dystrophy	N: Neuropathic
MyD:	Myotonic Dystrophy	M: Myopathic
BCH:	Benign Congenital Hypotonia (Amyotonia Congenita)	

progressive organization of motor control in the normal cephalocaudad direction, and independent walking is achieved at 2 years of age, on the average.

Distortions of Motor Function

Distortions in motor function are manifestations of release phenomena, i.e., release of inhibition or regulation. The disorders may be due to a general systemic condition, such as infantile tetany; to a local condition, as in the muscular spasm that occurs with fracture and scurvy; to abnormalities of the spinal cord; to lesions or defects of the nuclei or pathways of the motor cranial nerves; or to lesions of the upper motor neurons, including the motor cortex.

It has been customary to relate specific etiologic factors to specific types of disordered movement control (e.g., prematurity causes spastic diplegia, hemorrhage causes generalized spasticity and anoxia results in athetosis) and to relate specific sites of damage to specific disorders (e.g., spasticity results from pyramidal tract or motor cortex lesions, athetosis from extrapyramidal lesions). With the exception of postnatally acquired true hemiplegia (where there is involvement of the motor cortex of the opposite side) and kernicterus secondary to hyperbilirubinemia (with involvement of the basal ganglia), these etiologic and anatomic relationships do not obtain. Many children have mixed types of motor disabilities, as well as other findings of central nervous system dysfunction because of the diffuseness of involvement. Intellectual impairment occurs with about equal frequency in all types of brain pathology.

However, it is important to define the nature of the major involvement to determine which treatment will be most beneficial; conversely, it is just as important to decide there is no condition for which physical therapy or other specialized procedures are indicated. Management of patients with disordered movement control is complex, and a discussion in depth is outside the scope of this book. There are innumerable treatment systems, each with its strong proponents. In our experience, there are three prime considerations: prevention of contractures, supplying postural aids and provision of social and educational experiences appropriate to developmental level. All these are necessary for the child to be able to make maximum use of his potential, as compensation for the motor disorder occurs with increasing maturity.

The clinician should be acquainted with the clinical types of movement disorder and, more important, understand how they modify the normal development of motor control. Then he is alert to any exaggerated postural, prehensory, locomotor, articulatory and deglutitional patterns, and their abnormal elements are distinguishable.

SPASTICITY. This disorder is attributed to involvement of the motor cortex and its pathways, which are concerned with volitional movement. Thus it is stated that the signs of damage to the motor cortex are not apparent until the child is old enough to attempt voluntary movements. This is not strictly true. The cortex does not suddenly assume control over movement; the acquisition of control is a developmental process. Every organ is ready and able to function long before its functioning is apparent; every organ functions in some measure before it functions completely.

Marked spasticity becomes obvious when voluntary movements are attempted; it often is heralded earlier by hypertonicity and hyperactive reflexes. Mild forms of spasticity easily may pass unrecognized if the clinician is content with performance, regardless of its context and manner. How a child does a thing is as important as doing it, or not doing it. Indeed, hypertonicity in early months of infancy may present a fictitious picture of motor acceleration: "The baby extends his legs so well in standing," "His grip is so strong," "He tenses his body so vigorously when he is picked up." When more precise voluntary control of movement begins to emerge, it becomes apparent that the element of relaxation, so necessary to smooth muscular performance, is deficient or lacking. If one muscle group cannot relax, the opposing muscle group cannot do its work effectively. The spastic infant cannot perform with normal ease and control; effort becomes obvious; or he may not be able to perform at all, normal movement being so impeded by muscle spasm.

Spasticity involves predominantly the flexor muscles of the body, with the legs usually more affected than the arms. Movement is slow and explosive, but organized, and there is little or no overflow to other muscle groups with motion. Spasticity is characterized by increased resistance to *rapid* passive movement, i.e., there are increased stretch reflexes. Consequently, flexion at the elbow increases as the forearm is moved rapidly, but there is little effect from slowly imposed excursions; there also is increased resistance to full extension of the knee as the lower leg is moved quickly. The upper extremities are held flexed and adducted. The leg is swung around with circumduction in walking rather than showing normal flexion and extension at the knee and hip. Involvement of the hip adductors results in a narrow base or varying degrees of scissoring. Deep tendon reflexes usually are increased, and clonus may be present. Muscles of the mouth, tongue and pharynx rarely are affected in pure spasticity.

To illustrate, a 9-month infant with mild to moderate spasticity adducts his legs but holds his knees and hips flexed when he is placed in sitting on a flat surface. He is unable to maintain his balance unless his legs are dropped over the edge of the table or tailored, so he is able to erect his trunk. He has not yet coordinated his legs in creeping or in early attempts to walk. He may have great difficulty releasing his grasp of objects, although he can secure them. He develops wrist drop, contractures at the knees and hips and tightness of the Achilles tendons requiring surgery, if passive extension exercises are not instituted early.

DYSKINESIA. Discoordinate movement implies maldirected, maltimed movement complicated by accessory, superadded movement. It rarely is pure, but usually associated with tonal disorder of some degree. Tonal increase may contribute to discoordinations of movement by preventing the proper relaxation of antagonists, or just as often, tonal changes may be hypotonus and weakness. Thus, dyskinesia is a spectrum of disorder, involving the elements of change in tone and the presence of involuntary movements. Chorea and choreoathetosis are not common in "cerebral palsy"; they are characterized by many unwanted movements with little change in tone, except possibly for hypotonia. In athetosis there are both involuntary movements and tonal changes; tone is sometimes increased and sometimes decreased, depending on age, positional factors and the presence of mixed involvements. In dystonia there are dyskinetic posturings but much less involuntary movement. The clinical picture alternates between dystonia and athetosis at different ages, in different children, and is dependent on position as well—supine compared to supported standing, for example. Rigidity is rare, and involves both extensors and flexors, with so much change in muscle tone that movement is virtually impossible; even involuntary movements do not appear.

Athetotic movements are usually described as gross, purposeless, slow, tortuous and writhing. Athetosis distorts movements and deranges their normal course. Athetotic movements may appear spontaneously while the child is relatively motionless; they may appear on voluntary movement; they may be practically continuous except during sleep. They vary in intensity and scope from severe, generalized forms to mild, localized manifestations, although there is always a tendency for them to spread or overflow. When the child attempts to move a limb, its movement is at once distorted by gross, involuntary, accessory movements which spread to other parts of the body. In milder cases they may spread just to the face, producing grimacing; in more severe cases the overflow may be quite generalized—the head twists, the eyes roll; arms, legs and trunk are all involved.

The athetotic child may try to wait until the involuntary movements have subsided, only to have them begin again with his next attempt at voluntary movement. More successful is his device, when he can employ it, of controlling extraneous movements by bracing the moving part: he adducts the arms close to the chest, or attempts to keep his hands in contact with the table surface. In mild cases the child may conceal his difficulty quite successfully until he is induced to reach out into space. Sometimes the only discernible sign is an abnormal posturing of hands and fingers—a frozen section, as it were, of athetotic movement. When increased tonal changes predominate, there may be no involuntary movements apparent until enough control to move an extremity is gained.

Involvement of the muscles of the mouth, tongue, pharynx, larynx and diaphragm may affect swallowing, chewing and speech. Vocal expression and output are usually somewhat reduced, but jargon often is quite normal. When speech is attempted it may be quite impossible, or it may be produced only with great effort, explosiveness and indistinctness—dysarthria. The whole body may contort, and laryngeal movements may be so deformed that nothing intelligible is enunciated. With involvement of the diaphragm, respiratory, phonetic and articulatory movements may be so discoordinate that not even a whisper can be produced.

Discoordinate tongue and pharyngeal movement also is the basis of many "feeding problems." Gross movements of the diaphragm and abdominal muscles, particularly in the presence of an incompetent esophagogastric sphincter, may produce sudden vomiting, almost projectile in character. Such difficulties often are attributed erroneously to neurotic factors in mother or child; in many if not most instances, they have a pathologic neurologic basis. In some cases of dyskinesia the signs are almost completely limited to these oral patterns; in other cases they are but one aspect of a more extensive neuromotor impairment. The importance of feeding difficulties as neurologic indicators should not be underestimated.

In contrast to spasticity, dyskinesia affects predominantly the extensor muscles. There is more involvement of head, arms and trunk than of the lower extremities, and one of the major handicaps is difficulty with balance. Dyskinesia is characterized by increased resistance to *slow* passive motion; tone relaxes as the examiner increases the speed of manipulation. If the examiner holds the upper arm or the thigh and shakes the extremity, a previously stiffly held elbow or knee will virtually flail; the increased tone can be "shaken out." This is one useful technique for differentiating spasticity from dyskinesia. The positions assumed also are different. The arms are pronated and extended, the fingers often hyperextended or assuming clawlike postures. The gait is described best as "mincing," with knees and hips flexing and extending reciprocally; scissoring may be present if there is associated spasticity, but circumduction of the legs rarely is seen. Movement is unorganized, uncontrolled and repetitive, with overflow to other parts of the body; mouth and pharynx are involved frequently. Extensor thrust is common, whether the overall tone is increased or decreased, and may be almost forceful enough to throw an infant out of his mother's arms. Head retraction is common, but is combined with poor control, bobbing and sagging.

A 9-month-old with moderate dyskinesia has not yet achieved any sitting balance. His head still sags and his back is rounded. Reaching is maldirected, and he may even require head support before he can move his arms in space. While he may succeed in securing a larger object, it is virtually impossible for him to prehend a pellet. Sometimes grasp cannot be relaxed, but his chief difficulty is in retaining objects once they are in his hands; they fly out abruptly and uncontrollably. In prone he may be able to progress with creeping movements of the legs, but his head still droops and his arms may only get in his way. When supported under the arms in standing he makes reciprocal movements of his legs and even may succeed in "walking." In an erect position the pronated and extended arm positions become more obvious. In the absence of a significant amount of associated spasticity, the dyskinetic rarely develops contractures because he is always changing position, even if involuntarily.

Any significant degree of dyskinesia is always a serious obstacle. Performance is accomplished only with enormous effort, and a large percentage of efforts fail entirely. The extraneous movements bring in a flood of confused and disordered proprioceptive impulses which greatly confound matters for the developing child.

ATAXIA AND TREMOR. In *ataxia* there is incoordination and lack of balance. Organization of motion is poor; voluntary movements are large and slow, not rhythmic or regular, and are compensatory. There is no involuntary movement in the disorder. Muscle tone, if affected, is decreased; the entire body may be involved. *Tremors* are exceptional, in that direction and timing of movement may be relatively unaffected. Tremors are fine and rapid, with a regular rhythmic pattern; they may be constant, or appear or increase with voluntary activity. Posture, gait and tone are generally normal, since the disability usually is confined to the upper extremities. Mild tremors and ataxias usually permit performance but disturb its efficiency. The child accommodates and is not handicapped seriously in the development of function, even though the function may be poorly performed. However, more exaggerated tremors and ataxias interfere signally with successful performance.

Figure 10-1 summarizes the deviations of movement patterns that occur under the various conditions of abnormal neuromotor control discussed.

Disordered movement control is reflected in posture, locomotion, ocular and manual adjustments, swallowing, breathing, articulation, and also in modes of attention. Effort exhausts attention, repeated failure may eventually dampen initiative; extraneous movements and their accompanying proprioceptive sensations distract attention. Attention also undoubtedly is related closely to the maintenance of postural set, and particularly to ocular fixation; even small digressions and dispersions in ocular control tend to scatter or divert attention. In fact, ocular behavior is an integral part of a child's total behavioral complex and partakes of most of its attributes. A composed, slow-moving child tends to show

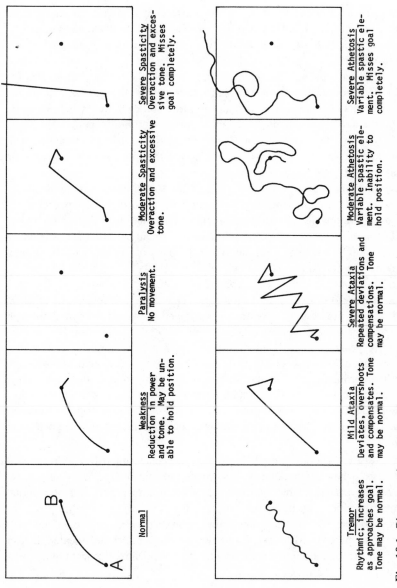

Fig. 10-1. Diagrammatic representation of a single movement from Position A (point of origin) to Position B (goal) under various conditions of neuromotor control.

slow, controlled eye movements and steady ocular and attentional fixations; a hyperactive child tends to show very rapid movements, fleeting fixations, and mercurial attention. A child with spastic, labored movements may have difficulty in bringing his eyes to bear on an object, holding his gaze and fixing his attention. The athetotic child, who shows extraneous discoordinate bodily movements, shows some degree of extraneous, discoordinate eye movements, and his attention often partakes of the same circuitous, irregular motion. Paradoxically, in the face of almost insuperable motor handicaps, sustained attention alone may be the clue to the presence of normal intellectual potential. Such an infant struggles valiantly, watches everything intently and wants to continue for hours, long after the examiner is exhausted.

An infant may be several months old before the exact nature of the discoordination of movements becomes clear. However, before then, abnormal postures, disorders of tone, exaggerated and abnormal reflexes and maldevelopment of function are apparent, and they are indicators of neuromotor pathology. Tonal changes alone, in the presence of motor behavior which is integrated and age-appropriate, suggest a search for an acute intercurrent process or a cause outside the central nervous system.

If environmental opportunities are equal and the child is not intellectually impaired, the motor-handicapped child maintains a chronic contest with his disability and develops devices for overcoming it. The athetotic child has such poor command of his effectors that he cannot imitate movement patterns; he has no latent neuromotor equivalents. Such equivalents are the basis of imitation in the normal child; lacking these resources to draw upon, the palsied child must become an innovator. This demands high intelligence and spirit. He becomes a kind of pioneer in his efforts to work out a communication code. This extra task constitutes an extra load, and normal progress of development is impeded. We have learned through clinical experience to have increased patience and some added optimism with respect to these early years, if interest and spirit are vigorous. The motor coordinations characteristic of the first year of life are probably easier for the child to approximate than are the coordinations of the years which follow. This should not be surprising; even for the normal child with an intact nervous system, the multitude of motor achievements peculiar to the second and third years of life are difficult to master. Sometimes as much as 5 years must be allowed before a motor-handicapped child finds himself.

The expression "finding himself" is somewhat vague, but it has a clinical and anatomic basis. When cerebral insult is so profound that it damages, even subtly, the deep-seated patterns which are at the basis of integration and attentional adjustments, the child may never find himself altogether. His personality problems will persist and reappear in changing forms, because they are so bound up with these attentional patterns. However, if the dysfunction is not so deep-seated, he can improve his integration and reward special efforts expended in physical therapy and special educational programs.

§4. ILLUSTRATIVE CASES

Devastating Dysfunction

Profound cases of mental deficiency are due most often to devastation by a variety of noxious events. Not infrequently, profound deficiency is associated with a relatively normal physique and comeliness of countenance. The contrast in physique and mentality adds to the pathos of the picture, and often increases the parents' resistance to an adverse prognosis. On the other hand, when they accept the diagnosis, the assurance that the defect was caused by insult to the brain rather than by an inherited disorder affords some comfort. When a careful genetic family history is negative, there ordinarily is no contraindication to further offspring, but the possibility of a mutation must be considered.

Case 1 illustrates the paradoxical association of some fragmentary normality and extensive defect from damage. At the age of *3 years*, she was brought to the clinic in a baby carriage and carried to the reception room. Our first glimpse showed her to be an attractive child. She was able to sit propped in a high chair, bent forward. She brought her hands close to her face and activated her fingers as though to look at them, sputtering the while. Occasionally she smiled, but the smile had no reference to anyone nearby. She seemed quite blind to them and heedless of sounds. She turned her head from right to left, but this was an automatic movement without adaptation. For short periods she sat quietly and then rocked back and forth with a weaving motion in her chair.

The examiner spoke to her in a natural voice and then with increasing loudness, but there was no evidence of attention. The examiner then tapped a cube on the tray of the high chair. The child responded with a movement of quiescence and then continued her spontaneous automatic activity. A cube was touched to the palm of her hand; the hand withdrew. She neither grasped an object nor retained it, even when it was pressed into her palm. She blinked when a bell was rung and turned her head responsively. The examiner brought a white enamel cup close to her eyes; she resumed her rhythmic self-activity and paid no regard to the cup. A formboard was brought before her eyes and moved back and forth; she paid it not even momentary attention. Briefly her hand activity ceased, and she seemed for a moment to be staring. Then she brought her hands up to her eyes, again lowered her head, and resumed her sputtering and fingering. The room was darkened, and a light was snapped on and off repeatedly. She may have had vague awareness of change, but she did not look at the light.

Placed in the supine position, she turned her head sharply to the right, inducing a momentary tonic-neck-reflex response. She turned her head to the left and back to the right repeatedly, with shifting symmetric and asymmetric attitudes. Her hands engaged in mutual fingering near the midline. Her leg activity was unintegrated with other reactions. There were no marked neuromotor abnormalities other than the persistence of the t-n-r and a moderately sustained plantar flexion of the toes. Her reflexes were normal; there was no spasticity, no flaccidity. When she was picked up, handled and held at the shoulder, her muscular tonicity seemed quite normal.

This description is brief, but it covers almost the entire repertoire of this child's behavior. We were dealing with cerebral damage of devastating proportions, associated with extremely premature birth (birth weight 2 lb, approximate fetal age 26 weeks). Delivery was normal, and the infant cried immediately after birth. There was a history of frequent minor convulsions, but without massive motor manifestations. Indeed, the relative normality of motor tonicity and coordination emphasized the severity of the general impairment. The apparent blindness presumably was due to lesions of the cortical sensory areas and not to receptor defect.

Brain structures were sufficiently spared to produce behavior suggestive of a 12–16 week maturity level. The tokens of behavior were partial and unintegrated, but they kept the behavior picture from appearing entirely random and formless. On occasion, while she lay in the crib, she raised her head momentarily, as if trying to sit up. She scratched the blotter on which she lay—a precursor, normally, of active grasp. She engaged her hands at the midline, a requisite for prehensory closing in. Periodically her apparently aimless self-activity was interrupted with a pattern which suggested hand regard: her eyes stopped their rolling and nystagmic oscillation; her head ceased its weaving; her eyes converged for a moment upon her hands, which at the same moment she held transfixed as though for inspection. Although we could detect no glimmer of visual perception in that fleeting moment, the attitude was the basic motor component of a perceptual pattern which by chance had been spared in the initial devastation.

In its entirety, this behavior was not comparable with that of a normal 12-week infant, whose innumerable patterns and initiatives are bound together and correlated within a unitary action system. Each day, each hour, the normally growing 12-week-old is organizing and integrating his behavioral equipment; he both learns and develops. This girl scarcely learned at all. There was a faint smiling response to her mother's touch, an almost infinitesimal result of 3 years of experience. There was no likelihood that she would learn much more or that she would elaborate the tithe of capacities which remained. More likely, her behavior would undergo relative deterioration; when noxious events annul the potentialities of development, there is no matrix for the formation of interests and for the progressive organization of patterns of behavior. That is the far-reaching result of drastic devastation.

Case 2 was born slightly prematurely, weighing 2500 g (5½ lb). Her birth was precipitate and occurred 1 hour after the mother suffered a fall. The infant had frequent attacks of vomiting, cyanosis and tonic spasms of the body, coincident with feeding, throughout the neonatal period. Her respirations were irregular.

At the age of *12 weeks,* the child apparently was blind and showed marked spasticity of all the extremities. The tonic-neck-reflex position was assumed with exaggerated intensity. Her eyes roamed, and although ocular movements were usually coordinate, there was no fixation or following, no blink on visual threat and only occasional narrowing of the eye slits under the stimulus of a bright flashlight. Responses to auditory stimuli, on the other hand, were fairly well defined: there was prompt blink to a hand clap and cessation of activity on bell-ringing. Objects placed in the hand were held with exaggerated reflexive grasp without manipulation or exploitation. No social responses were obtained. Behavior was at a neonatal level, but qualitatively abnormal. She presented a picture of diffuse cerebral dysfunction with generalized spasticity.

At *36 weeks* the infant showed some evidences of vision, following a light fairly competently, the ring through a small arc and apparently regarding a toy in hand briefly. Development was not at a standstill, and her maturity level had risen unevenly to approximately 12 weeks. Social responses remained deficient. At 40 weeks convulsions supervened; behavior regressed slightly and remained practically unchanged since that date. At *2 years* of age her nutritional status was good, and she gave little trouble to her devoted parents. She was able to eat semisolid food and remained quiet and happy in her crib all day, vocalizing in a monotonous sing-song, and mouthing her left hand. When handled or talked to, she smiled faintly. At *3 years* the story and the picture were virtually unchanged; there was no developmental progress.

As in Case 1, 3 years of experience had almost no effect upon the patterning of behavior. Case 1 had a relatively intact motor system; she sat, rocked and sputtered through her fingers. Case 2 was spastic and lay rigidly, mouthing her hand. The adventitiousness of insult produces a variety of behavior pictures, but in both these children the developmental potentials were laid waste. The value of sensory experience, whether visual, auditory or tactile-motor, depends upon the integrity of the associational areas and motor effectors.

Selective Dysfunction

There is an element of selectivity even in devastating injury. We use the term *selective* to designate those cases in which there is considerable survival of behavioral capacities, offset by serious defects and deficiencies. There is extreme variation in intact capacities and defined disabilities. Selective cerebral injury is most perfectly exemplified in patients with dyskinesia. These children are gravely incapacitated, and yet cortical mechanisms may be relatively unharmed in many instances. This clinical type is of special importance because it may simulate mental deficiency so strongly that a child is denied physical therapy and educational measures by which he may benefit. It is especially important that these cases be recognized in infancy to avoid misunderstanding and mismanagement.

Case 3 was born prematurely by easy version and extraction. His birth weight was 1690 g (fetal age 31 weeks). He appeared fairly vigorous but had frequent cyanotic attacks during the first day. He did fairly well for the first 2 weeks but then became jaundiced, showing opisthotonus and head retraction. Vomiting and diarrhea were severe, and there was despair for his life. However, after 3 weeks he began to improve. Opisthotonus and head retraction disappeared about the 40th day, jaundice on the 48th day; weight gain began on the 56th day. At the age of 28 weeks (corrected age about 20 weeks) his weight was 12 lb 13 oz; he was well nourished, but the extremities were stiff and abnormal movements of the arms were noted.

The first developmental examination was made at the age of 40 weeks (corrected age about 32 weeks). A total of nine developmental observations were made up to the age of 9 years. The findings of these examinations indicate the diagnostic difficulties and the selective effects of the injury on behavioral development and educational progress.

At *32 weeks,* the child presented a picture of extreme motor disability. Tone in arms, trunk and legs was increased; the arms were in almost constant gross athetotic activity. He was unable to sit up without support; voluntary movements of the arms and hands were performed only with the utmost difficulty and with fantastic distortions. In spite of the severity of his neuromotor symptoms, his behavior was remarkable for its vigor and force. During the entire examination his drive was directed with marked intensity toward the examination materials. He succeeded in approaching the cube and prehending it with a palmar grasp. He regarded the pellet for prolonged periods with recurrent intensity. Personality characteristics were vivid: he displayed eagerness and determination and showed undoubted emotional satisfaction in regarding his own hands, in manipulation of the toys which were put into his hand, and in his attempts to exploit them. This satisfaction in achievement was displayed most dramatically in the rattle situation. He seemed to be trying to bring the rattle to his mouth. The harder he tried, the more rigidly extended his arm became. All at once flexion broke through, so suddenly and with such intensity that he struck himself a smart blow in the face, hard enough to produce emotional upset in an ordinary child: this boy was delighted. He was stimulated by the novelty of the examination situation and responded eagerly and without fatigue to the whole experience. He vocalized abundantly, squealing, cooing, crowing and laughing. Making every allowance for his motor disabilities, his behavior approximated a 24-week developmental level. This in itself constituted a considerable degree of retardation, but his extraordinary drive, his favorable personality characteristics, and his perseverance strongly suggested the possibility of normal mental development. We recommended more social and experiential stimulation. Because of his early difficulties and his motor disabilities, it had been assumed too freely that he should not have normal experience; he was treated as a bed-ridden child. He responded so eagerly to the test table situations that a program to give him similar opportunities at home was recommended.

At the corrected age of *52 weeks* he showed only a slight degree of progress. Descriptively, his developmental level had risen to about 30 weeks. He exhibited the same persistence, vigor and drive and the same promising personality traits. We were particularly disappointed that he had not made more gains in the field of language and comprehension.

At *18 months,* he propelled himself about on the floor by lying on his back and pushing with his heels. He still could not sit without support. Although neither the increased tone nor the athetosis had in any way abated, his prehensory approach was somewhat more direct, and grasp was frequently successful. He actually prehended the pellet, and he poked at the clapper of the bell. He managed to combine two objects in exploitive play, and he could vocalize "da-da." His general level was approximately 40 weeks. The retardation was apparently greater than the first examination had indicated, but perhaps the greater retardation was an expression of the enormous difficulty in learning and performance imposed upon him by his handicaps. During the next year progress seemed hopelessly slow, but it did continue. Because he continued to strive so valiantly and because his original showing had been so good, we continued to hope that this boy would find a competent effector that he could use in solving his developmental problems.

At *3 years,* he had begun to find the answer in language. With great difficulty he began to enunciate words and even to use short sentences. He named seven pictures, could give his own name and answer a few simple questions. His comprehension and insight were not deficient. He adjusted to rotation of the formboard and succeeded in imitating a crude circular scrawl in spite of his great difficulty in handling a crayon. His developmental level was 24 months, with several successes at the 30-month level. Persistence, effort and drive were so impressive that they definitely indicated still greater latent capacities.

By *4 years,* there was no longer any doubt that the higher centers had been spared. He had won his way through his handicap and gave the best performance of his career. Speech, though dysarthric and produced only by great effort, was readily understandable. He recited several nursery rhymes and earned a developmental rating of only a little less than 4 years.

Between *5 and 9 years,* the steady progress continued, and the basic intelligence of this boy was very close to average expectations. He could maintain the sitting position in an armchair, and he was able to get about in a specially devised wheeled contrivance that he propelled with his feet. He had extensive muscle training to achieve this degree of control; he may walk eventually. His craving for school experience and his capacity for education was met, first by visiting teachers in the home and later by an hour a day in public school. He was learning to read with notable success and undoubtedly would be able to use a typewriter. He amused himself very well with tinker toys and erector sets as do normal boys of his age, and he enjoyed the children of the neighborhood.

The neonatal history of this child was more disturbed and abnormal than that of many cases of devastating injury. However, the end results showed that much was spared. The child realized his intellectual potential in spite of extreme motor incapacity. He did not retain the complete neuromotor equipment necessary to satisfy all behavioral propensities, but he retained the insight to perceive the normal goal of his neuromotor striving and to notice his shortcomings. He saw the difference between himself and other children, his handicap was explained to him, and he knew that everything was being done to help him. Most important, he helped himself; he accepted his disabilities, not passively but actively.

He showed some of his promise on his first developmental examination; only a guess can be hazarded to explain why the promise seemed to decline during the second year. Examination performance and indeed development itself during the first 2 years is tremendously dependent on motor function. It is our interpretation that he had sufficient motor control to take the first steps in development. Development was then almost blocked until the time when language and comprehension assumed the lead; through this channel, normal experiential intake and normal outlets of achievement could flow and pervade his total reaction system. The motor handicap became less important; he could grow and develop and take his place in the family and neighborhood circle in spite of his motor handicap. Thus, it is wise to place a favorable prognostic interpretation on all evidences of adaptive drive and perseverance.

Cases 1, 2, and 3 illustrate that there is *no simple one-to-one relationship between motor capacity and mental development.* Profound mental deficiency may be associated with almost intact motor ability; or profound palsy may be associated with high intelligence. Cerebral injuries may be selective.

Case 4 was seen at annual intervals from 3 to 6 years of age. Delivery was instrumental, and the child's condition during the neonatal period was poor. She was given several blood transfusions and had to be fed by medicine dropper. Several convulsions occurred during this critical time.

When she was *3 years old,* she presented a definite picture of bilateral spasticity, the right side more seriously involved than the left. She could use her left hand to point, manipulate objects and handle a crayon well enough to carry out examination requirements, when motor abilities were all that were necessary. She was able to sit when tied in a chair, she could walk leaning back against her mother for balance, and she progressed independently by rolling on the floor. Articulation was not affected, but her vocabulary was limited to 3 or 4 words, and she relied upon a shake of the head for a "yes" or "no" response. She filled a cup with cubes, pushed two cubes in imitation of a train and differentiated the stroke and circular scribble. She fed herself, played imitatively with a doll and helped her mother in simple household tasks. The developmental examination showed an uneven adaptive function at the 18–21 month level, with DQ about 55.

Physical therapy was continued faithfully, and at 5 years a tendon release operation was performed with successful results; she mastered independent walking very promptly. Developmental examination at the age of *6 years* showed uneven slow progress but no improvement in outlook. She walked but was unable to attain the standing position independently; she seated herself in a small chair but needed assistance to get up. She even was able to go upstairs holding the banister. Her motor abilities were rated at about an 18-month level; her abilities in the adaptive, language and personal–social fields were slightly below the 30-month level. Attention was poorly sustained but was readily and repeatedly recalled. She was an amiable and docile child, defective and handicapped; her DQ was about 45.

The insult in this case inflicted obvious damage to the motor areas. However, in addition to this the child suffered an irregular, diffuse insult, in spite of the facts that her motor equipment for speech was relatively intact and that her motor equipment for locomotion, prehension and exploitation, while impaired, was adequate for successful performance. This child had competent effectors, but the damage to the higher centers prevented her from realizing any great benefit from this advantage. She was a much less competent child than Case 3, who had much more serious motor handicaps. With normal speech mechanisms, she still could join only 2 words ("go bye," "call daddy") and could identify only 8 pictures at 6 years of age.

Interestingly, her behavior showed increasing integration as she grew older. Therefore, she seemed somewhat more mature without being fundamentally any more advanced in her capacities. This modest but constant gain in poise and integration was an expression of her original normal potential, an indication of the child she should have been.

Figure 10-2 illustrates this child's deficiency in organization. It reproduces diagrammatically the recording of her examination behavior. The record is stripped of its context and reduced to its simplest terms: a solid cell represents an established behavior pattern, and an open cell represents the lack of an ability. The irregularities in her performance are characteristic of damage.

Case 5 is an unusual example of selective cerebral damage. The child's motor disabilities were considerably less than in the two previous cases, but the disabilities were too severe to be classed as minimal. This child was delivered after a normal gestation by low forceps. The cord was coiled about the neck. Crying was spontaneous; the birth weight was 7½ lbs. She was a very good-natured baby, but while her parents considered her alert and responsive, they also recognized that her behavioral development was very retarded.

She was referred for developmental examination at the age of *40 weeks* because of her failure to sit and hold up her head. She was a large, well-nourished infant. Her face wore an extraordinarily bland and sober expression due to excessive relaxation of the facial musculature. Muscles of the back and neck were similarly relaxed so that she needed firm support in the sitting position, and her head drooped forward. Arm and leg muscles were hypertonic: the arms were held in flexion, the hands fisted; the legs in extension, the toes in tonic plantar flexion. The deep reflexes were hyperactive. At the test table her prehensory movements were slow, labored and leaden, as though she were perpetually embarrassed by the force of gravity. She never lifted her hands from the table surface, but she seized the cube with a radial palmar grasp, and the pellet with raking flexion followed by an inferior scissors grasp. Her prehension had an asynergic stilted character without smooth blending of the component parts.

Motor coordination difficulties characterized her entire development. Maturation continued at a sure though retarded pace, and she mastered, in her own way, many of her motor problems as she went along; however, she never caught up with the most recent problems. She suffered from a selective dysfunction of the neurologic equipment governing tone, synergy, timing and coordination of voluntary movement. Her handicap showed itself in retardation and distortion of

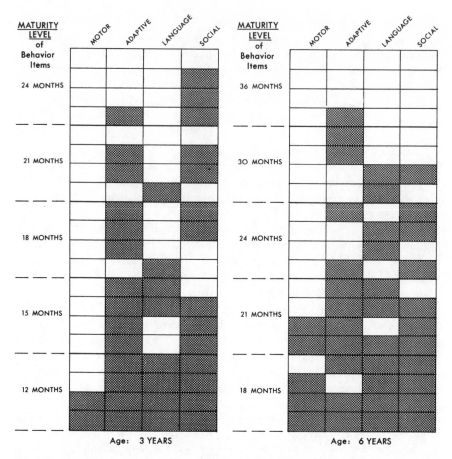

Fig. 10-2. Diagrammatic representation showing the behavioral organization of Case 4 at 3 years and at 6 years of age. Solid cells represent an established behavior, open cells lack of behavior in a given field. The behavior at 6 years is somewhat better integrated, but relative to age, not more advanced.

posture, locomotion, manipulation, articulation and the motor aspects of adaptive behavior. Even her attentional and emotional characteristics reflected this central lack of control. However, in insight and intelligence this girl was distinctly normal and above rather than below average in caliber; even on her first developmental examination at 40 weeks, her adaptive behavior was well above the 32-week level.

The general course of her later development can be summarized briefly:

Adaptive behavior: From the beginning, this girl showed undeniable evidences of normal intelligence and even of advanced potential ability. She had a good sense of form and balance, despite her failures to achieve these qualities in her own movements. She was fond of books and liked to be read to. Reasoning ability and intellectual curiosity were well-developed.

Motor behavior: At 1 year she sat alone, leaning forward on her hands, and she could stand holding the crib rail. At 15 months she crept, but in an extraordinary manner, without rearing her head, and she cruised about furniture. At 24 months she walked, her head hanging down. At 30 months she walked with head retracted, looking at the ceiling. This uneven reciprocal imbalance of flexors and extensors was characteristic of her neuromotor development. At this time her manipulatory and locomotor movements first showed true though relatively mild athetosis. At 3 years she was able to run unsteadily and heavily. At 4 years she stood waveringly on one foot. At 5 years her drawing of a man was correctly detailed but very crudely executed due to the aberrancy of her movements; hand movements were uncertain and poorly controlled.

Language behavior: Comprehension of language was far in advance of her ability to express herself. For a period she relied heavily on highly expressive gestures. At 15 months she said "da-da"; at 30 months she had a vocabulary of 25 words and was beginning to combine them. At 5 years she defined a chair with superior analysis: "A chair has legs, a body and a top." Articulation was explosive, and she stuttered.

Personal–social behavior: In basic temperament this girl was amiable, reasonable and sociable. As an infant she showed a quiet unexcited perseverance in attempting to overcome her postural and manual difficulties. However, as she grew older and social adaptations of increasing difficulty became necessary, she demonstrated another aspect of her disability: She was unable to meet normal life situations; behavior problems arose on all sides. She was overexcitable, silly and "naughty," or even destructive and aggressive under quite normal social pressures. She indulged in strange fantasies, strange emotional attachments to objects and equally strange fears of inanimate objects. She failed to adjust to kindergarten.

The path of this child's development was not and will not be an easy one. Her motor disability was relatively mild; but injury was so pervasive that the entire complexion and patterning of personality were affected. The organization of personality is closely dependent upon the integrity of neurologic structure. Even if we call this girl's conduct an inferiority reaction, we are only saying the same thing in another way.

§5. SUMMARY

It is not possible to discuss in detail all the abnormalities which arise under various types and degrees of neuromotor handicap at all ages. Their detection comes with experience and—a point which cannot be emphasized too often—a firm knowledge of the normal. The Developmental and Neurologic Evaluation Form in Appendix A-5 includes provision for recording the quality of the behavior and the neuromotor patterns. Under various functional and anatomic headings it lists the abnormal signs encountered most frequently, and specifies the pertinent ages at which they take on pathologic significance. The form itself does not yield a diagnosis; it enables the examiner to assay functions, skills and behavior patterns in terms of maturity and adequacy. The clinician then uses the form in the context of the total behavior complex.

The diagnostician also is called upon to define etiology as precisely as possible, to distinguish between gene-borne defects and exogenous damage. Disturbances in the neonatal period may occur in either case. The presence of other major or minor congenital anomalies does not differentiate the two situations; however, these physical abnormalities do place the time of the insult early in gestation, at conception if they result from chromosomal disorders. The question of etiology has practical importance for genetics counseling and for the detection of metabolic errors.

These problems are solved by historic data and by investigations which supplement the behavioral observations. The answers may influence the attitudes of the parents toward the child and the feelings of guilt they may harbor. Aside from these considerations, the matter is almost academic. It is far more important to determine the extent and seriousness of the handicap and its effect on development; the essential thing is to appraise the child in terms of his sensory receptors and motor effectors, his developmental potentials, and his social adequacy.

11

Minimal Brain Dysfunction

For many medical conditions, terminology and concepts undergo changes with the swings of time's pendulum. Minor and even major disorders of behavior have been attributed to parental mismanagement entirely, on the one hand, or "brain injury," on the other. In the latter organic category, literally dozens of different terms have been employed—cerebral dysfunction, choreiform syndrome, diffuse brain damage, minimal chronic brain syndromes, minimal cerebral damage, organic brain disease, to name but a few. They all carry the connotation of a disturbance in central nervous system function; the confusion is frustrating. The situation is not helped when minimal brain dysfunction is discussed in the literature as if it were a single disease entity, and as if brain damage invariably results in a particular constellation of behavioral symptoms. Reaction to these implications has led many pediatricians, neurologists, psychiatrists and psychologists to say that minimal brain dysfunction does not exist. Purist clinicians maintain that brain dysfunction cannot be diagnosed without demonstration of independent physiologic, biochemical or anatomic alterations.[6]

Rationally, we should anticipate that minor degrees of impairment exist. We know that a wide variety of traumatic, and more importantly, hypoxic lesions in the brain and spinal cord are found in the vast majority of infants who die in the neonatal period—even when the central nervous system lesion is not primarily responsible for the death. We know also from observation of their behavior that gross brain dysfunction exists in some children who survive, and that various disabilities and combinations of disabilities occur, depending on the areas of the central nervous system affected. Pathologic examinations of the brains of individuals who die weeks or even many years after birth have demonstrated the existence of various stages of subacute and chronic lesions which have evolved from the acute hypoxic lesions found in newborns.[74,75] Neonates also show subacute and chronic lesions, acquired prenatally. The problem becomes one of quantity, or perhaps of the strategic locations of the damaged neurons. We long have known that significantly different degrees of quantitative alterations can give rise to qualitative changes. Hypoxic cerebral damage is not an all-or-none phenomenon; the conclusion would seem inescapable that lesser lesions occurring in the gestational and neonatal periods would be responsible for lesser degrees of clinical disability. Anatomic proof for this thesis has not been forthcoming because the affected children do not die primarily from their central nervous system disease; when death occurs from other causes, detailed pathologic examination of the brain is not done or correlated with the clinical picture.

At this time in the history of the discipline, we are warranted in considering minimal brain dysfunction in infants and young children as a syndrome worthy of separate classification. Discussion of signs and symptoms, management and prognosis is indicated. The etiologic factors in children with minimal dysfunctions are similar to those which result in the variety of major disabilities, but their prognoses are different. There are a sizable number of cross-sectional and longitudinal studies which support the existence of the minimal syndrome, and we will present data from those in which we have been involved. Although we have used the word syndrome in the singular, there is a multiplicity of disabilities in varying combinations, just as there is a multiplicity of causes which can give rise to similar clinical pictures. Hopefully, in time, we will be able to identify specific disorders with specific etiologies, give them distinctive names and place them in a proper classifactory scheme.

Any consensus which now exists can be summed up best by the statement that the *minimal brain dysfunction syndrome* refers to children with intelligence in the normal range who have various combinations of impairments in perception, conceptualization, language, memory and control of attention, impulse or motor activity, generally associated with minor neuromotor abnormalities.[13] Most of the current literature on minimal brain dysfunction is concerned with the school-age child. It is not within the scope of this volume to enter into an extensive discussion of the problems of diagnosis and terminology in the school-age group, but data will be presented on the relationship of the abnormalities in infancy to later function.

§1. MINIMAL BRAIN DYSFUNCTION (MBD) IN INFANCY

With minor editorial changes, the indented paragraphs which follow were written in the first edition of this volume almost 35 years ago. They indicate the pioneering thinking of Gesell and Amatruda, before the term minimal brain dysfunction became so confused and abused:

> The concept of minimal damage has been forced upon us gradually by our clinical experience with atypical infants. Definitely defective and definitely palsied infants were readily classified on the basis of conventional categories. There were other infants whose behavior deviations could be ascribed, for want of specificity, to inborn temperamental characteristics, to external environ-

mental factors or, in rare instances, to faulty management. However, there remained a sizable group of cases which presented atypical syndromes that could be accounted for only on the basis of mild or resolving injury.

The diagnosis of minimal cerebral impairment is not always supported by the paranatal and neonatal history. The diagnosis rests upon the nature and the historic development of the neuromotor and sensory deviations and deficits. Here, as elsewhere, one must take the total behavior picture into account and must reconcile the findings of successive examinations. Even when there is a portentous history which would seem to point unmistakably to devastating or selective injury of severe degree, it is well to place the utmost reliance on the behavior picture. . . . . .

On the other hand, an entirely negative prenatal history and an uneventful neonatal period may nevertheless demand a diagnosis of minimal damage because of persisting or gradually diminishing neuromotor signs. In obscure or doubtful cases the following is a safe rule: Do not assume that there has certainly been a cerebral injury, but assume that every child who is born alive has run the universal risk of such injury.

The vast majority of infants have mechanisms of adaptation which result in prompt recovery from insult to the brain. The minimal dysfunction group consists of those infants who make a slow and delayed recovery and present unmistakable signs of behavioral disorganization in infancy. Because prognosis and management are different, minimally damaged infants warrant a separate category from those infants with mental deficiency and those with qualitative changes in movement control ("cerebral palsy"), who continue to show impairment of varying degrees. While most infants with minimal dysfunction do compensate completely, they form the core from which the children who show learning and behavioral aberrations at school age are drawn. Other conditions being equal, the risk for persistence of abnormalities is least for children with more mature performance and good integration in infancy. The consequences of slight impairment are greatly aggravated by disorganization and emotional sensitivity in the child and by faulty environment and care. The presence of convulsions at any time greatly increases the risk of failure to compensate.

Much of the confusion, disorganization and skepticism about the existence of minimal brain dysfunction stems from the fact that most professionals concerned with school-age children have not seen them in infancy. They have not been involved in longitudinal studies and are unacquainted with the manifestations of central nervous system dysfunction, almost never missed in the first year of life. They do not conduct their neurologic examination in a developmental framework. Many questions about diagnosis at school age might be answered by reference to past records and by obtaining a detailed history (Appendix A-5).

It must be stressed again that children in whom a diagnosis of minimal brain dysfunction is made must have normal intelligence. The tacit assumption is made, correctly, that when mental deficiency is present there is major impairment of central nervous system function. At school age, diagnosis also is complicated by the fact that many children who exhibit some aberrations similar to those found in minimal brain dysfunction do so as a result of suboptimum learning opportunities and adverse environments. Such children comprise the bulk of the population of the mildly mentally subnormal, and they have no neuromotor abnormalities or organic brain disease.

In infancy, differential diagnosis of mental deficiency from mental retardation and from minimal brain dysfunction does not present the same problems that it does at school age. Except for those from extremely adverse circumstances or environments, infants who have not suffered any cerebral impairment function normally. The discussion in Chapter 10 indicated that the neuromotor abnormalities which signify central nervous system dysfunction in infants with normal intellectual potential usually are present also in those who have mental deficiency; the degree of abnormality diagnosed depends on the adaptive maturity level and the extent of the abnormal signs. Consequently, the terminology of *abnormal neuromotor signs* of minor or marked degree leads to a more fruitful diagnostic conceptualization. Fundamentally, abnormalities can be called minimal only if they are unaccompanied by mental deficiency or by qualitative changes in movement control ("cerebral palsy").

§2. DIAGNOSIS OF MINOR NEUROMOTOR ABNORMALITIES IN INFANCY AND EARLY CHILDHOOD

In Chapter 10 we described the continuum of neuromotor dysfunction and pointed out that assignment to a diagnostic category depends on the frequency, severity, pervasiveness and quality of the abnormal neuromotor deviations, as well as on the degree of interference with function they produce. We also referred to the detailed tabulation of abnormal patterns on pages 7-10 of the Developmental and Neurologic Evaluation Form in Appendix A-5. Diagnosis would be simplified enormously if we could state that combination A of abnormal patterns signified minimal brain dysfunction, combination B, cerebral palsy, etc. Unfortunately, the variable nature of the disabilities produced by diffuse damage to the developing nervous system prevents neat categorization. Diagnostic skill in this complex area comes only with clinical experience; however, certain principles can be outlined to provide a frame of reference.

The primary consideration in neuromotor diagnosis has been referred to in previous contexts: except for qualitative changes of spasticity, dyskinesia, ataxia and tremor which are encompassed in disordered movement control, the significance of any abnormal pattern can be interpreted only in relation to the maturity level attained by the child. Associated disturbances in neuromotor integration which accompany the qualitative derangements of "cerebral palsy" are the same ones found in those infants and young children who have lesser degrees of impairment. Each disturbance must be considered in light of what is to be expected in a normal child of comparable maturity, and in the context of the total behavior picture. Failure to appreciate this fact is inherent in the kinds of statements that appear frequently in describing behavior—"This 15-month old uses his hands well; he transfers objects." Equally uninformative is "This 5-month infant does not sit alone." The first is normal for 28 weeks, the second for 40 weeks. Many of the problems in detection of minor degrees of neuromotor disability in older children arise because the tasks employed are expected to be equally discriminating over an age range of 3–10 years.[73] In contrast, a list of deviations can be compiled for adults and applied to all adults.

The second important consideration is that the greatest neuromotor impairment generally is discernible in those parts of the body where active organization and individuation is taking place, and which are coming under voluntary control at that particular developmental stage. Even though progressive compensation in a cephalocaudad direction occurs, findings at early ages may persist into the later stages. The following details provide a general guide to the kinds of minor abnormalities seen at each stage; they are not a rigid categorization. Difficulties may be in fine motor control, without gross motor impairment, or an admixture.

In the first 3 months of life, basic vegetative functions are being integrated, and one sees disturbances in sucking, swallowing and respiration. Movement at this age normally is not coordinated and still is dominated by reflex behavior; neuromotor disorganization manifests itself by an increase or decrease in muscle tone. Growth failure may be present. Vomiting may occur from inadequate peristaltic control, or there may be excessive crying, startling and tremulousness. These behavioral problems, and others which will be discussed in the following section, may persist throughout infancy and beyond.

By 16 weeks the head and eyes have come under voluntary control, symmetric postures predominate and there are beginnings of eye—hand coordination and arm control. Dysfunction manifests itself in poor head control—in prone, supported sitting and on pull-to-sitting. True strabismus replaces the imperfect eye coordination that is normal earlier. The tonic-neck-reflex, particularly a side position of the head, continues, and the arms may not approach the midline unless the head is cradled in midposition. Hands often remain fisted, with cortical thumbs, and muscle tone changes may persist. Although the legs usually are passive, increase in tone in supported sitting may be manifested by varying degrees of hip flexion, or by a narrow base with leg extension and adduction.

By 28 weeks, difficulty with head control has diminished or disappeared; it may be evident only in a dynamic context, such as on pull-to-sitting. Abnormalities of upper trunk and arms are most prominent. The upper trunk remains rounded, there is little or no ability to sit propped leaning forward on the hands and the abnormal narrow base persists. The direct one-hand approach does not appear; reaching remains bilateral and is maldirected. No radial specialization for grasp of the cube has occurred, and there is difficulty retaining and persistence of fisting. If muscle tone is decreased, inadequate shoulder girdle support is present. Legs withdraw or the infant collapses on attempts to induce supported standing. If tone is increased, there is a narrow base in standing and some persistent extension of the legs, which interferes with grasping the feet. The earliest independent locomotion of rolling to prone may not be possible.

At 40 weeks, legs, lower trunk and fingers normally are being integrated. The achievement most routinely inquired about in developmental histories, sitting independently, is not achieved, and a narrow base or rounding of the back persists. Progress is made by rolling or pushing with the feet (arching) in supine rather than by coordinated quadripedal prone progression. The abnormalities of the arms seen at 28 weeks persist and may appear exaggerated. Difficulty in retaining often permits exploitation of only a single object at a time, and smooth transfer is delayed or absent. Failure of digital differentiation results in persistence of palmar grasp of cubes, and pellet prehension may be impossible or achieved only by curling all the fingers into the palm. Poking and tipping of objects may replace grasping; exaggerated casting may substitute for retention. A supported erect posture is maintained only by locking knees and hips in extension on a wide base, if muscle tone is decreased. If tone is increased, the 28-week postures persist, and the infant may stand on his toes consistently.

By 52 weeks the difficulties may be confined only to the most distal body parts. Finger and hand problems may reveal still-incomplete radial specialization, and persistence of accessory support of the arms as a prerequisite for pellet prehension. Controlled release is not yet acquired. Static erect posture may be reasonably well integrated, but alternating coordination of the legs has not appeared. Hypotonicity of the facial muscles may prolong drooling.

Toddlers have delay in the acquisition of independent walking, and it is poorly coordinated and wide-based when achieved. Finger use still is imprecise and release and placement are inaccurate, requiring assistance from the examiner. Manipulation of objects remains awkward. This awkwardness persists with cubes, pellets, crayons and books; perceptual—motor problems may become apparent as the complexities of tasks increase at 2 and 3 years of age.

If the difficulties are chiefly unilateral, the infant or child may be able to achieve the behavior appropriate to his age with the normal hand, in spite of clear distortions on the affected side.

Two final aspects of minimal brain dysfunction suggest corollaries to the preceding principles and descriptions: First, compensation for disabilities occurs with increasing maturity, as already pointed out. The older the child, the more subtle the manifestations and the more precise and specific the tasks must be to elicit imperfections in neuromotor integration. Second, the active participation of the infant must be evoked, and he must be examined in all positions, not merely placed in supine and manipulated. Performance may be adequate when accessory support is provided, and aberrations brought out only when position is changed —e.g., a move from supine to sitting or standing, or inducing reaching out into space, in tower building as opposed to putting cubes into the cup.

"Maturational lag," "temperamental" differences and other hypotheses, rather than brain dysfunction, have been offered as explanations for the developmental delays seen above. These are tautologies, not explanations; they are as inappropriate for distortions of neuromotor integration in infancy as for such things as reading disability (dyslexia) at school age.[72]

§3. OTHER ASPECTS OF MINIMAL BRAIN DYSFUNCTION

Movement of some kind underlies virtually all behavior, so deviations in motor patterns are the most prominent feature of neurologic impairment in early life. However, they are not the only manifestations of central nervous system dysfunction. Convulsive seizures—*prima facie* evidence of brain dysfunction—are covered in Chapter 13; sensory and psychotic abnormalities are discussed in Chapters 14–16.

Three other aspects of behavior considered to be classic reactions in children with minimal dysfunction warrant further discussion: attention, hyperactivity and emotional instability. Normally, when a stimulus is presented, the examiner literally can "see the wheels go round" as the infant perceives it and makes an appropriate response. Attention is one aspect of the integration and organization of behavior. This, too, is age-dependent: at 16 weeks attention focuses on people; at 28 weeks it is directed more restrictively to objects; after 40 weeks both can be borne in mind simultaneously. Appropriate responses can be distorted by extremes of environmental impoverishment, but the normal infant is interested and stimulated by the examination situation. When integration is impaired, attention may be described as variable, fleeting, distractible and capricious, or alternatively, as perseverative and unduly fixated. Concomitantly, exploitation may be designated haphazard, impulsive and disorganized, or in contrast, stereotyped. Rarely do these distortions appear in the absence of motor, sensory, intellectual or convulsive manifestations; if they do, environmental causes should be sought.

Hyperactivity requires very precise definition. The essential qualities of hyperactivity are its inappropriate, nondirected and irrelevant nature and the inability of the child to control it. Hyperkinesis must be distinguished from gross motor overactivity, from normal motor activity bothersome to parents because of their unduly high expectations for control and from lack of appropriate play opportunities available to the child. Also, evaluation must be made in a structured situation. In an ordinary office or examining room, when parents and examiner are engaged in conversation, a curious child understandably explores drawers, wastebaskets and other objects if he has nothing else to do, or has obtained attention at home only when he does something that elicits a reprimand. In the context of a developmental examination, with firm control and proper pacing of the situations by the examiner, this overactivity disappears, and the child settles down. A diagnosis of hyperactivity should be reserved only for the individual who continues to show tangential responses in circumstances which normally elicit organized behavior.

Emotional stability, or lack of it, is more difficult to evaluate as a manifestation of brain dysfunction, because there are great individual differences. Some infants make an immediate, sociable and absorbed response to the examiner and the examination. Others are fragile, labile, irritable, uninterested or tentative, and withdraw to their mothers. In the ordinary course of events, even the initially suspicious infant usually succumbs, and by the end of the session may permit the examiner to pick him up or perform a physical examination. Whether persistent emotional fragility in the absence of any other abnormalities indicates brain dysfunction or not, it certainly can interfere with adjustment to life situations.

Since the infant does not develop in a vacuum, there is an inevitable interaction and feedback mechanism with the environment. It is easy to be consistent in the management of a predictable and stable child. However, when a child is disorganized and his behavior capricious, his parents have difficulty in knowing how to behave. Their actions inexorably set up reactions; data from examination of nearly 1000 infants in the Study of Prematures over 20 years ago (Chapter 8), suggest that the initial focus of such a vicious circle resides in the infant. Table 11-1 demonstrates that many of the behaviors delineated here and in the preceding section, and inquired about independently from the examination of the infant, correlated with the neuromotor diagnosis.[40] The frequency of abnormal behaviors in the first month of life and up to the time of examination at 40 weeks of age increased as the degree of neuromotor abnormality increased. Convulsions, crankiness, feeding difficulties, illnesses, muscle tone changes, sucking difficulties and twitching occurred more often in infants with increasing degrees of central nervous system dysfunction. In turn, these behaviors, with the addition of sleeping problems and vomiting, also were associated with tenseness and uncertainty in the way mothers handled their infants—a judgment made independently of knowledge

Table 11-1. Significant Associations of Some Abnormal Behavior in Infancy with Infant Abnormal Neuromotor Status and Tenseness in the Mother

INFANT BEHAVIOR	ABNORMAL NEUROMOTOR STATUS	MOTHER TENSE
Convulsions	+	+
Crankiness	+	+
Feeding Difficulty	+	+
Illnesses	+	+
Muscle Tone Changes	+	+
Sleeping Problems	-	+
Sucking Difficulty	+	+
Twitching	+	+
Vomiting	-	+

After: Knobloch H, Pasamanick B: The developmental behavioral approach to the neurologic examination in infancy. Child Dev 33: 181-198, 1962

Table 11-2. Relationship between the Emotional
Stability and Quality of Integration of 40-Week
Infants and the Emotional Behavior of the
Mother

INFANT STATUS	NO.	PER CENT OF MOTHERS TENSE
Emotional Stability		
Normal	904	3.3
Abnormal	88	12.5
Quality of Integration		
Normal	899	3.7
Abnormal	93	8.6

Data from Study of Prematures, Baltimore, Maryland

of birth weight or neurologic impairment. That the infant with difficulties may cause the tension in his mother requires serious consideration.

Support for this proposition also is gained from the data in Table 11-2. Significantly fewer mothers were judged tense if the infant was considered to have normal emotional stability (3.3% in the normal infants, 12.5% in the abnormals), and if the quality of the infant's integration was normal (3.7% compared to 8.6%). Central nervous system dysfunction, as well as disturbances in maternal behavior, are more common in infants of low birth weight (Chapter 12). Prolonged separation of mother and infant in the neonatal period has been postulated as causative; however, Table 11-3 shows that the mother's behavior was related to the infant's neurologic status, independent of his birth weight. Significantly more mothers of low birth weight infants are tense and uncertain, because more such infants have central nervous system dysfunction. The percentage of mothers termed tense and uncertain increased, from 3, to 6, to 17%, as neuromotor status progressed from normal, to minor abnormality, to marked abnormality, whether the infant was categorized as premature or fullterm.

It is appropriate to comment briefly on the problem of child abuse. Parents who abuse their children—often only one particular child—are supposed to have suffered similar experiences in their own youth. Rarely is consideration given to the contribution the battered child makes to his own battering. The brain-injured child

Table 11-3. Relationship between Birth Weight, Infant Neuromotor
Status and the Mother's Emotional Behavior

INFANT NEUROMOTOR STATUS	MOTHERS TENSE AND UNCERTAIN					
	Prematures		Fullterm		Total	
	No. Infants	% Mothers	No. Infants	% Mothers	No. Infants	% Mothers
Normal	367	3.8	434	2.3	801	3.0
Minor Abnormality	87	5.7	50	6.0	137	5.8
Marked Abnormality	46	17.4	8	12.5	54	16.7
Total	500	5.4	492	2.8	992	4.1

Data from Study of Prematures, Baltimore, Maryland

who exhibits aberrations of behavior may be responsible in part for provoking his parents. The danger of abuse also is increased if he suffers from psychomotor convulsive seizures, resulting in unprovoked and uncontrollable crying. Exposed to equivalent risks of brain damage, some parents may replicate their own early treatment because they themselves have some degree of organic dysfunction. The possibility that their rage reactions may be psychomotor seizures also must be considered. The physician must be alert to these possibilities when he suspects child-battering, make a diagnosis and institute appropriate therapy.

§4. QUASIRETROSPECTIVE STUDIES

The concept of a continuum of reproductive casualty (Fig. 5-1) as one of the etiologic factors for brain dysfunction has evolved because of the relationship between abnormalities of pregnancy and pathologic evidence of central nervous system damage during the fetal and neonatal periods. Brain lesions are the most frequent cause of fetal and neonatal mortality. We undertook a series of investigations to determine if associations were present between these same abnormalities of pregnancy and a variety of clinical disorders. The conditions representing major disturbances of central nervous system function included autism, "cerebral palsy," mental deficiency and epilepsy. Those which were manifestations of lesser degrees of brain dysfunction were behavior disorders, reading disabilities, strabismus, hearing disorders, school accidents and tics. Details and ramifications of these studies have been summarized and reported elsewhere; only a few highlights will be presented here.[61] The basic design of all of the investigations was similar. Cases were obtained from clinics and child care agencies, the group sizes ranging from 50 to 725 for the various conditions. In the behavior disorder and school accident studies, the control was an uninvolved matched child in the same classroom. For other studies, the control was the next surviving infant in the birth certificate file, matched on several important demographic variables, and not known to have developed any disorder. The studies are only quasiretrospective; although the data on complications of pregnancy, birth weight and neonatal complications were gathered after the clinical abnormality was diagnosed, collection did not depend on parental recall, with all the biases inherent in that procedure. Information was obtained from perusal of hospital records, without knowledge by the abstractor of the status of the child. The physician recorded his observations at the time of birth, and could not have been influenced by what the future outcome would be.

A pattern of associations emerged. There was an increased incidence in the cases, compared to the controls, of complications of pregnancy, low birth weight and neonatal abnormalities. The more severe the clinical impairment, the greater the disparity in rates of abnormalities between cases and controls. There were no significant differences in the incidence of mechanical complications of labor and delivery; the important factors were the chronic anoxia-producing complications of toxemia, hypertension and bleeding, with their associated low birth weight and neonatal problems. In any given clinical syndrome, the number of patients was too small to demonstrate significant differences for single prenatal complications, each of which alone had a low frequency. However, when all of the cases and the respective controls were pooled, the contribution of specific complications became manifest. Differences were demonstrated separately for toxemia, third trimester bleeding of unknown cause, placenta previa, premature separation of the placenta and miscellaneous complications—almost entirely infectious processes. Breech delivery was significantly increased in black cases.

Among the many byproducts of the studies, four other aspects relevant to the question of minimal brain dysfunction should be mentioned. First, all the clinical conditions were more common in males. Second, 40% of school referrals for behavior disorders were for children who were hyperactive, confused and disorganized. In whites, associations with the antecedent abnormalities were present only for this subgroup (hyperactive, confused and disorganized); in blacks, associations were highest for this same subgroup but still present for all the aberrations. Cerebral injury in blacks may be so pervasive that it infiltrates all types of behavior disorders. Third, adolescent referrals to courts for juvenile delinquency did not fit the pattern found in the other conditions; these boys had the lowest rates of complications observed in any group, including the controls, and less than average rates of low birth weights. A logical hypothesis for this finding is that disorganized, clumsy children are not acceptable members of delinquent gangs. Fourth, speech disorders unassociated with the major manifestations of cerebral impairment did not conform to the patterns found in the other aspects of the continuum.

We are not proposing that adverse conditions of pregnancy, which are associated highly with low socioeconomic status, account for all impairments of brain function; nor do all infants exposed to the risks manifest clinical symptoms. Nevertheless, broad health and social welfare programs—which are not primarily the responsibility of the physician in his narrowly defined and specific professional role—would do much to prevent the disabilities found.

§5. LONGITUDINAL PROSPECTIVE STUDIES: VALIDITY AND PROGNOSIS

If causal relationships rather than associations are to be derived, individuals at risk must be identified and their subsequent course determined. The effect of one of the major factors discussed in Section 4, low birth weight, is covered in considerable detail in the next chapter. A few aspects of the relationship between infant neuromotor status and behavior at 3 years of age are included here; they are of interest because they cover an intermediate level before school age.

Three hundred of the infants examined at 40 weeks in the Baltimore Study of Prematures were reexamined at 3 years of age.[40] Differences at this age appear to emerge only in those aspects of behavior which have a neurologic substrate, and not in the areas of peer relations or intrafamilial interaction patterns. Bowel, daytime bladder and nighttime bladder control, in that normal developmental progression, were achieved by a greater percentage of 3-year-olds diagnosed as having normal neuromotor status in infancy than in those with minor neuromotor abnormalities; lowest rates of success were found for those infants markedly impaired at 40 weeks. It is of interest that almost 40% of 3-year-olds who were normal in infancy still wet the bed at night more often than once a week; enuresis must be considered normal at this young age. Full lateral dominance probably is not achieved until 8 or 9 years of age; at 3 years, persistence of ambidexterity was observed in almost 30% of the normal infants, in 40% of those with minor abnormalities, and in 70% of the markedly impaired infants, with no differences between low birth weight and fullterm infants. Likewise, the quality of behavioral integration at 3 years correlated positively with abnormality in infant neuromotor status, the percentage with disorganization increasing from 15 to 20 to 60 across the three diagnostic categories normal, minor and marked.

The ability to maintain an average intellectual potential is probably one of the most crucial aspects of development. A significant relationship between this ability and preexisting impairment in infancy already is apparent at 3 years of age. Table 11-4 indicates that the percentage of infants who fail to maintain a low-average or better intellectual potential increased from 6% in those with normal neuromotor status, to 14% in those with minor abnormalities, to 33% in the small number who had marked abnormalities in infancy. In Section 2 of Chapter 10 data presented for another sample we followed longitudinally indicated that, at school age, rates of failure to maintain normal intellectual status were 5% in normal infants, 25% in those with minor neuromotor abnormalities and 45% in those markedly impaired. Such findings suggest that most infants who will deteriorate will have done so by 3 years of age; any further decline with increasing age will occur mostly in those

Table 11-4. Relationship between Neurologic Status at 40 Weeks and Change in Intellectual Potential between 40 Weeks and 3 Years

INFANT NEUROMOTOR STATUS	INFANT INTELLECTUAL POTENTIAL LOW AVERAGE OR BETTER	
	No. Infants	% Failing at 3 Years
Normal	224	6
Minor Abnormality	36	14
Marked Abnormality	9	33
Total	269	8

After: Knobloch H, Pasamanick B: The developmental behavioral approach to the neurologic examination in infancy. Child Dev 33: 181-198, 1962 children showing evidence of impairment as infants. Part of the lowering of IQ test scores for children with antecedent impairment may be due to their inability to respond to the stress of structured classrooms and psychologic testing situations.

The interrelationships between infant DQ, neuromotor status and school-age IQ, and the influence of socioeconomic status and subsequent seizure activity were discussed in Section 7 of Chapter 5. Table 11-5 lists the battery of tests employed at school age, designed to evaluate as many different functional areas as possible.[46] There was a significant direct relationship between infant neuromotor status and adequate performance on all of these tests: the more impaired the infants, the greater the proportion with impaired performance on each test at school age. The IQ test score correlated highly with almost all other tests; it appears to be a major factor in all aspects of function. Accepting the stipulation that minimal brain dysfunction syndromes at school age include only those children with near average or better intelligence, further analysis is necessary to determine if the infant neuromotor diagnosis has other influences on later behavior, independent of its effect on IQ test score. Of the 136 children whose IQ was above 75, 93 had a normal infant neuromotor status, and 43 had minor or marked infant neuromotor impairment. Each of these groups was subdivided into those children who had IQ scores of 96 or more and those with IQs between 76 and 95. Twice as many of the 93 who were normal in infancy had a school-age IQ over 95, while only half of the

Table 11-5. TEST BATTERY USED IN SCHOOL-AGE FOLLOWUP OF CHILDREN EXAMINED IN INFANCY

1. Audio-Visual Integration Test (Birch)
2. Bender Visual-Motor Gestalt Test
3. California Achievement Tests: Selected Tests of
        Arithmetic
        Handwriting
        Reading
        Spelling
4. Finger-Tapping Speed
5. Garfield Motor Impersistence Test
6. Illinois Test of Psycholinguistic Abilities: Subtests
        Auditory Decoding
        Auditory Vocal Automatic
        Motor Encoding
        Visual Motor Sequencing
7. Kinsbourne-Warrington Test of Finger Agnosia: Subtests
        In Between
        Same-Different
8. Language Function Tests (Strong)
        Auditory Associative Learning
        Ideational Fluency
        Inductive Reasoning
        Speech Discrimination
        Speech Mimicry
        Verbal Fluency
9. Oseretzky Test of Motor Ability (Gollnitz Revision)
10. Perceptual-Motor and Perceptual-Motor Sequencing Test (Birch)
11. Prechtl
12. Stanford-Binet Form L-M
13. Wechsler Intelligence Test for Children: Subtests
        Coding
        Mazes

43 previously impaired infants did. The total number of children involved was relatively small; nevertheless, infant neuromotor status had an influence independent of IQ. Significantly fewer children whose IQ scores were 96 or better, but who had demonstrated neuromotor abnormalities as infants, had average or better performance in the following areas: The Oseretzky Test of Motor Ability, the California Achievement Tests in Reading and Spelling, the Bender Visual–Motor Gestalt Test, the Auditory Vocal Automatic and Auditory Decoding Subtests of the Illinois Test of Psycholinguistic Abilities, the Garfield Motor Impersistence Test, the Same–Difference Subtest of the Kinsbourne–Warrington Test of Finger Agnosia and the Analysis and Synthesis Subtests of the Birch Perceptual–Motor and Perceptual–Motor Sequencing Test. Trends on other tests were in the same direction, but did not reach statistical significance. The behaviors sampled by these tests correspond to the kinds of difficulties which are considered components of the minimal brain dysfunction syndrome, in part because any diagnosis at school age often is made on the basis of performance on these or similar tests.

§6. MANAGEMENT

The general principles of management and guidance are discussed in Chapter 18. As for other developmental deviations, special attention must be paid to recognition by the parents of the organic substrate of the child's problems, but without neglecting how parental responses interact with and affect his behavior. At times there is no alternative to negative reinforcement for undesired behavior, but reward is always preferable to punishment. Simplifying the environment and reducing the number of impinging stimuli and choices of activity are probably helpful in decreasing disorganization and distractable attention. School-age children require early detection and remediation of specific learning deficits; small classes and specially trained teachers are recommended for fostering improved behavior and enhanced learning.

Drug therapy with amphetamines, imipramine or methylphenidate rarely is employed or required in infancy. It begins to have a proper role about 3 years of age, but is used most often in school-age children. These drugs can have dramatic effectiveness in modifying hyperactive and destructive behavior and improving performance in properly selected children. In large part, failures are due to overuse, consequent to overdiagnosis and misinterpretation of hyperactivity. Studies with more rigidly specified criteria, including detailed pharmacologic investigations, undoubtedly will do much to clarify the issues.

Scientific parsimony would support the existence of minimal brain dysfunction syndromes, based on the accumulated evidence of paranatal etiologic factors, pathologic examinations of the brain and the communality of neuromotor abnormalities with infants having mental deficiency and "cerebral palsy." The continuum of neuromotor dysfunction is most dramatic when lesser disabilities are found at school age in infants diagnosed as exhibiting abnormal neuromotor signs of minor degree, compared to infants with the major disorders. Absolute precision of diagnosis always is preferable, particularly on an etiologic and/or pathoanatomic basis; however, we must be realistic. We must be prepared to deal with things as they are at the moment, particularly when current information is useful to the physician, and benefits the patient and his family.

§7. ILLUSTRATIVE CASES

Case 1 presents a severely abnormal history with evidence of rapidly resolving cerebral damage. The birth was at full term, weight 7½ lb. High forceps were applied with difficulty, resulting in fractures of both parietal bones and of the occipital bone, confirmed by x-ray and by bleeding from the ears. The head was extremely contused. Two days after birth the infant was apathetic, listless, flaccid and hypersensitive to handling. She was almost completely unresponsive during the first month of life.

She was referred for developmental examination at the age of *34 weeks.* At this time she showed well-maintained interest and attention to the demands of the examination. She was slightly retarded in postural control and somewhat advanced in her adaptive behavior. She rated at a full average level in maturity of performance; however, there were several residua of cerebral insult. Her sitting was of the narrow base adductor type. She showed excessive unilateral preference in her use of the right arm and a tendency toward tonic plantar flexion of the toes. Her deep reflexes were hyperactive, especially those of the left arm, which was weak. Supine performance was superior to her behavior at the test table, a discrepancy of significance. There was a tendency to hyperextension with overreaching before grasp, and also after release. In her approach to the pellet she pushed it with her index finger, approximating the thumb but without flexing the conjoint digits, an anomalous pattern noted in several other cases of suspected cerebral dysfunction. Although her eyes wore an alert expression, there was a definite tendency to blanking out of facial expressiveness, strongly suggesting weakness of the facial muscles.

Reexamination at *52 weeks* again showed a full average level of maturity. She was then a big, healthy, happy vocal infant, deliberate, poised and self-controlled. She made excellent adjustment to the examination. With the exception of slight retardation in gross motor control, the behavioral residua of cerebral damage had almost completely disappeared. She no longer sat on a narrow base; she used both hands equally well; there was only a slight tendency toward plantar flexion of the left toes; her expression was continuously alert, no longer blanked out. At 52 weeks her prehension, grasp and release were virtually normal, with only a slight exaggerated tendency to poke with the index finger. She walked at the age of $16\frac{1}{2}$ months, and there was no abnormality in her gait.

This case serves as a striking example of the importance of the infant's initial central nervous system integrity in determining the response to physical trauma.

Immediate neonatal difficulties are better withstood if there are no prenatal abnormalities. We have no means of knowing to what extent trauma in this instance affected the cerebral substance. In all probability, edema associated with the obstetric injury produced some of the behavior symptoms. It would not have been surprising if the infant had shown physical and behavioral residua of her early difficulties for an indefinite period. However, the minor behavioral residua noted at the age of 34 weeks were so minimal at 52 weeks as to be practically inconsequential. It is almost certain that within another year they will have disappeared entirely. It also is conceivable that in a few other restricted areas they might reappear, under stress or in school performance, because this child undoubtedly suffered cerebral insult.

Case 2 was born following premature rupture of the membranes and a difficult labor. The second stage lasted for 10 hours, but instruments were not used. The infant cried spontaneously and immediately, but weakly. The head was markedly molded, the circulation poor; generalized twitching of the left side was present for 3 days after birth.

The infant was referred at the age of *12 weeks* to determine whether there were any residua of cerebral insult. She proved to be an alert, reactive infant, up to the standards for her age, and advanced in her adaptive behavior. Her ocular coordination and perceptual behavior were distinctly superior. She showed a slight overactivity of the extensors; the reflexes were quick, brisk and easily elicited; she startled very readily. There was a history of feeding difficulty with frequent refusal and spilling over, suggesting imperfect swallowing mechanisms.

These almost microscopic deviations had clinical significance. They were the expression of a slight but genuine cerebral impairment which became even more obvious on the next examination at *24 weeks,* the age at which the arms are normally coming under control. At that age there was an obvious difference between the efficiency of her ocular fixation and the awkwardness of her prehension. Her arm movements were abrupt and angular. In prehending an object, she tended to withdraw her hand just prior to contact and to extend her fingers sharply immediately after grasping. Often her grasp failed or was ineffectual. Her exploitational activity in the supine position was better than her exploitation when seated; her supported standing was superior to her sitting ability. She gagged on semisolid food. We interpreted this as an expression of motor discoordination rather than a neurotic reaction, and we also suspected that it was a minimal and possibly transient symptom of underlying damage.

Examination at *40 weeks* strengthened the previous clinical impression of generally advanced behavior, but again performance in fine motor adjustments was relatively poor. The accentuated release pattern previously noted had developed into an overindividuated casting type of exploitation. Marked sensitivity to sounds again was observed. Her tendency to drool and to gag on solid foods continued.

At *18 months* her performance remained advanced in most fields, and she showed a mature quality of attention. She had great spirit combined with sensitivity. However, she had not yet overcome her relative deficiencies in motor performance. She still showed a tendency to exaggerated extension in prehensory release, she assumed atypical everted postures of the hand, and her grasping was not adept. She pointed to objects with a circuitous outward deviation. In tower building she flexed her hand sharply at the wrist just prior to releasing the cube, imparting awkwardness to her otherwise creditable performance. The oral musculature was still sufficiently relaxed to cause slight drooling. Her speech was definitely less developed than her language comprehension.

All told, these motor deviations were not in themselves very serious, yet they were highly significant. They suggested some slight but fairly pervasive impairment in the mechanisms of coordination. In spite of the uniform excellence and energy of her performance in all other fields of behavior, she had not thus far overcome the motor crudities which revealed themselves in manipulation, body posture and mouth posturing. These crudities can scarcely be classified as congenital eccentricities or inborn idiosyncrasies; they are the residua of cerebral insult. We classify them as minimal dysfunction because they are so mild. They may prove to be more permanent than those which were described in Case 1. If permanent, they may interfere with easy acquisition of motor skills in later life. In a sensitive child under adverse social conditions, they might have an influence on the course of personality development. They are minimal, but they are not negligible.

Case 3 was the ninth child, born at term after a normal pregnancy, with a weight of 10 lb 10 oz. Oxygen was given at birth for a short time, and vomiting was present for 5 days, attributed to the presence of a cleft palate. The infant was examined first at *37 weeks* because the parents had been concerned, since she was 6 months old, about the generally slow development in comparison to her siblings. She made an immature and undiscriminating adjustment to the examination, attention and interest were hard to attract and ill-sustained, but there was little disorganization. The infant often stared into space, but she appeared to be in contact, and the episodes were not considered to represent seizure activity at that time. There were abnormal neuromotor signs present. The infant showed moderate hypotonicity of the back and extremities, but only mild hypotonicity of the neck, and tendon reflexes were increased. She sat supported with a rounded back and slight flexion of knees and hips, and moved about by rolling. Arm posturings showed slight pronation, wrist flexion, fisted hands and thumb adduction. Approach remained two-handed, with maldirected reaching and difficulty retaining, especially on the left. In spite of the fact that the adaptive maturity level was only about 28 weeks, the quality of behavior was normal rather than defective. Motor behavior was at 25 weeks; in relation to the adaptive level of maturity, the abnormal signs were of only minor degree. The parents accepted the infant's problems. Although restricted financially by the large family, their standards were high. The mother was a high school graduate, and the father had some college education. We anticipated that the child would continue to function in at least the dull normal range, with gradual compensation for her motor problems.

The cleft palate was repaired at 1 year of age, and the infant reexamined at *61 weeks.* Behavior had integrated markedly. She was friendly, entered into the examination spontaneously, showed sustained interest and attention and had entirely adequate exploitation. Her general maturity level was 61 weeks, and a full average development was indicated. Motor behavior still lagged, at 57 weeks, with persistence of mild hypotonia and flexion of knees and hips in sitting. Hand use was adequate for performance, but a scissors grasp persisted on the previously weaker left side. The abnormal neuromotor signs no longer were of clinical significance. In retrospect, the staring episodes, which had been dismissed at the first examination, probably were abortive grand mal seizures which had disappeared spontaneously. Undoubtedly they had depressed adaptive behavior below its true potential and may also have influenced motor behavior.

A followup study was conducted at $7\frac{1}{2}$ *years* of age. In the interval the child had recurrent otitis media with insertion of drainage tubes on five different occasions because of some degree of bilateral hearing loss. She demonstrated immature and somewhat erratic behavior in school and had to repeat kindergarten. She had received dextroamphetamine for hyperactivity, with only temporary effectiveness, and had been placed in a special class for neurologically handicapped children in a lower middle class public school. There was no history of any further convulsive seizures. On examination she was cooperative and motivated throughout, but restless, insecure and anxious about missing schoolwork during the long testing sessions, and falling behind her classmates. Except for a slight nasal twang, speech was normal and clear. Her Stanford-Binet IQ was 97, with verbal ability better than performance. Neurologic examination revealed slight tremulousness of both arms, difficulty with standing balance on the right, inability to hop and some difficulty with finger-to-nose and heel-to-shin tests. There was mild but definite impairment on almost all of the tests employed (Table 11-5). At home the child was happier playing alone, resented the authority of the older children and was an irritant to them. The parents felt that there were no major management problems, although the hearing impairment had recurred. They were satisfied with her school progress, and hoped that she would continue to hold her own. They would have liked her to go on to college, but felt that this was an unrealistic goal.

Case 4 was considered a normal infant, examined for teaching demonstration. He was born at term with a weight of 7 lbs. His mother had gained 35 lbs, had edema of her hands and feet and was treated with diuretics. There were no other problems during pregnancy. At *44 weeks* he was a tiny infant, a familial growth characteristic, but was friendly and stable. Interest and attention were well-channeled and exploitation persistent. In sitting, his back was markedly rounded, the base narrow and knees and hips flexed. He almost fell over a few times and cried when he could not get to prone. In standing, he locked his knees and hips to maintain his posture. The right arm was held abducted, with fisting and a cortical thumb. There was mild difficulty retaining and persistence of a whole-hand grasp. He had great difficulty with the pellet, which he attempted to secure by curling his index finger against the dorsum of his flexed thumb. His general maturity level was 44 weeks, and a full average development was indicated. Motor behavior scattered from 35 to 46 weeks; the abnormal signs present were of minor degree. There was no history of seizures, behavior was well-integrated, and prognosis was felt to be favorable.

He was *6 years and 9 months* at followup, and was in the first grade of an above-average school. His father was president of a building firm and had some college education, and the mother had graduated from high school. He was still a tiny child, spontaneous, highly verbal, gregarious and with a sense of humor. His IQ test score was 127, and his other performance was entirely normal, with the exception of some difficulty with eye-hand coordination giving rise to poor handwriting. His mother reported that he became upset and cried when he couldn't form his letters well, but he was improving and she wanted to delay any special remediation programs. He had no other problems. In a good home, and subsequently in a good school, this stable and organized infant without seizures had compensated almost fully for his early disabilities and was continuing to improve. He should be able to realize his parents' expectations that he go into a profession, "if he wants to."

Case 5 presents a contrast to the previous two cases. She was born 16 days before the expected date after an uncomplicated pregnancy, with a weight of 4 lbs 11 oz. She did well for the first month until she developed an upper respiratory infection. Four days after its onset she had two episodes of apnea and cyanosis at home and three more in the hospital emergency room. During her first day of hospital admission she had approximately 24 attacks of respiratory arrest accompanied by cyanosis and stiffening. Dilantin was given, and the episodes stopped after three days. Investigation revealed an abnormal electroencephalogram, but no evidence of hemorrhage or space-occupying lesions, and the infant was discharged after 14 days. She was readmitted 3 days later for recurrence of seizure activity. The apneic and cyanotic episodes again subsided after the first hospital day, and the infant was sent home on the fourth day. Dilantin was discontinued after a few days.

The infant was examined at a corrected chronologic age of *36 weeks.* While the mother had been concerned in the first few months about possible "brain damage," she felt the child was making satisfactory progress, and brought her for evaluation only because the outpatient clinic suggested it would be advisable to be certain about the infant's status. The infant was alert and active and made a prompt adjustment to the examination situation, showing well-maintained interest and attention, and integrated exploitation. No seizures were observed, but abnormal neuromotor patterns were present. There was mild hypotonicity of the legs, with increased deep tendon reflexes. Supported sitting was on a narrow base, with flexion of knees and hips, and she stood supported with legs adducted. She had difficulty retaining, excessive abruptness of release, incoordinated transfer, a whole-hand grasp and curling of her fingers into the palm in her attempts to secure the pellet. The general maturity level was 39 weeks, and a full average intellectual potential was indicated. Motor behavior was at 31 weeks, but it was anticipated that compensation for the abnormal neuromotor signs of minor degree would occur. In view of the early history of seizures, it was recommended that regular anticonvulsant therapy be instituted, but the suggestion was not followed.

There was no further contact until the age of *7 years and 5 months.* The family situation had always been bad, and continued to be so. The father had a violent temper and frequently was physically abusive to his wife and children, especially to the first child who was not his. He had a fourth-grade education, while the mother had completed the eighth grade. All five living children had been delivered prematurely, with low birth weights. The last pregnancy terminated at 6 months with the birth of a $1\frac{1}{2}$-lb infant who survived for 23 days. Although the home was adequately large and reasonably neat, no reading material was in evidence. Income was limited. The next older child had suspected meningitis at 9 months of age, was a behavior problem and was failing in school. Our patient also was very difficult. The mother described her as hostile and aggressive, hitting out at all children at home or in school, regardless of their size. She screamed and kicked if she didn't get her own way and did not mind or respond to spanking and punishment. She also was failing in school, and the mother was worried that neither child could learn. She felt both children should be in slow-learner classes. The father disagreed and thought that all the children needed was a medical study.

At the time of examination, the child was thin, pale and unhealthy looking. Her clothes were worn, tattered and dirty. She was tense, anxious, displayed self-doubts, sought support from the psychologist, and seemed fearful of being censured for failure. Her Stanford-Binet IQ score was 86. She was a nonreader and could not spell, but did well with arithmetic. She had considerable difficulty with all the other tests administered. Neurologic examination revealed slight tremor of the hands and mild incoordination. The psychologist felt that the child's potentialities were better than her performance, in spite of the difficulties encountered, and thought that some individual attention and remediation was indicated. The mother was referred to the social service department for assistance and planning, but it is unknown if she followed the advice.

Cases 3, 4, and 5, as infants, had similar neuromotor impairments, but differed in the organization of their behavior and in their associated characteristics and complications. All three made gross compensation for their early motor disabilities, but their subsequent courses were divergent, influenced not only by their individual variability, but also by the diversity of their home and school environments.

12

The Low Birth Weight Infant

Low birth weight is a problem of far-reaching importance for medical practice and for the field of developmental diagnosis. In current usage, the concept of the low birth weight infant is defined by both gestational age and weight at birth. The term *immaturity* has been discarded, but *prematurity* remains a valid concept.

Do those surviving infants born before term, or with a lower than expected weight for the duration of their gestation, pay a developmental penalty for their survival? Do they gain an advantage from being expelled from the uterus before their time? Do they suffer from deprivation? Uncomplicated preterm delivery apparently exacts little or no developmental penalty. However, a host of complications are associated with low birth weight—toxemia, maternal bleeding, infections, chromosomal and metabolic abnormalities, congenital malformations, neonatal diseases and intracranial hemorrhages. In turn, all these complications have associations with poor maternal nutrition and other sequelae of low socioeconomic status. More than any other factor, weight at birth is inversely related to the continuum of reproductive casualty, i.e., mortality, *in utero* and throughout infancy, immediate and subsequent morbidity, congenital anomalies, chronic diseases and the whole spectrum of neuropsychiatric disabilities. The survival and developmental fate of a low birth weight infant is determined by the number and severity of these complications and by the initial integrity of the central nervous system.

§1. BIRTH WEIGHT AND GESTATIONAL AGE

As with all biologic phenomena, there is normal variation in both birth weight and duration of gestation. Infants of a given weight are not homogeneous in regard to duration of pregnancy, and for a given gestational age there is wide variation in weight at birth. A birth weight of 2500 g and a gestation period of 37 weeks have been adopted as conventional dividing lines between mature and preterm infants, because of increased mortality and morbidity and a need for special medical and nursing care below these cutoff points. More meaningful information is obtained when both age and birth weight are taken into account.

The risks of low birth weight are demonstrated most easily by the criterion of *perinatal mortality,* regardless of what gestational ages or neonatal periods of survival are included in the definition of this term. (As we shall see later, similar relationships to birth weight and gestation obtain for the risk of sequelae in the survivors.) Lowest mortality occurs in infants weighing over 2500 g with gestational ages over 36 weeks. The rate triples if the duration of gestation is less than 37 weeks. When birth weight is between 1500 and 2500 g with a gestational age of 37 weeks or more, there is a sixfold increase in mortality; the rate is 20 times higher if the gestation period is shorter than this. When birth weight is less than 1500 g, mortality rate is almost 100 times greater than that found for the mature reference population, regardless of the duration of gestation.[83]

These relationships are expressed by another set of terms encompassed in intrauterine growth and neonatal mortality risk charts, the best known of which are those of Battaglia and Lubchenco.[2,55] Percentile curves are plotted from the distribution of birth weights for given gestational ages. An infant is classified as appropriate for gestational age (AGA) if birth weight is between the 10th and 90th percentile, large for gestational age (LGA) when it is over the 90th percentile and small for gestational age (SGA) when it is below the 10th percentile. The term small-for-dates infants also is used for the latter group. Newborn mortality and morbidity are increased in both the LGA and SGA groups; the birth weight is most important—the lower the weight, the greater the risk.

§2. DEVELOPMENTAL DIAGNOSIS AND POSTCONCEPTIONAL AGE

There are numerous physiologic handicaps even for a low birth weight infant who is otherwise healthy—imperfect temperature regulation, inadequate development of enzyme systems for handling both normal catabolic products and administered foods and drugs, reduced surfactant in the lungs impeding expansion, decreased renal function, small gastric capacity and impaired sucking and swallowing ability, to name but a few. In addition to parameters of size, other physical criteria also vary with postconceptional age—skin and hair texture, nail development, dermal ridge patterns, genital and breast tissue development, and a variety of tonal and reflex responses. There is a voluminous literature on physiologic handicaps, medical problems and treatment of low birth weight infants. Our concern is with his developmental status.

What of the maturation of the central nervous system when an accident of birth has made the fetus an extrauterine infant? Is there a deleterious effect from the isolated atmosphere of the incubator, where he misses the joltings, jarrings, impacts, changes in position and travel consequent to the activities and comings and goings of the mother he would have experienced were he still in the uterus? Is there any benefit from early birth? Prematurity in itself does not appear to either retard or accelerate the inherent sequences of behavioral maturation. With increasing age his central nervous system matures, just as do other physiologic and anatomic aspects of development. Several weeks after birth he might exhibit an apparent precocity in a few forms of behavior, such as eye following. But his fundamental behavioral maturity is not advanced and he gains no real advantage from his head start; neither does he suffer any setback, provided that the premature delivery was not caused by or related to other fetal or maternal abnormalities.

The developmental status of a low birth weight infant always must be appraised in terms of his *corrected* or *postconceptional* age rather than his chronologic postnatal age. Technically, the infant born before term is always "premature" and never "catches up" in development. Since corrected chronologic age, not time of birth, is the important variable, the proportion of the total life span that the weeks of prematurity represent determines whether a premature infant should be expected to behave as does his fullterm brother of the same postnatal age. The effect that preterm delivery has on observed behavior depends on the infant's chronologic age at the time of his examination and the duration of the pregnancy: the younger the infant and the greater the prematurity, the larger the percentage of apparent retardation. By 40 weeks of age, or even earlier, differences in behavior of an infant 2–3 weeks premature would be within the normal range of variability. But 12 weeks of prematurity might still affect the judgment of the child's potential at 36 months of age. At 28 weeks of age, failure to consider these 12 weeks would lead to an erroneous diagnosis of mental deficiency.

Calculation of the Corrected Chronologic Age (CCA)

In determining gestational age, the neonatologist has both the history and the infant to aid him. Rarely does the developmental diagnostician have the objective newborn observations available. How, then, should he solve the often knotty problem of the amount by which he should correct the chronologic age of a low birth weight infant? He begins by obtaining *specific* historic information. What *day* did the *mother* expect the baby to be born? How sure is she of this date? Were her last two menstrual periods entirely normal? Asked this way, precise and useful information is obtained. He must not assume that a discrepant history is unreliable. Even if the mother does not know the precise date of her last menstrual period, she does know if her pregnancy was shorter or longer than expected. Thus, the first two important variables in the calculation are obtained: birth weight and the *observed* length of gestation.

The third variable in calculation is derived from distributions of birth weights by gestational age; these tabulations vary with the character of the population on which they are based, but all are more or less similar. Table 12-1 is derived from the Baltimore Study of Prematures (Chapter 8) by plotting birth weight against length of gestation and using the 50th percentile as the basis for the regression line. It is easy to remember and clinically adequate. For a given birth weight, obtain the

Table 12-1. Days of Prematurity Calculated
for Given Birth Weights

BIRTH WEIGHT (Pounds)	CALCULATED DAYS OF PREMATURITY
5-8	22
5-0	32
4-8	43
4-0	53
3-8	64
3-0	74
2-8	85
2-0	95
1-8	106

Data from Study of Prematures,
Baltimore, Maryland

corresponding calculated days of prematurity from Table 12-1, and assume a normal variability of 3 weeks on either side; call this 21-day range the *limit*. Use the observed length of gestation if it falls within the 3-week limit. When a discrepancy exists, compromise by taking the 21-day limit, in the correct direction, as the assigned amount of prematurity, in the absence of specific contraindications. If no history is available, the only choice is to use the *calculated* number of days of prematurity in the table.

Two illustrative cases follow:

Birth weight: 2041 g (4 lb 8 oz); birth date: 6/1/68; expected date: 7/1/68

Calculated days of prematurity:	43 (Limit of 21: 22–64 days)
Observed days of prematurity:	30
Difference:	13

The observed 30 days agrees, within 3 weeks, with the 43 calculated days for the birth weight. Thirty days are assigned, and a corrected birth date of 7/1/68 is used for determining the corrected chronologic age.

Birth weight: 2280 g (5 lb); birth date: 6/1/68; expected date: 8/13/68

Calculated days of prematurity:	32 (Limit of 21: 11–53 days)
Observed days of prematurity:	73
Difference:	41

In this instance, the 41-day difference is outside the 3-week limit. Bring the duration of gestation to this limit by adding 21 to the 32 days calculated. Therefore, 53 days of prematurity are assigned, with a corrected birth date of 7/24/68 to be used in calculating the corrected chronologic age. If the history indicated delivery 7 days before the expected date, 11 days of prematurity would be assigned as the limit by subtracting 21 from 32.

Practical Corollaries

A variety of possible errors in assigning the length of gestation and the *consequences* of such errors in evaluation of the infant must be considered.

FAILURE TO CORRECT FOR PREMATURITY. The diagnostic importance of making this age allowance is shown concretely in the case of a 28-week infant brought for examination. He was a surviving twin; the pregnancy had been terminated 12 weeks before term. The parents were somewhat concerned about the possible effects of the prematurity, the stormy neonatal course and the early retardation in physical development. From a birth weight of $2\frac{1}{2}$ lbs, the infant had attained a weight of 14 lbs. He was vigorously reactive without, however, showing any desire to sit up.

He was examined in the supine position with the following findings: He lay with head in the midline and maintained this midposition for prolonged periods. He rotated the head freely and turned it fully from one side to the other. Only traces of the t-n-r were seen. His arms were symmetrically active; they were predominantly flexed and the hands were loosely closed. He rolled freely to the side. He regarded his surroundings and brought his hands to the midline where they engaged. He perceived a dangling ring when it was presented in the midline and gave it immediate and prolonged regard. While he inspected the ring he brought his hands together over his chest, but he did not attempt to prehend the ring. He followed it repeatedly with his eyes through an arc of 180° and shifted his regard to the examiner's hand holding the string. When the examiner placed the dangling ring in his hand, the infant regarded it and carried it to his mouth. When pulled from supine to the sitting position he tensed his shoulders and showed no head lag.

Unquestionably, these patterns are less mature than those we expect in an average 28-week infant. In fact, they are highly characteristic of the 16-week level of maturity. Retardation of 12 weeks in an infant born 28 weeks ago would mean a DQ of approximately 60, indicating a mild degree of mental deficiency. However, the quality of the behavior was vigorous and attention was excellent. The corrected chronologic age was *16 weeks* and the retardation was spurious. The parents were assured that the developmental outlook was favorable, that the child had suffered no ill effects from his "bad start," and that his behavior was entirely normal for his true age. The subsequent history of the child justified the assurance; at the age of 6 years he had maintained a full average level of development and intelligence. Failure to correct for prematurity may lead to an erroneous diagnosis of mental deficiency.

POSTMATURITY. The upper range of normal pregnancy is accepted as 42 weeks. Cases are reported to be prolonged beyond this point, with or without signs of dysmaturity associated with placental failure. In practice, nothing is gained by adding to the chronologic age for pregnancies lasting longer than 40 weeks. In the absence of dysfunction, failure to increase the chronologic age can result only in some degree of acceleration, particularly at early ages. Such acceleration is of no concern to the clinician. Postmaturity should be borne in mind as an explanation for some apparent deceleration in developmental rate in later infancy, but function will always be in the normal range, providing there are no central nervous system abnormalities.

LARGE FOR GESTATIONAL AGE INFANTS. Consider a baby who weighs 7 or 8 lb after a gestation of 32 weeks. If the mother is diabetic, the birth date must be corrected by 8 weeks; this clinical association of diabetes with high birth weight is well known. If she is not diabetic, the most likely explanation is that bleeding occurred at the time of the expected menstrual periods; a history of some deviation from the mother's normal periods will provide the clue. In this instance no correction is made for prematurity, but the development of such large infants should be watched closely, since there is an increased risk of abnormality. Correction would cause only spurious acceleration.

SMALL FOR GESTATIONAL AGE INFANTS. If the mother insists her pregnancy lasted 40 weeks, even though the infant weighed only 3 lb 12 oz, there is an increased risk of abnormality which calls for careful supervision. In the absence of dysfunction, assigning 8 weeks of prematurity could result only in marked acceleration in early infancy, and is unnecessary. If abnormality is present, only serial observations will provide answers about prognosis and the true postconceptional age. No correction is made when the birth weight is over 2500 g, unless there are specific indications for doing so.

In summary, virtually all neonates suffer repercussions, mild or severe, temporary or permanent, from the process of birth and its antecedents. Diagnostic differentiation may be difficult in the neonatal period because of the complexity of all the variables and the amorphous character of newborn behavior. The most frequent error when the development of a low birth weight infant is assessed at later ages is failure to make allowances for preterm delivery. Consequently, there is undue concern about the development of an infant who is progressing normally if his true chronologic age is considered. On the other hand, low birth weight infants have a higher incidence of neuropsychiatric disabilities. As a group, they require closer supervision for the early identification of those who might present problems. The converse error is equally dangerous—failing to recognize dysfunction of the central nervous system and obscuring true deficiency with vague terms such as immaturity.

§3. BEHAVIORAL DEVELOPMENT OF THE FETAL INFANT

The preterm infant comes within the scope of developmental observation, and it is profitable to appraise not only the vitality but also the patterning of his behavior.

To indicate in the ensuing discussion that he remains in the gestational period of development, the preterm infant is called a fetal infant from the time of his birth until the 40th postconceptional week. After 40 weeks of gestation he is referred to as a premature infant throughout the period of infancy.

The infant's basic equipment is laid down in the first half of the fetal period. Behavioral development is already under way at a gestational age of 8 weeks, when the fetus is a scant inch in length. At that age stimulation of the oral region of the surgical fetus results in unilateral body flexion. At $9\frac{1}{2}$ weeks a similar stimulus produces bilateral flexion—a kind of body swing. At 11 weeks hand stimulation evokes finger flexion. At 14 weeks the fetus can wink (with fused lids), sneer and swallow; at 16 weeks it can make a single gasp. At 20 weeks torsion of the head arouses movement of the arm on that side. This marks the genesis of the important tonic-neck-reflex. At 25 weeks the fetus is capable of shallow but rhythmic prerespiratory movements, which prepare him for the crisis of birth.

If birth is delayed another week or two beyond this age he may survive. His survival depends on the maturity and integrity of his central nervous system, on the absence of abnormal complications and on the sophistication of the medical care available. Among other things, modern methods of intensive care can compensate for deficiencies in the tonal elasticity of his thoracic musculature and in the efficiency of his nasopalatopharyngeal aparatus so essential to successful feeding. His behavioral capacities, of critical importance in this early period, will display progressive developmental changes in the patterns of his behavior throughout the period of fetal infancy.

The spontaneous and responsive behavior of a sizable group of fetal infants has been reported in *The Embryology of Behavior*.[26] The observations, supplemented by cinema records, were sufficiently systematic to establish well-defined growth trends of behavior typical of three levels of maturity:

1. Early stage of fetal infancy (fetal age: 28–32 weeks)
2. Midstage of fetal infancy (fetal age: 32–36 weeks)
3. Late stage of fetal infancy (fetal age: 36–40 weeks; from observations of the early and midstage infants 2–3 months after their birth)

A brief summary of these three stages indicates behavioral characteristics which have significance for developmental diagnosis and methods of care and management of the preterm infant.

Early Stage Fetal Infant (28–32 Weeks)

At the beginning of this stage the fetal infant weighs only about 2 lbs. He is so diminutive that he can be held in the palm of an adult hand. He is fragile, scrawny and wizened, with underdeveloped buttocks and legs. There is no adipose under the thin dusky skin that covers his bony frame. Occasionally he stirs, but even when he is a few weeks older the distinction between activity and rest is not clearcut. He really neither sleeps nor wakes, but only drowses, with brief ripples of bodily activity. Even his torpor is fluctuant and shallow. Muscular tone is minimal, flaccid and uneven. Movements are so poorly sustained that their terminations are more evident than their beginnings.

Nevertheless, behavior is steadily organizing and taking shape. His complex facial musculature is busy: he moves his eyeballs conjointly, laterally and vertically; his eyelids flutter; eyebrows lift; the frontal brow corrugates (sometimes only half the brow, for bilateral integration is not yet firmly achieved); the tongue protrudes and lips purse, munch and mince. Breathing is shallow and irregular. Rarely he emits a faint bleat or squeak; his cry may be soundless and is never prolonged.

His postural movements are sporadic and meager. In the supine position he lies with head turned to one side; head rotations are slight. He may extend his legs bilaterally or scissorswise and may even roll to the side, reverting to a curved attitude reminiscent of the rounded walls of the uterus. He straightens by mild stretching and relaxes into indifferent positions. Sometimes he arrests his arm movement into a transient catatonic pose, or he slowly elevates a flexed arm in a "floating" (t-n-r) pose.

He reacts to sensory stimuli: His fingers flex feebly on the tactile pressure of a rod inserted in the palm. He reacts with a small wave of activity to vibration and to sound. He blinks and frowns to a bright light, but he is heedless of a dangling ring. He can swallow, and under certain feeding conditions, he can even register satiety, but he is usually fed by gavage at frequent intervals night and day.

The young fetal infant is busy with innumerable bits of behavior, which are not as detached as they seem. They are symptoms of a maturational process; they are incorporating within a growing, unitary action system.

Midstage Fetal Infant (32–36 Weeks)

In physical appearance as well as behavioral capacities, the midstage fetal infant is definitely more mature. His anatomy is more compact, less molluscous. His skin is less loose and wrinkled; it fits him more tightly because adipose has gathered beneath, except at the buttocks, where the skin still falls in folds. He seems slender rather than scrawny (he has nearly doubled his weight), and he is less flaccid, less apathetic.

All things considered, the most important developmental advance achieved by the midstage fetal infant is his capacity for brief periods of wakeful alertness. He is still an indisputably drowsy individual, but recurrently during day and night he pricks the surface of mere being with small acts of awareness. He keeps his eyes more widely open, and opens them more often. He shows more vivid distaste for bright light. He does not fixate upon a dangling ring with true inspectional regard, but when the ring is moved slowly he reacts with visual awareness; his eyes move saccadically in brief afterpursuit. He flexes on a rod placed in his palm with active grasp.

He shows increased responsiveness and adaptivity in his postural control. When he is picked up for bathing or feeding, his body tone increases, at least momentarily, to meet the challenge. His head station is palpably firmer, and his head is functionally more united to the trunk. Changes in trunk position induce active, rather than passive, changes in head posturing. In the prone position his head averts adaptively as though to reduce the hazard of suffocation. A vigorous infant, when prone, may even make a convexing movement like the hunch of an inch worm. When supine, he readily assumes the t-n-r attitude. He holds it quiescently; at times he activates it, flourishing the extended arm in a windmill orbit. He is capable of a larger amount of spontaneous postural activity, even though he generally husbands his energy in drowsy quiescence. When a gross motor action does occur, it tends to be more configured. It has lost some of the fading inconclusiveness of the early stage.

His feeding and language behavior also are more robust and better defined. He can register hunger with a fairly lusty, though brief, cry. He is capable of mild grunts, mewing sounds, yawns and sneezes. His suck and swallow pattern is sufficiently advanced to allow him to take food from a bottle.

Having noted his positive behavioral increments, it must be remarked that his total behavior resembles more that of a fetus than a fullterm neonate. In general, he is weak, indifferent and unresponsive. Even his sleep is indecisive, despite the promising punctuations of wakefulness. He is still a fetal infant, unripe and unfinished. He must be granted his drowsiness; he is under no compulsion to exercise behavior patterns which are undergoing their dormant maturation.

Late Stage Fetal Infant (36–40 Weeks)

Compared with his earlier stages, the late stage fetal infant presents a somewhat finished appearance. Adipose tissue has rounded his contours, and he may be almost chubby. He is physiologically more robust, and his behavior patterns are more clearly configured. Breathing, heart rate, blood pressure and temperature regulation are better correlated; the internal environment likewise is steadier. In general, he functions more smoothly. His body has acquired some homeostatic wisdom.

Accordingly, his behavior has more character. Rhythms of activity and rest are taking shape. His sleep is more expert and has more structure. A month or more ago it was shallow, variable, fluctuant and not always distinguishable from wakefulness. The mature fetal infant falls off to sleep more decisively, sleeps more deeply and clings to sleep more tenaciously. He awakes spontaneously at intervals and stays awake, although his emergence from sleep is much less decisive than his dropping off to sleep. All this reminds us that sleep is a complex function which needs intricate developmental organization, both at cortical and subcortical levels.

During wakefulness there are lengthening periods of visual and auditory awareness and heedfulness of internal states of being. Prone, he can lift his head momentarily. Supine, he can rotate his head through a quarter arc. He indulges in short cycles of spontaneous arm and leg activity, usually in the framework of the tonic-neck-reflex posture. His eye slits widen, and he immobilizes on hearing a sound. For brief moments he immobilizes his eyes in a primitive kind of fixation, as though drinking in visual impressions in a diffuse and passive manner. His eyes move very sketchily in a seeking kind of inspection, and they follow a moving ring some 30°. At times his regard seems to be halted by the face of nurse or examiner. He cries more crisply. If fussing, he tends to quiet when picked up. Thus, he shows the effect of experience as well as of his greater maturity.

It is instructive to compare his behavior to that of the fullterm newborn, who at a postconceptional age of 40 weeks has had no extrauterine experience whatsoever. The fullterm neonate begins his postnatal life with all the advantages which accrue from a normal period of gestation. He has relatively mature behavioral equipment and is therefore more ready for the transition to independent existence.

It takes the fullterm infant about a week to recover from the physical insults of being born. This is a period of adjustment. Breathing may be irregular in depth and rate. Pulse varies widely in strength and rhythm; blood pressure is low after a prolonged labor. For several days the intestinal tract is hyperactive, and there may be a tendency to reversal of peristalsis. Control of body temperature is unsteady and flighty. Current practice is to recognize and prevent some of these problems by warming, early feeding and better obstetrics to decrease prolonged labor.

The autonomic and central nervous systems are called upon to establish co-operative functional interrelations. The segmental and the suprasegmental portions of the central nervous system must achieve a vast complex of coordinations within a single integration. During the first week after birth both the neural and humoral systems are in a state of imbalance and irritability—hence the tendencies to trigger response, to tremor, to clonus; to wide and sometimes erratic fluctuations in physiologic and behavioral adjustments. One might say of fullterm and preterm neonate alike that neither is fully born until these excessive fluctuations are delimited to a more fixed and moderated range.

The late stage fetal infant has had some weeks in which to refine his adaptations to an extrauterine environment. For a brief period he may appear to be better organized and more expert than a newborn equivalent. He functions more smoothly, is less irritable and a little more responsive. However, any behavioral differences which favor the mature fetal infant are temporary and superficial. By the time the fullterm infant is 4 weeks old, he is physiologically more stabilized, and his behavior patterns are comparable to those of a premature infant without neonatal complications who has attained a corrected chronologic age of 4 weeks.

§4. GROWTH TRENDS IN THE BEHAVIOR OF THE FETAL INFANT

The foregoing outline demonstrates once again the essential orderliness of all behavioral development. The circumstances and contingencies of birth are so numerous, and some complications so obscure, that great caution must be exercised in appraising developmental outlook at the time of birth. Nevertheless, an infant will display certain growth trends even in the first weeks of his postnatal behavior.

These trends, within limits, have import both for diagnosis and for the care of the newborn, whether preterm or fullterm.

Growth trends become apparent in each of the five major fields, and they are continuous with the growth trends charted in Appendix B for age levels from 4 weeks through 3 years. This continuity is well illustrated in the developmental history of the tonic-neck-reflex, which is summed up in Fig. 12-1. At the

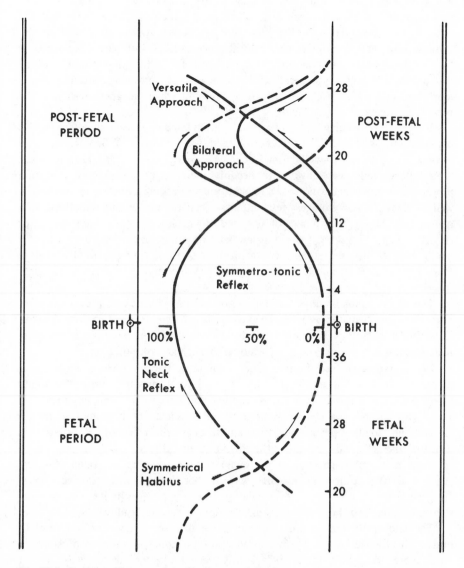

Fig. 12-1. Reciprocal interweaving of prehensory behavior.

gestational age of 16 weeks, the postural habitus of the fetus is symmetric. The fetus is capable, on stimulation, of approximating the hands toward the midline. At a fetal age of 20 weeks, rotation of the head to one side tends to produce extension of the arm on that side. This foreshadows a well-defined t-n-r attitude, which is manifested by the fetal infant at a gestational age of 28 weeks. The t-n-r is a conspicuous feature of spontaneous supine behavior of a fullterm infant until about 12 weeks of age, when it begins to wane. By 16 weeks of age the head is more labile, preferring the midline, and tonic symmetry takes the place of the t-n-r which had held sway. This symmetric attitude also is a tonic reflex—the symmetrotonic reflex (s-t-r). Like the t-n-r, the s-t-r holds temporary sway and is displaced by versatile unilateral coordinations, smoothly incorporated into varied postural sets for purposes of prehension and manipulation. Thus, the t-n-r should not be regarded as a stereotyped reflex; it is a complex growing pattern, whose morphogenesis traces back to early fetal life, and which advances well into the period of infancy.

Most of the behaviors of a fetal infant undergo a similar progressive organization, as indicated by Table 12-2. Motor activities, at first fluttery and inconclusive, advance to well-defined flexions and extensions. Grasp, head rotation, head lifting and eye movements become increasingly decisive. Vocalization progresses from squeaks and mews to a lusty cry. Feeding gains in competence as well as vigor. In the youngest fetal infants, sleep is shallow and undefined. In a mature fetal infant, four phases of sleep are distinguishable: (a) going to sleep, (b) staying asleep, (c) waking, (d) staying awake. The embryology of sleep consists of a developmental differentiation and organization of these four phases. The mature fetal infant is most advanced in phases (a) and (b)—he falls off to sleep and he clings to sleep.

Like sleep, tonus is subject to embryologic elaboration. Tonus is a condition of muscle tension mediated by both the autonomic and cerebrospinal nervous systems. However, it is not a generalized quality or quantity which simply increases in magnitude; it is behavior, and it is patterned through growth processes.

In the youngest fetal infants tone is minimal, flaccid, uneven, patchy and precarious. It rises, falls and shifts above its low level. It may be comparatively high in one region, and low in another. As tonus tires, it seems to "wander" to fresher areas. This meandering characteristic is probably related both to morphogenetic factors and to the physiologic mechanism of recruitment. Muscle fibers are recruited and activated in squads rather than in their entirety.

Even in the midstage fetal infant, tonal responses are more integrated. His gross postural activity comes in configured waves rather than in small localized ripples. His general tonus increases on manipulation and rises to meet limited emergencies. He is not as fragile as he seems, although his tone does wane readily.

The late stage fetal infant has more tone in reserve; he does not need to husband his tone as before. The whole substratum of tonus is more consolidated; he seems more firmly knit into a single, sturdy piece. He is more nearly ready to meet the buffetings of fate. This progression toward organized tonus represents the

Table 12-2. GROWTH TREND CHART:FETAL AND CIRCUMNATAL INFANCY

(The growth trends for any given behavior are ascertained by reading horizontally across the chart from age to age. The lines of continuity are represented by leaders ....)

	I (28-31 Weeks)	II (32-36 Weeks)	III (37-41 Weeks)	0-4 Weeks
Motor				
Supine—Small head movements (side position)			Turns head 90°	
T-n-r				
Floating t-n-r]				
Shoulder—Head droops	Slight retraction		Erects head briefly at shoulder	
Prone—Minimal head rotation	Returns head to side		Lifts head Zone I briefly	Crawling movements
Tone—Minimal, flaccid	Moderate, increase on manipulation		Good, sustained	
Rod—Brief, feeble closure	Active closure and grip			Hands fisted, clench on contact
Adaptive				
Dangling ring—No response	Ocular pursuit movements		Follows 30+°	Follows 90°
Bell ringing—Wave of activity			Attends, quiets	
Percussion—Wave of activity	Startles			
Regard—Eyes open at times	Eyes open more widely		Pseudo-fixation	Indefinite regard
Language				
Vocalization—Squeaks, mews	Soundless or brief cry when disturbed		Lusty, newborn cry	Small throaty noises
Expression—Small, twitchy face movements	Impassive face		Fusses or cries with waking	
Personal-Social				
Sociality—No response			Passive regard	Attends, quiets
Feeding—Gavage or dropper	Breck feeder or bottle		Bottle or breast	
Sleep—Undifferentiated	Brief periods of wakefulness		Differentiated	

essence of the neuropsychology of the fetus and of the fetal infant. His mental life is mainly one of kinesthesia and tactility; it has less to do with seeing and hearing, and much to do with the satisfactions of bodily movement, the sensorium of skin and mucous membrane, and his basic muscle tonus and patterns of tonal behavior.

§5. NEUROPSYCHIATRIC SEQUELAE OF LOW BIRTH WEIGHT

The literature has indicated a major effect of birth weight on subsequent behavioral development. This is not to say that every low birth weight infant demonstrates signs of central nervous system dysfunction; the prognosis for any individual infant can be determined only by a careful evaluation of his behavioral status. However, there is no question that group predictions demonstrate a wide range of later disabilities—from gross mental deficiency to learning disorders—the incidence of which increases as birth weight decreases.

There is one exception to this general rule. Paradoxically, the infant with a birth weight of 1000 g or less tends to have a better prognosis, if he survives, than if his weight had been between 1000 and 1500 g. His very survival apparently indicates a basic central nervous system integrity. With modern neonatal intensive care units and advances in medical techniques, survival rates may be increasing. Reports are appearing which indicate that in some centers there also has been a concomitant improvement in outlook for those infants under 1500 g whose lives are saved. These reports offer some possibility of altering the following rather dismal picture presented by past experience.

Adequate longitudinal studies of large numbers of subjects all demonstrate the same general picture of neuropsychiatric sequelae. Differences between investigations result from differences in sampling and methods of presenting the data. In addition to a higher proportion of smaller infants in twin pregnancies, twinning *per se* is associated with an increased incidence of abnormality. When a sample includes relatively few small infants, the overall incidence of impairment is decreased. When infant status, birth weight and socioeconomic factors are all taken into account, interrelationships otherwise obscured are clarified; a few studies will illustrate the general findings.

Alm[1] showed that even in adulthood low birth weight infants have not compensated. Data, primarily from military service records, for approximately 1000 low birth weight infants and a comparable number of controls indicated that mortality rates in the first 2 years of life had been higher, and that mean height and weight was lower. A significantly higher proportion of the prematures required institutional care or were receiving pensions for spastic paralysis, epilepsy or educational and medical mental deficiency. Drillien[17] has reported extensively on longitudinal studies which correlate weight at birth with a variety of environmental indices and later function; sequelae are similar and interrelationships important.

Interesting information is contained in later reports from the 1952 Baltimore Study of Prematures, which was based on the examination of 500 infants weighing

2500 g or less at birth and 492 matched controls. At 9 years of age, twice as many prematures as controls had IQs in the range of 50–79. The percentage of children with an appropriate grade placement for age was 45% if birth weight was less than 2001 g, 57% when it was between 2001 and 2500 g, and 72% when the child weighed over 2500 g.[79] At 12 years of age, when 85% of the original sample was located, 6.2% of the prematures but only 0.9% of the controls were in a variety of special care and educational settings.[78]

A closer look at some of the data for this group of infants at two points in time is instructive. Figure 12-2 shows a factor analysis of the 40-week data for 841 of

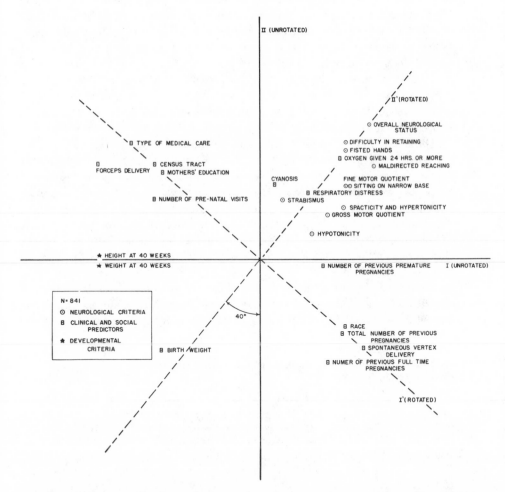

Fig. 12-2. Factor analysis of clinical and social predictors, physical growth and neurological consequences of birth weight. Two unrotated factors were graphed, and rotation through an angle of 40° accomplished by visual inspection and manual rotation.[63]

the 992 infants.[63] Simple rotation of two orthogonal factors can be done by inspection. First, the analysis indicates that the matching of the prematures and controls for socioeconomic status was good, and the independent effect of birth weight is demonstrated clearly. The comparison does not negate the association between low birth weight and socioeconomic status. Second, an inverse relationship between overall neurologic status and birth weight can be demonstrated, with abnormal neuromotor patterns and neonatal precursors of central nervous system dysfunction contributing in varying degrees to the overall neurologic status.

Table 12-3 shows in greater detail the relationship in infancy between birth weight and both neuromotor and intellectual deficits. Half of infants weighing under 1501 g at birth were impaired; 17.5% had minor neuromotor deficits, and 31.5% had either a major neuromotor defect or mental deficiency. Between 1501 and 2000 g, 30% of the infants had impairment, while those between 2001 and 2500 g fared only slightly better. Even within the fullterm control group, there were differences related to birth weight. The lowest rate for neuromotor abnormality of marked degree and mental deficiency combined, less than 1.5%, was found in the infants with birth weights over 3000 g. As a whole, 85% or more of infants weighing over 2500 g at birth showed no significant neuromotor or intellectual abnormalities at 40 weeks of age.

The relationship between birth weight, infant central nervous system integrity and later function, shown in Table 12-4, is far more revealing in alerting the clinician to groups at risk. The children diagnosed in infancy as having mental deficiency were excluded from the table; *abnormality* refers to those with neuromotor deficits with a normal intellectual potential. There was no differential loss in the sample, and the percentage of infants abnormal by birth weight was not different for the 85% of the original sample reexamined at 6–7 years of age. Clearly, birth weight still played a role; more children whose birth weights were less than 2001 g were untestable or had IQs less than 80 at school age, whether they were impaired or not in infancy. The infant neuromotor status is even more important. For all but one of the birth weight groups, the abnormal infant had roughly $2\frac{1}{2}$–3 times the risk of failing to perform adequately at early school age.

Table 12-3. Distribution of Intellectual and Neuromotor Deficits at 40 Weeks of Age, by Birth Weight

Birth Weight	No.	STATUS AT 40 WEEKS Per Cent			
		Without Significant Deficit	Minor Neuromotor Deficit	Major Neuromotor Deficit	Mental Deficiency
<1501 grams	57	51	17.5	17.5	14
1501–2000	84	71	14	12	2
2001–2250	103	75	20	4	1
2251–2500	256	77	16	6	1
2501–3000	153	85	10	2	3
3001+	339	87	12	<0.5	1

Data from Study of Prematures, Baltimore, Maryland

Table 12-4. Children Untestable or with Stanford-
Binet IQ Below 80 at 6-7 Years of Age, by Birth
Weight and Infant Central Nervous System Integrity
(Infants with Mental Deficiency Excluded)

Birth Weight	INFANT STATUS			
	Normal		Abnormal	
	#	Per Cent Untestable or IQ <80	#	Per Cent Untestable or IQ <80
<2001 grams	79	15	39	44
2001-2250	69	11	22	27
2251-2500	167	13	49	30
2501-3000	112	10	16	12
3001+	243	7	33	18
Total	670	11	159	29

Data from the Study of Prematures, Baltimore, Maryland

Almost half the impaired smallest infants, who had an initial intellectual potential in the normal range, had function at school age which indicated that special care or special education might be necessary.

In the preceeding discussion, the term *premature* sometimes is employed loosely, as though it were entirely synonymous with low birth weight. The influence of the length of gestation can be studied by dividing any given birth weight group arbitrarily into two segments, above or below a percentile of weight for gestational age. This was done using the 50th percentile and the 10th percentile. The Lubchenco Denver charts,[55] the New York City percentile charts,[82] and the 50th percentile derived from the Baltimore data were used. Whichever combination of percentile and chart was applied to the 500 Baltimore infants under 2501 g, birth weight is the most important factor. The incidence of dysfunction is comparable within each birth weight group, no matter how the division is made, and it increases as the birth weight decreases. Similar findings obtained for 70 infants and children with hypoglycemia, a condition known to be associated highly with small-for-gestational-age pregnancies.[49] Major central nervous system handicaps were twice as high in those children whose birth weights were less than 2000 g.

In simple terms, an infant weighing $3\frac{1}{2}$ lb at birth whose gestation lasted 40 weeks is likely to have endured more adverse intrauterine influences than infants of 5–7 lb with the same gestational period. Conversely, an infant weighing $3\frac{1}{2}$ lb is more likely to have been born before term. Both types of infants, regardless of gestational age, risk poor outcome because of low birth weight.

These data present only part of the picture. Illnesses and convulsions after the infant examination have not been taken into consideration. The sociocultural environment also plays an important role, and data relative to the effect of the mother's socioeconomic status, as indicated by her education, in fostering adequate performance have been presented in Chapter 8. Twenty years ago it was apparent that methods of care conforming to recommended standards decreased mortality rates significantly for infants weighing between 1001 and 2000 g at birth, precisely those with the greatest degree of subsequent central nervous system dysfunction.[64]

In summary, the handicaps of low birth weight infants persist. They are not due to low birth weight and prematurity *per se* but to the fact that such infants are more apt to be impaired because of the associated abnormal paranatal factors. Clinical experience in a neonatal intensive care nursery indicates that major efforts still need to be directed towards the prevention of preterm and low birth weight deliveries. Developmental diagnosis has a key role in the supervision of the low birth weight infant, to identify the infant who has suffered neuropsychiatric impairment and who will need careful medical and sociopsychologic intervention to maximize his developmental potential.

13

Convulsive Seizure Disorders

Seizures figure frequently in the case histories of developmental defect and deviation. A convulsive seizure must be regarded as one of the most important symptoms in childhood. It reflects a pathologic state, and in turn may interfere directly with the normal course of development. Seizures vary enormously in immediate gravity, from a single benign episode in a fleeting infection to severe status epilepticus, a medical emergency which may terminate in death, the seizures occurring in such rapid succession that the patient does not regain consciousness. Seizures, *per se,* do not necessarily cause mental deterioration, but when there is loss of substrates such as glucose and oxygen, and alterations in other biochemical homeostatic mechanisms, they do cause damage and may have a devastating effect. Their recognition is vitally important because they are one of the few conditions in which proper treatment almost always is effective. The most frequent error in diagnosis is failure to consider the possibility of seizures as an explanation for aberrant behavior, whether or not there are other signs of central nervous system dysfunction present.

Etiologic factors are similar to and as numerous as those of other developmental neuropsychiatric disabilities. In addition to the effects of changes in glucose and oxygen, convulsions can result from alterations in calcium, phosphorus, magnesium, copper or pyridoxine, to name but a few possible biochemical disturbances. A seizure clearly is an indication of some basic impairment of central nervous system integrity. The precise mechanism producing convulsive seizures still is unknown; recent careful microscopic study of brains has demonstrated the presence of damaged neurons which probably are responsible for initiating the abnormal electrical discharges.

The purpose of this chapter is to concentrate on those aspects of seizure disorders where our experience differs from commonly held views, to emphasize some often unrecognized manifestations of seizure disorders in infancy and childhood and to present a treatment regimen which we have found effective. A brief description of the common types of seizure disorder is included for completeness. The reader is referred to standard texts listed in the general reference section of Appendix E for more details.

§1. DEFINITIONS

The simplest all-inclusive definition of a *clinical seizure* is a paroxysmal, recurrent, stereotyped alteration of brain function. The duration, number and location of the abnormal neuronal discharges produce the different manifestations. The exception to this definition is the occurrence of but a single convulsion. Otherwise, no qualification is needed for the wide variety of clinical manifestations; neither convulsive movements nor loss of consciousness is necessary in seizure disorders. Recurrent episodes in which retention of consciousness is associated with complete absence of movement should make one suspicious of another process such as drug intoxication or one of the periodic paralyses.

The term epilepsy is falling into disfavor because of its unfavorable connotations in the mind of the layman. Epilepsy is an archaic synonym for any recurrent seizure disorder, regardless of cause or clinical manifestations.

Seizures vary enormously in frequency, type and severity. Pediatric and neurology texts contain extensive, although often conflicting, descriptions of the common types. *Grand mal* seizures with no electric or clinical lateralization are characterized by a sudden loss of consciousness followed by generalized tonic-clonic spasms of the muscles, often associated with urinary and fecal incontinence and followed by a postictal state of lethargy of varying degrees. *Petit mal* seizures consist of brief absence attacks, lasting 10—40 seconds, with or without accompanying motor automatisms, and usually without loss of postural control. The diagnosis depends on the presence of 3-per-second spike and wave patterns in the electroencephalogram. The disorder very rarely occurs before 3—4 years of age or has its onset after puberty. Similar clinical manifestations prior to or after these ages are not accompanied by the characteristic EEG pattern. Status epilepticus may occur in both grand and petit mal seizures. *Myoclonic* seizures consist of sudden involuntary massive contractions of muscle groups with brief or no apparent loss of consciousness; they must be distinguished from *akinetic* seizures which are characterized by loss of postural tone with almost immediate return of consciousness. *Psychomotor* seizures are organized, complex, involuntary episodes, either motor, mental or sensory in nature, and usually identical from one episode to the next; often they are followed by postictal states. As the name implies, *autonomic* episodes are manifestations of a variety of autonomic disturbances—focal or total body changes in color, vomiting, sweating and borborygmus. *Infantile spasms* or *hypsarhythmia,* peculiar to infancy and with onset between 3—6 months, and *febrile* seizures, usually restricted to the first 5—6 years of life, are discussed in Sections 3 and 4. In the first few months of life, focal seizures do not have the same connotation of a localized structural lesion that they have at later ages.

Seizures occur in three different groups of individuals, those who have:

1. Seizures and other manifestations of organic brain disease.
2. Seizures alone.
3. Apparent mental deficiency secondary to a seizure state.

In the first group, the seizures can be treated and controlled, with great benefit to the patient and the family, but the accompanying disorders such as mental deficiency or "cerebral palsy" are not altered, although the behavioral organization may be improved. When seizures are the only demonstrable evidence of central nervous system dysfunction, treatment is vital, episodes can be controlled and potential deterioration prevented, but the developmental rate is not necessarily accelerated. In the third group, the patients appear to be mentally defective because they are out of contact as a result of their almost constant seizure activity. Often a clue is present in the observation of fragments of age-appropriate behavior, or in a history of normal developmental milestones prior to the onset of symptoms. Although there is only a small number of patients in the third category, treatment is rewarding, since it results in a "cure" of the seeming mental deficiency.

In the presence of uncontrolled seizures, no predictions regarding intellectual potential can be made until adequate therapy is instituted and the episodes abolished. Moreover, one must exercise caution in evaluating a patient following any serious seizure episode; postconvulsive confusion may take time to dissipate.

§2. CLUES TO ATYPICAL SEIZURE MANIFESTATIONS

Any unexplained behavior always warrants careful investigation for the possibility that it may derive from a seizure state. A list of situations to which the clinician should be alert in infancy follows; some manifestations occur in later childhood and are not unknown in adults:

1. Developmental failure of any kind—in adaptive, motor or language behavior, or in growth.
2. Discrepancies between different areas of behavior, either reported by the parents or observed during the examination, particularly when language is significantly advanced over adaptive behavior. For example, the mother of a 9-month-old may report the infant says "dada" or waves "bye-bye" but isn't interested in toys and plays briefly with only one at a time.
3. Discrepancies within areas of behavior, either reported or observed. For example, a 6-month-old may be reported to support himself in sitting but not have good head control.
4. Generalized disorganization of behavior interspersed with integrated responses appropriate for age.
5. Any recurrent episodic behavior where there is alteration in the usual pattern

of responsiveness of the child. The parents often will report that they can tell by the "look in the child's eyes" whether the day will be one of normal alertness and responsiveness or whether the behavior will be inexplicable. The child may sit apathetically for long periods wherever he happens to be placed; he may be irritable, whiny and dissatisfied no matter what is tried; he may walk about the house with his hands above his head, heedless of sound and unaware even if he burns his hand on a hot stove.

6. A suspicion of blindness, deafness or insensitivity to pain. When these phenomena are intermittent they almost invariably represent seizures, except in the rare instance in which the child appears deaf only when he is not facing his parents.
7. Staring and being out of contact with the environment, again particularly when episodic in nature.
8. Twitching, tremors, apnea and cyanosis, especially in the newborn.
9. Temper tantrums, unprovoked crying, paroxysmal laughter (with or without associated running), colic, nightmares and sleepwalking.
10. Episodes of limpness, stiffening, eye-rolling or breath holding.
11. Episodic stridor, dysphagia, vomiting, sweating or other autonomic disturbances.

Two of these behaviors warrant more detailed discussion. They are among the most common manifestations of seizure disorders in infancy.

STARING EPISODES. If an individual who appears to be staring is actually fixating and in contact with his environment, he responds to obstruction of vision by avoidance. Waving a hand in front of his eyes does not interfere with looking; obstruction must be achieved by *placing* and *holding* a hand in front of his eyes. Even at 2 months, an infant turns his eyes or his head; an older infant may smile, laugh or reach for the intruding hand. Visual obstruction is the most reliable method of arousing a reaction, since turning to sound or touch may not occur during this "daydreaming." Some abnormal children seem perpetually heedless of auditory or tactile stimulation, yet they object vigorously to interference with vision.

The examiner is acutely aware of these episodes during the course of a developmental examination because he is watching the infant's behavior so closely that interruption of responsiveness is striking. Complete suspension of activity does not occur always during the periods of staring; various automatisms may be seen. Eye deviation, aversion of the head, chewing, mouthing movements and aimless movements of the hands probably are associated with lateralized lesions, particularly those arising in the temporal lobe. Failure to respond to pain or absent corneal reflexes in association with the staring episodes often convinces the skeptic of the convulsive nature of the attacks.

Descriptively, these episodes resemble petit mal seizures. In older children with petit mal it is common to see eye blinking and a slight rhythmic jerking of the arms at a rate of about 3-per-second, consonant with the abnormal electric discharges; rarely, abrupt falling to the floor occurs. In younger children, when the automatisms are not due to petit mal, the characteristic EEG changes are not present and the manifestations respond to treatment with phenobarbital, a drug usually ineffective in petit mal.

Staring episodes perhaps should be classified as psychomotor seizures. We have labeled them *abortive grand mal seizures;* they are comparable to stiffening or loss of consciousness with eyes rolling back, manifestations which are seen at the onset of a grand mal attack but which may never progress to tonic-clonic convulsions.

CRYING EPISODES. Most discussions of convulsions state that psychomotor seizures are rare in infants and young children. This conclusion probably results from failure to recognize that crying is one of the earliest forms of organized behavioral response, which continues well into childhood. So-called colic is a common form of episodic crying in young infants. In the toddler and preschooler, crying spells often are called temper tantrums, the implication being that the crying is but another expression of temper. Parents often say that a child has two kinds of temper tantrums: "At times he is 'just mad'; at others he is mad at me about a specific thing I have or have not done." During nightmares the mother reports that the infant's eyes are open but he keeps right on crying in his sleep and she says "Once I really get him awake, then he recognizes me and I can comfort him."

If all infants and young children cry, isn't the behavior merely a voluntary expression of emotion? Why not just faulty management of the child? Sometimes it is, but the crying episodes most suggestive of psychomotor seizures are characterized by an abrupt onset, without any, or with only a trivial, precipitating cause. They cannot be assuaged no matter what is done, and there is alteration in the usual responsiveness of the child. Admittedly it is extremely difficult to decide in the first 2 or 3 months of life if a crying infant is in contact with his environment, but mothers usually are quite skilled at making a distinction between ordinary crying and spells in which neither holding, feeding, walking nor anything else comforts the infant. The episodes may last a few minutes or several hours. They terminate abruptly with resumption of the previous activity, only rarely subsiding gradually. They often are followed by a postictal phenomenon which may look very much like the exhaustion following prolonged normal crying.

An entire episode of this type of seizure may be seen in the course of a developmental examination: The infant is alert and friendly, busily exploiting a toy, when he beings to cry suddenly. He does not cling to his mother and look balefully at the examiner, as an emotionally upset infant does. He pushes back in her arms and cries whether he is held or put down, whether he is given his bottle or it is taken away, whether mother, father or the examiner tries to comfort him. Regretfully, the examiner may suggest that another appointment will have to be scheduled. Suddenly, the episode terminates, and the infant resumes participation as though nothing had happened; an entirely satisfactory examination is obtained.

One is not always fortunate enough to see the end as well as the beginning of an attack.

Even before a child is able to walk and talk, psychomotor seizures may involve a variety of complex acts. In many instances, episodic deviations in behavior may subside without treatment; however, we have innumerable documented cases in which there was a subsequent onset of typical grand mal attacks. Whenever there is any doubt, differential diagnosis by the therapeutic trial discussed in Section 6 should be undertaken.

§3. INFANTILE SPASMS (HYPSARHYTHMIA)

Infantile spasms usually have their onset from 3–6 months of age. Diagnosis is based on finding a combination of a specific EEG abnormality and characteristic clinical picture. In a typical case of the idiopathic form, pregnancy and neonatal periods are normal and the infant does well. He begins to smile, coo, laugh, play with his hands and a rattle, and engage in social play; he is described by his parents as being alert and reactive. Between 3 and 6 months, seizures begin. These myoclonic spasms are sudden, brief, massive involuntary contractions of the body, usually flexor but occasionally extensor in nature. Characteristically the initial episodes are single, but within a week they begin to come in showers, perhaps as many as 50 times a day. Within a week or two after the onset of seizures, behavior regresses, previous function is lost and the infant becomes inert and unresponsive, or irritable and equally unresponsive. In the awake state, his EEG shows a persistent diffuse abnormality with high-voltage, irregular, slow delta waves and spike discharges which occur independently in all leads; rarely, the discharges may be generalized and synchronous. The spike and wave are unlocked; that is, they are random rather than sequential. If the infant is sedated, as often is the case in this age group, the malignancy of the record is reduced and the slow, irregular, unlocked spike and wave may be depressed or abolished.

Occasionally the initial seizures do not show the typical pattern of massive flexion or extension, but any seizures which occur in showers are suspicious. If the EEG is typical, the classic convulsions usually appear soon. Myoclonic episodes are often mistaken for colic because of the episodic nature and the sharp flexion or extension movements. They also are seen in infants with other developmental deviations and other types of seizures. In the absence of the typical EEG these seizures probably are not hypsarhythmic, but they may have an equally grave prognosis.

The etiology of infantile spasms is obscure, but there is some evidence that the idiopathic type is an autoimmune phenomenon. The microscopic picture is very similar to the pathology seen in experimentally produced allergic encephalomyelitis. The autoimmune process probably is the main reason for central nervous system neuronal cellular damage. In the absence of interference with an adequate blood supply, the seizures themselves are unlikely to contribute to brain damage.

Even without treatment, the seizures tend to change in form and disappear with time, usually between 3 and 6 years of age. However, the cerebral damage is reversed in only about 15% of untreated patients, the rest remaining mentally defective—usually markedly so.

According to Sherard,[68] the chief difficulty in the treatment of idiopathic infantile spasms is that therapy must be initiated in the first 2 or 3 weeks after the onset of symptoms, before any central nervous system damage has occurred. Otherwise, seizure control is achieved, but for 85% of the patients, the cerebral function that has been lost is not reclaimed. Delay in the institution of therapy probably is why many investigators feel that treatment has not changed the course of the disorder.

When ACTH treatment is started early, seizure control and reversion of the EEG to normal occurs within 48—72 hours. There is little evidence that ACTH is more efficacious than prednisone, and ACTH has the disadvantage of requiring injections. The 9-fluorinated compounds, such as Decadron, should be avoided, because the enzymes necessary for degradation of the corticosteroids are markedly inhibited by fluorination. After 48 hours, Valium or phenobarbital treatment should be started. These medications may be discontinued at the end of a year, provided that there is absolutely no evidence of any abnormality in a properly obtained EEG.[68]

§4. FEBRILE SEIZURES

Febrile seizures are restricted almost entirely to the first 6 years of life. Opinion is divided in regard to the definition of the term and the method of treatment. Some neurologists consider febrile seizures to be a distinct clinical entity. Regardless of whether or not this is so, a *febrile seizure* should be defined as a generalized convulsion occurring with an upswing of temperature to above 102 degrees and lasting less than 5 minutes; the temperature usually is higher and the duration shorter than just stated. Affected children clearly have a decreased threshold for seizures, since the overwhelming majority of children with fever—as high as 90% according to pediatric texts—do not convulse. About 80% of children with febrile seizures have sufficient central nervous system maturation to resist the stress of the fever by the time they are 4 years old. Immaturity of the brain probably explains the marked difference between children under 4 and adults in the incidence of seizures accompanying bacterial meningitis due to pnemococci or H. influenza bacilli (45% compared to 8% for adults).[60]

Other neurologists consider febrile seizures to be part of a continuum, in which the first episode may be followed by recurrent seizures, then status epilepticus and finally acute toxic encephalopathy, resulting in major damage to the central nervous system or death. Pediatric texts indicate that 20—40% of children with a febrile seizure conforming to the restricted definition develop other seizures without fever. There is some evidence to show that this is more likely to occur when there is a positive family history of febrile seizures at an early age, particularly when such early seizures were followed by a chronic convulsive disorder. In any given instance, it is impossible to predict the subsequent course with confidence. Therefore, there is no logic to withholding preventive medication because there has been only one seizure. This is of prime importance after a known infection of the central nervous system or in a child with other signs of neuropsychiatric impairment.

We support the increasing consensus toward recommending continuous medication to maintain an elevated seizure threshold until 6 years of age, because of the possibility of irreversible damage. Beyond this age susceptibility to febrile seizures is past for virtually all children. There is no value to giving phenobarbital by mouth with the onset of the fever, since its action is not rapid enough to be effective in stopping a convulsion, in spite of the fact that it may inhibit heat production. Further, by chance alone, the fever will occur half the time at night when both child and parents are asleep. Other appropriate steps to decrease the fever and investigate the nature of the infectious process are indicated.

§5. DIAGNOSIS

A diagnosis of seizures *is made* by an adequately obtained history of paroxysmal alterations of brain function. In general, the clinician will be able to observe only those episodes which occur many times a day. Further investigation for etiologic conditions amenable to specific therapy, in addition to anticonvulsants (outlined in Chapter 5, Section 8), always is necessary. The family history is important in detecting associated underlying diseases known to have a hereditary basis, but is of little help regarding a particular child. Tuberous sclerosis is an example of a disease in which recognized seizures in one child could indicate previously unsuspected manifestations in other family members. The role of genetics in the etiology of seizure susceptibility still is controversial; familial aggregation is not always synonymous with inheritance.

Techniques of electroencephalography constantly are improving and becoming more sophisticated. Any single record is a small time sample of the total behavior, but repeated recordings eventually yield a 95% correlation between an abnormal EEG and clinical evidence of seizure activity. Moreoever, the type of EEG abnormality most often correlates with a particular type of seizure. In infants and young children, considerable patience is required to obtain natural awake and sleep records without artifacts. The diagnosis cannot be rejected and treatment withheld because of failure to demonstrate an abnormal EEG at any one time; conversely, therapy should not be given for an EEG abnormality in the absence of any evidence of recurrent paroxysmal alteration of brain function. The EEG is specific for a diagnosis of petit mal or infantile spasms. Except in the latter condition, it is not useful as a guide for altering or discontinuing therapy.

Finally, a diagnostic trial of treatment is warranted, particularly in the situations discussed in Section 2 where much controversy exists about the implications of the observed behavior. Ideally, a double-blind program should alternate placebo and active drug, because any medication or suggestions for management can modify the behavior of both parents and child. Two clinicians are required, one to prescribe and one to evaluate the response in conjunction with the parents. When two physicians are not available, the parents should engage in a blind evaluation under the clinician's direction, particularly when behavior such as crying episodes could be the result of emotional upset. Most parents are willing to cooperate if time is taken to explain the situation in detail. A positive response to phenobarbital over placebo may still leave doubts in the minds of skeptical clinicians, but the treatment benefits both the child and his family. We conducted a double-blind study of only 19 patients and demonstrated a highly statistically significant superiority for phenobarbital over placebo in infants and children with these manifestations.[38]

§6. SUGGESTED REGIMEN FOR LONG-TERM CARE

The objective of anticonvulsant therapy is to maintain full doses of medication for a minimum of 2, and preferably 4, seizure-free years (Section 7). Resistance to long-term medication comes less often from parents than from physicians, who seem to strive to discontinue medication quickly.

Treatment with one drug at full dose is preferable to multiple drug therapy. Phenobarbital in our experience is the drug of choice in treating *almost all* seizures, particularly in the age range with which this volume is concerned. It is virtually nontoxic, inexpensive, has a relatively rapid onset of effect and has an observable endpoint by which the dose can be regulated for each individual. At all dosages below lethal levels the body adapts to phenobarbital, probably by increased liver enzyme activity, and the blood level falls even though the same dose is continued. Adequate dosage is indicated when the initial drowsiness which occurs disappears and the seizures are controlled. Clinical judgment is necessary in regulating the dose, but empirically the starting doses outlined in Table 13-1 have been found highly effective.

For infants up to 21–24 months of age, *10 mg per kg per day is the starting dose;* this amount is necessary before one can consider having given phenobarbital an adequate therapeutic test. This dosage may increase the sleeping time by 25–30%, with a peak 3–5 days after starting treatment. There may be no increase in actual sleep, but the child may be groggy and cross and want to lie down; an ambulatory child may try to fight off the drowsiness and stagger about irritably. *On the same dose*, the drowsiness usually disappears in 7–10 days, but it may last 2–3 weeks. Then the child is awake and more alert than he was previously when seizures were present. He has achieved a full therapeutic dose with adequate seizure control and no side effects.

Most young children show the desired result with 10 mg/kg, but there is

Table 13-1. Recommended Starting Dose of Phenobarbital, by Age
of Patient*

	STARTING DOSE mg/Kg/24 hr.
Newborn	10-15
1-24 months	10
2-4 years	8-7
4-6 years	6-5
7+ years	4-3

*Clinical judgment, as described in
the text, must be used in regulating
the dose for each child.

individual variation. If 10 mg/kg produces no appreciable increase in drowsiness or irritability or no evidence of seizure control in 2 weeks, the total dose should be increased by 15 mg; if the child's reaction is to stay awake for most of each 24 hours, a further increase may be tried. Conversely, if adaptation does not begin by 14–21 days or the child is becoming increasingly drowsy, half the total dose should be omitted for 36 hours to allow partial excretion, and then the 24-hour dose decreased by 15 mg. This procedure may be repeated at 14–21-day intervals as needed.

One important word of warning must be given: If adaptation to drowsiness has occurred but the child continues to have seizures after 2 weeks, then it is unlikely that significantly larger doses or the addition of other medication will control the convulsive seizures. In such circumstances appropriate investigations for the detection of space-occupying lesions or degenerative diseases should be undertaken.

Above the age of 21–24 months a smaller dose is necessary, as outlined in Table 13-1; as age increases, dose per kilogram of body weight decreases. These empiric starting doses must be adjusted according to the individual child's response. At school age the 3–4 mg/kg dose often must be supplemented by dextroamphetamine to enable the child to continue to function and still maintain seizure control. Newborns tolerate and sometimes require more than 10 mg/kg. Infants generally need in increase of 15 mg for every 3–4 lbs of weight gain. An older child should be challenged every 6–9 months by 15 mg increases until drowsiness occurs, followed by the adaptation procedure outlined above.

The "paradoxical" reaction of excitement and insomnia is produced most often when the dose of phenobarbital is too small, but it can occur at any dosage. This response is an indication for increasing the amount given, not for discontinuing medication. Some children continue to be stimulated until increasingly large doses cause persistent sleep; the percentage of patients with such a response increases with age. These undesirable results often can be eliminated by replacing phenobarbital with Mebaral at twice the dosage. Occasionally, substituting Mysoline for half the phenobarbital in a ratio of 10 mg Mysoline for 1 mg phenobarbital will eliminate the drowsiness, when high doses are needed to control seizures. However, just as often, low doses of Mysoline can produce a rather startling degree of drowsiness, which increases as the proportion of Mysoline substituted is increased.

Phenobarbital is excreted relatively slowly and tends not to show wide daily fluctuations if given at least every 12 hours. Approximately one-third the dose is given in the morning and two-thirds about 12 hours later, before bedtime. If there is any excessive drowsiness, it occurs at night. Occasionally a more effective schedule is morning, afternoon and bedtime, divided $\frac{1}{4}$, $\frac{1}{4}$, and $\frac{1}{2}$. Even in very small infants, *tablets* crushed in a teaspoonful of juice, fruit or other food are easier to administer and better accepted than the elixir. When less than 15 mg is needed for small infants, the liquid may be necessary since tablets are too small to divide. When an intermediate dose is appropriate for the weight of an older child, it can be achieved by giving 15 mg additional on alternate days. (The mother can remember what she is to do by giving an even number of tablets on even-numbered days, odd on odd.)

These procedures to be employed and the effects to be expected must be explained to the parents in careful detail. Close contact must be maintained with them during the first weeks of the adaptation period to ensure successful results.

Figure 13-1 is a graphic illustration of the theoretic adaptation to phenobarbital. No blood levels appear on the abscissa because they increase for any given

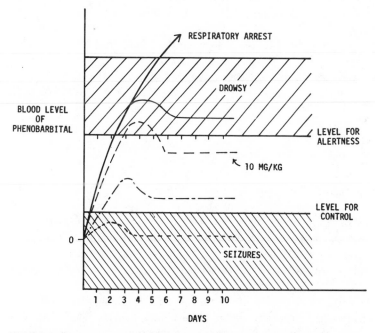

Fig. 13-1. Theoretical representation of adaption to phenobarbital. No blood levels appear on the abscissa because they increase with increasing age, for any given dose. Therapeutic levels are 3–5 mg/ml.

dose with increasing age. Therapeutic levels are between 3 and 5 mg/ml, higher than those usually given in texts. The curves demonstrate the concept that adaptation in blood level occurs at all dosage levels. The dose may be too small to control seizures or so large that continuing drowsiness or even respiratory arrest occurs. The ideal is a combination of alertness and control of seizures. If this state can be achieved at lower doses than the empirical 10 mg/kg, as the next-to-the-bottom curve illustrates, why should a dose this high be employed? There are three reasons for doing so. First, a therapeutic effect is obvious if 20 seizures a day are eliminated on a smaller dose. However, if the child's pattern is one episode every 6 weeks or 6 months, and the dose is not titrated for weight and age, there is no logical basis for selecting any one of the possible smaller amounts. More important, there is no assurance that the next seizure will not be severe enough to cause irreversible damage. Second, under the stress of fever or other unusual circumstances, escape may occur. Third, weight gain may be more rapid than anticipated; the dose can be outgrown and seizures of unpredictable severity can recur.

Petit mal does not respond often to phenobarbital. Myoclonic seizures which are not hypsarhythmic are difficult to control on any medication. Control can be acheived in the vast majority of other seizures on the recommended regimen of phenobarbital *alone*. If convulsions persist, other medication can be added, but the likelihood that the seizures will be controlled is doubtful. Dilantin and its derivatives have possible serious toxic effects, including immunologic defects and permanent cerebellar damage. In young infants they produce drowsiness if blood levels are in excess of 3–4 mg; at levels in excess of 2 mg, ataxia is common. It is often difficult to distinguish the toxic signs from seizure manifestations, and occasional idiosyncratic reactions occur on low doses. Use of hydantoins has no advantage, and many disadvantages, over phenobarbital, and should be avoided under 10 years of age.

§7. PROGNOSIS

Data for large groups of unselected patients treated systematically or in controlled studies are not available. Consistent followup is difficult. A recent survey of 148 patients whose seizures had been controlled for 4 years reported relapse in one-quarter after discontinuation of therapy; febrile seizures were not excepted.[31] The numbers were too small to draw conclusions about the various seizure types, but the relapse rate appeared least for grand mal seizures. The best prognosis seemed to be for patients whose seizures started early in life and were brought under control in the first year of treatment.

Prognosis depends, of course, on the nature of the underlying disease process. Any major seizure can cause irreversible devastating damage. The danger in inadequate treatment is the inability to predict the occurrence of another episode or to determine which subsequent attack might result in brain damage. By and large, mental deterioration does not occur. However, untreated and unrecognized seizures can cause deterioration in function, as the followup at early school age of 200 children which was presented in Chapter 5, Section 7, demonstrated. How much of the loss found was irreversible, how much was secondary to ongoing seizure activity could not be determined in most of the children, since we were not in a position to reinstate therapy. Deterioration was more common if other evidences of central nervous system impairment had been present in infancy.

There are a small number of infants with frequent abortive seizures, particularly in association with hypotonia, abnormalities in visual organization or "autistic" behavior, in whom deterioration occurs in spite of adequate therapy. These children do not have a true degenerative process; they do not lose already acquired function but rather fail to make progress. Whether the seizures cause the lack of progress or whether both are the result of an underlying disease process has not been established, and an adequate explanation so far has eluded the clinicians who have seen these infants.

These results emphasize the importance of striving for early diagnosis and treatment. The parents must be informed fully about seizure manifestations and the necessity for long-term therapy. The attitude of the family should be one of intelligent optimism. They will need to assist in the education of the child when he is old enough to understand, and they should know of the resources for help that are available.

§8. ILLUSTRATIVE CASES

Infantile Spasms (Hypsarhythmia)

Case 1 was born after an uncomplicated pregnancy to a young woman who lived with her parents. She was the delight of the family and made rapid progress until $4\frac{1}{2}$ months of age, when myoclonic seizures began. They were thought to represent attacks of colic until the pediatrician observed one of the many episodes that were occurring. Rapid deterioration set in, and by *26 weeks* she had lost all interest in her environment. EEG was characteristic of hypsarhythmia. On examination she still retained good muscle tone, had good head control and sat leaning forward on her hands. She retained placed objects briefly without regard, did not follow them and only occasionally immobilized to bell ringing.

Phenobarbital did not affect the episodes appreciably, although they had decreased in frequency by *52 weeks.* The only behavioral change was loss of the ability to sit, and she continued to function at an atypical neonatal level. The seizure episodes stopped eventually, but she made no developmental progress and died at 2 years from bronchopneumonia. An autopsy was not done.

Case 2 was born at term weighing 7 lb 3 oz, after a pregnancy complicated by spotting and elevated blood pressure. His developmental progress was quite normal until 6 weeks prior to hospitalization, at which time he developed frequent episodes of myoclonic seizures. The family was traveling abroad at the time, and the nature of the problem was unrecognized. At the time of hospital admission he was having as many as 40–50 episodes daily and his behavior had regressed; the EEG was characteristic.

When examined at *35 weeks* he was markedly irritable and totally disinterested. He had no regard for the examiner or his parents, and exploitation was extremely meager. Occasionally he reached for an object held in front of his eyes or grasped one on contact. His only vocalization was crying. His hands were held semifisted; he sat erect but unsteadily for brief periods and stood with hands held. No maturity levels could be assigned.

After the institution of ACTH therapy, the EEG began to improve and became normal after 4 weeks; seizures decreased and stopped entirely after 2 weeks of treatment. At *40 weeks* he was a somber infant with well-sustained interest who exploited toys actively and had appropriate social relationships. His behavior was moderately impulsive and disorganized. Adaptive behavior scattered from 32–39 weeks, centering at 36, and low average development was indicated. He sat alone indefinitely but with legs extended and adducted, and pulled himself to standing at the crib rail. He had some maldirected reaching, and his hands still fisted intermittently. Fingers had not yet differentiated, grasp was palmar, he had difficulty retaining and he could not secure the pellet. ACTH dosage was being tapered slowly.

Whether his minor abnormal neuromotor patterns were secondary to his seizures or related to the complications of pregnancy could not be determined. At *21 months* he was making steady progress, and seizures had not recurred.

Case 3 had been taken into her adoptive home from the newborn nursery. She was delivered 2 weeks prematurely, weighing 5 lb 7 oz, and had respiratory difficulty at birth. She fed slowly and was stiff when handled. At 3 months of age she developed frequent daily attacks of jerking.

At a corrected chronologic age of *17 weeks* she was hyperactive and disorganized, with fleeting interest and attention. Behavior was immature, adaptive behavior was at 13 weeks and a dull normal development was indicated. She exhibited hypertonicity of all four extremities and had persistence of a tonic-neck-reflex and fisted hands. At least one myoclonic seizure was observed during the examination. The parents were advised of the guarded prognosis, but they elected to proceed with permanent adoption.

The infant was treated with phenobarbital for a short period under the supervision of the family physician, and the seizures eventually disappeared. At a corrected age of *14 months* she had compensated fully for her neuromotor difficulties. Exploitation was vigorous and varied, interest was well maintained, adaptive behavior was at 16 months and above average development was present. At *7 years and 10 months* her Stanford–Binet IQ was 130. She was well above average in all areas of functioning.

These three cases demonstrate the varied outcomes in this disorder. Unhappily, the first child is more typical of the usual prognosis. The adopting parents were fortunate indeed. Faced with similar circumstances, we would again have to give an unfavorable prognosis.

Psychomotor Seizures

Case 4 weighed 6 lb 4 oz at birth. Pregnancy was complicated by spotting for 3 weeks in the first trimester, treated with hormones until the 5th month, and by hypertension starting in the 7th month. At 10 days of age the infant began to have crying spells lasting as long as 3 hours, which could not be assuaged, and she lost weight. Frequency increased, so that by *18 weeks* of age she cried for 20 out of 24 hours. Milk intake was about 14 oz per day, and weight was below the third percentile. A variety of formula changes and medications did not alter her behavior. The consulting pediatrician noted hyperextension of the back and mouthing of the nipple without any real awareness or effective sucking. On examination she exhibited frequent crying episodes, poor head control, increased muscle tone and hyperactive reflexes. Periodically she cooperated briefly, and adaptive behavior was felt to be within normal limits. She was started on phenobarbital at 10 mg/kg.

A week later, at *19 weeks,* the crying had stopped, she was taking 32 oz of formula plus solid foods and had gained 18 oz. The hypertonicity had disappeared and behavior was well organized, with a maturity level of 21 weeks. At *30 weeks* and again at *15 months* she had continued to gain weight, remain seizure-free and demonstrate slightly above average development.

Her last examination at *28 months* followed two unfortunate experiences—a gastric lavage a few weeks before because she had swallowed some of her father's cardiac medication, and stranding overnight in a snowstorm encountered during the long drive for the appointment. Phenobarbital tapering had been completed a month previously. She had a fairly long period of initial inhibition and then remained very active and demanding of her mother's attention. Adaptive behavior was adequately organized at 28 months. Gross motor behavior was 27 months, with some incoordination, and manual dexterity was clumsy. In her academically oriented family, one would have expected more advanced behavior, and the parents were disappointed that she was not doing as well as her older brother. However, they were reluctant to continue medication for a longer period, a course which we felt was advisable. We did not feel the motor behavior could be explained by the upsetting experiences she had undergone; consequently, her less than anticipated adaptive behavior might also have had an organic basis. There was no further contact with the family, and we do not know if seizures recurred at a later date.

Case 5 also was an adoption candidate. Birth weight was 8 lb 14 oz. In the newborn period she was tense and jittery, sensitive to noise, had recurrent vomiting and lost 12–14 oz. At 3 months of age she began to have daily staring spells of 20–30 minutes' duration. At her first examination at *21 weeks,* one of these episodes lasting 1–2 minutes was observed. In spite of an immature adjustment, interest and attention were fairly well maintained, but there was considerable scatter in both adaptive and motor behavior from 11–21 weeks. She exhibited moderate hypotonia, head retraction and sagging and fisting of the hands. Treatment with phenobarbital was instituted.

At *41 weeks* she had been free of seizures. Interest and attention were well maintained, and exploitation was of good quality. Adaptive behavior was at a 39-week level. Gross motor behavior scattered over 27–38 weeks, and there were many minor abnormal neuromotor patterns involving legs, arms and hands. Compensation for these problems was anticipated, and adoption placement was recommended because of good drive and the integration of her behavior in response to anticonvulsant therapy.

She was not seen again until $39\frac{1}{2}$ months of age. Adoption had been effected, and she had done well until 29 months of age when she began to walk into walls and not recognize her parents. Phenobarbital had been discontinued, but was reinstituted when an abnormal EEG was noted. Behavior returned to normal until 4–6 months prior to her reevaluation, at which time she developed a variety of episodes of bizarre behavior—hysteric crying for no reason; emptying out all the drawers and closets in her room in frantic haste; clawing, striking and biting in a frenzy. On examination her behavior was disorganized, she was easily distracted and exploitation was haphazard. Adaptive behavior was at 34 months, still in the normal range. The only neuromotor abnormality was some perceptual motor difficulty in reproducing what she saw. The phenobarbital dosage was increased, with resultant disappearance of her bizarre behavior.

Her last examination was at *7 years* of age, when she was given a battery of tests. She had developed a transient hemiparesis following a seizure, but had been maintained on phenobarbital without recurrences for the past 3–4 years, except for one possible episode a few months before being seen. Development had decelerated, but the rate at which this had occurred was not known. She had been attending community classes for the retarded since 5 years of age and was making a satisfactory adjustment there. On examination she was shy, insecure and lacking confidence. She had a serious speech defect, gave inappropriate answers and had problems with visual—motor coordination. There was moderate retardation in all areas of function, with a Stanford—Binet IQ of 53. The etiology of her deterioration was unknown, and no further information was available on whether she had a true degenerative process with continued loss of function and the development of major motor difficulties. One can only speculate whether consistent maintenance of anticonvulsant medication adequate to prevent any seizures would have altered her course.

"Cure of Mental Deficiency"

Case 6 was born at term with a weight of 5 lb 14 oz, after a normal pregnancy. At 5 weeks of age she had an onset of vomiting and diarrhea, which responded to a short hospitalization but then recurred. She was readmitted to the hospital at about 10 weeks of age with dehydration, hyponatremia and acidosis. She made a poor response to therapy, developed anemia requiring transfusion, and showed fluctuation in weight, dropping as low as 5 lb 6 oz, but generally remaining at about her birth weight.

At *17 weeks* she was a scrawny, wizened irritable infant. Fleetingly, she showed a 20-week pattern of grasping an object held near her hand, but for the most part behavior was amorphous and stereotyped, with episodic attention. Staring with failure to respond to visual obstruction was a frequent occurrence. Head control was poor, there were moderate t-n-r positions, cortical thumbs, flexion of the knees and hips in supported sitting and maintenance of the hands fisted at the occiput. Gross motor behavior scattered over 6–13 weeks; adaptive behavior centered at 12 weeks. DQ was approximately 70, and borderline dull development was diagnosed—the presence of some normal behavior and probable constant seizure activity mitigating against a diagnosis of mental deficiency. She was started in a double-blind program of treatment with phenobarbital and placebo.

Ten days later, at *18 weeks* of age, she had gained more than a pound and had changed to an alert and attentive infant who exploited enthusiastically and maturely. Gross motor behavior had not altered materially, but adaptive behavior was 19 weeks, DQ 106, with a full average intellectual development indicated.

The mother had used up her supply of medication 4 days before the next scheduled examination at *23 weeks,* and the infant again was irritable. Interest and attention were fixed intermittently on the test objects, but were interrupted by crying and vomiting. Although behavior was disorganized, adaptive function was at 23 weeks, and DQ still 100. Abnormal neuromotor patterns persisted, but gross motor behavior had advanced to 15–23 weeks. She was changed to medication #2 in accordance with the study protocol.

At *30 weeks* weight gain was still continuing, and she had advanced to the third percentile. Exploitation was lackluster and of poor quality. The examination was punctuated by frequent crying which could not be assuaged, even on her mother's lap. Staring and loss of contact was observed, but she always responded to pinprick. Adaptive behavior was approximately 25 weeks, and the DQ had dropped to 83. Abnormal neuromotor patterns persisted, but motor behavior was organizing at about 24 weeks. She was returned to medication #1, as dictated by the study protocol.

The mother was relaxed and content with the infant's behavior for the first time at the *34-week* examination. The infant again was stable, interested and alert; behavior was well organized and of excellent quality, with no loss of contact. Adaptive behavior was 37 weeks, DQ 109 and a full average development was indicated. The abnormal neuromotor patterns were beginning to resolve but still were present. Weight gain was continuing, and she was almost chubby.

When the study protocol code was broken, it was determined that medication #1 was phenobarbital, as the clinical response had led us to expect. She was maintained on therapy, with appropriate increases for weight gain. At *52 weeks* she had reached the 20th percentile for weight, and excellent organization of behavior continued, with no evidence of seizure activity. Adaptive behavior was at 54 weeks, language at 58 weeks and the only abnormal neuromotor pattern was persistence of a scissors grasp.

When the child was 15 months old the mother discontinued the phenobarbital because she thought it had given her diarrhea. The last examination was at $18\frac{1}{2}$ months. The child had continued to gain weight and had reached the 30th percentile. Behavior was not quite as well organized as it had been 6 months previously. No clear seizure episodes were observed or reported, but attention was easily distracted. A scissors grasp was still present, but again was the only abnormal neuromotor pattern. Adaptive behavior scattered from 14.5–21 months, centering at 18; DQ was 97, and average development continued. Our strong recommendation was for continuation of phenobarbital for at least another year, but the mother was unwilling to reinstitute therapy.

The further course of this child is unknown, and it is possible that she would have recovered spontaneously. However, review of this interesting case indicates that, after 7 weeks of no weight gain, there was an immediate response and consistent progress with the institution of anticonvulsant therapy—possibly because the infant was sufficiently in contact to consume adequate calories. The relationship between phenobarbital therapy and development was equally striking. In 10 days there was an increase of 36 points in DQ, from borderline mental deficiency to full average. On placebo therapy, the aberrant behavior returned and the developmental rate decelerated, with prompt reorganization of the behavior when phenobarbital was reinstituted.

Case 7 was a patient for whom a greater number of abnormalities existed. Pregnancy was complicated by spotting throughout and bleeding 2 weeks prior to and at delivery because of a partial placenta previa. Birth weight was only 4 lb 8 oz, although gestation was fullterm. At birth the infant was cyanotic and did not cry immediately. Seizure episodes began at 3–4 months of age and were characterized by arching of the back, crying out as if in pain and then generalized rigidity. The attacks lasted 5–30 minutes and increased in frequency until they were daily occurrences. Development was consistently slow in all areas, with some improvement after he was fitted with glasses 4 weeks prior to his first examination.

At *52 weeks* he showed very disorganized behavior with undiscriminating exploitation and numerous stereotyped mannerisms. Interest and attention were difficult to elicit and fleeting, and he was extremely irritable, even on his mother's lap. There was hypotonia, and neuromotor abnormalities of the hands, as well as nystagmus and a marked strabismus. Adaptive behavior was approximately 28 weeks, DQ 50–55 and he was functioning at a level of mild to moderate mental deficiency. There was little in his history to suggest a normal intellectual potential, but a prognosis was withheld because of the presence of uncontrolled seizures. Treatment with phenobarbital was recommended to the pediatrician.

The child was started on 15 mg of phenobarbital twice a day, and at $18\frac{1}{2}$ months he showed considerable improvement. The seizures were less frequent and had changed in character. They were primarily episodes of crying, but there was also falling with loss of consciousness. Behavior was adequately organized, with an adaptive level of 15 months, DQ 80. He was still hypotonic, with persistence of other neuromotor abnormalities, and gross motor behavior was at a 13-month level. It was recommended that the phenobarbital be increased, and the pediatrician added another 15 mg.

At $25\frac{1}{2}$ *months* the seizures had stopped, and behavior had improved further. The child was friendly, alert and stable. Interest and attention were well maintained and exploitation was quite discriminating. Minor neuromotor abnormalities persisted. Adaptive behavior was at 21 months, DQ 85 and development was considered low average because it was well integrated.

The final examination was at *7 years and 8 months.* The strabismus had been corrected, but he had a complex visual problem and was wearing corrective lenses. Phenobarbital had been discontinued without recurrence of any known seizures. The child had entered kindergarten at 6 years and 10 months and was being placed the next school year in a small class for neurologically handicapped. He was a fairly well motivated and outgoing child, immature in many ways, and quite dependent on his mother. Poor visual—motor coordination was present, and gait was atypical and awkward. Verbal surpassed performance abilities, and his Stanford—Binet IQ was 83. He was still a handicapped child, particularly in his academically oriented professional home, but he could not be considered mentally defective. He had the advantage of understanding and accepting, although disappointed, parents, and of special educational facilities. In less favorable circumstances, he probably would not have been able to function as well as he did. Again, it is pure speculation whether earlier and more adequate anticonvulsant therapy would have improved his behavior more.

14

Communication Disorders

Communication with verbal symbols is one of man's most distinctive characteristics. Normal development of communication depends on the intactness of the mechanisms for hearing, language comprehension and motor expression.

Hearing is a specialized form of tactile sense which makes the organism aware of vibrations of distant origin and enables him to get into *touch* with what is spatially remote. To a profound degree, the child who cannot hear or understand language is "out of touch" with his surroundings. He suffers from lack of contact with what is happening all about him. Hearing loss isolates the child even from himself, for he does not sense fully the vibrations which he produces with his own larynx or through his manipulations of the physical world. There is no resonance in his inner life—no echo to reflect mirrored images of sound. He is wrapped in silences.

§1. FAILURE TO DEVELOP SPEECH

The most common reason for failure to develop language at the appropriate age is mental deficiency. Speech production is only one facet of language development. Often the clinician is faced with a 2- or 3-year-old who uses no words; he then must determine three things by developmental assessment. Does the child have normal intelligence? Does he hear? Does he understand what is said to him? If the answers to these questions are "yes," the child will talk when what he wishes to communicate cannot be transmitted adequately by means of gesture and pantomime. The parents must avoid pressuring the child to talk and emphasize intercommunication instead. Any congenital anomalies which could involve the motor mechanisms for producing sound would have become apparent before this age. Formal speech therapy for articulatory defects which might become manifest will be more effective if delayed to 4 or $4\frac{1}{2}$ years.

However, the situation is quite different if the child's speech difficulty results from a sensorineural hearing loss or a central communication disorder. In these two conditions, recognition in early infancy is vital for subsequent normal or near-normal development of communication. The remainder of this chapter deals with the early diagnosis and management of these two types of hearing impairment.

§2. THE ROLE OF HEARING IN NORMAL INFANT DEVELOPMENT

Hearing includes both the perception of a sound stimulus and its interpretation by complex cortical and subcortical mechanisms. To appreciate the meaning of a hearing handicap, it is necessary to trace briefly the role of auditory experience in the early development of human behavior. Neurologically, the mechanisms for hearing are prepared well in advance. There is good evidence that the fetus responds with sudden movements to loud sounds. This reaction may be regarded as an auditory reflex, or as a tactual reflex if it is mediated by the skin of the fetus rather than the organ of Corti. In the absence of muffling fluid in the middle ear, it is certain that prematurely born infants with a fetal age of 30 weeks or more will react to the sound of a tinkled bell, either by positive movements or by immobilization of movement. Shortly after birth, the fullterm neonate assumes listening attitudes to the sound of a human voice.

The normal infant passes through successive growth stages with respect to his sensitivity to speech vibrations. Auditory discrimination, like visual discrimination, comes by gradual degrees; it is dependent upon complex mechanisms of attention and perception, not merely the simple capacity to pass on movements of the ossicles of the middle ear. It is possible that ontogenetically the infant is at first most susceptible to the fundamental laryngeal tones with a vibration frequency of 100–400 per second, the frequency of the vibrations of his own vocal cords. It is the low fundamental range which is so important for modulations of tone which express moods, attitudes and shifting emphasis. Later the normal infant becomes sensitive to overtones of the laryngeal sounds, whose frequencies range from 400 to 2400 vibrations per second. These frequencies correspond to some of the consonants and to special vowel characteristics. Still later he attends to the third band of frequencies, from 2400 to about 8000 per second, which includes the fricative sounds *v, s,* and *z* made by placing the tongue close to the teeth or the palate. The normal infant of adequate maturity is sensitive to all ranges of frequency.

Hearing is a social as well as an intellectual sense. Sounds acquaint the infant with important events in the physical world. Through audition he also establishes primary social contacts and acquires the cultural meaning of what occurs in the course of his everyday living. The sound of approaching footsteps awakens anticipations. The clicking of a spoon in a bowl comes to mean food. At first, the click is made by the adult who cares for the infant. Later the infant executes the click himself; this self-produced sound adds to his insight into the constitution of the physical world. The whole web of the child's environment is permeated almost continuously with sounds: episodic sounds, routine sounds, occasional sounds, emergency sounds—they form the substance and patterning of the psychologic environment.

A mother talks to an infant long before he understands articulate words. By such talking she conveys moods and emotional values which contribute to the infant's organization of personal attitudes and social patterns of behavior. This is not a one-way communication system. The normal infant has a capacity to produce vocalizations himself. Even in the neonatal period he makes small throaty sounds in the low register of tonal speech. By the middle of the first year he is making polysyllabic vowel sounds and beginning to penetrate the higher band of vibration frequencies by articulating consonants which begin with *m* and *d*. In the third quarter of the first year he is beginning to put these powers to socialized uses. When the "ma-ma" he produces acquires specific meaning, it is the beginning of speech. During the second year he imitates—often with musical fidelity—the auditory syntax of speech, exercising in variegated jargon the phonetic framework of conversation.

In the last quarter of the first year, the normal child begins to listen to and readjust discriminatingly to words. He learns to inhibit an action on a verbal cue. He uses vocal signs and words in situations highly charged with social values. He continues to use gestures, even total response gestures, but words comprehended and words spoken begin to function as labels for simple generalizations and as expressions for personal mental states. Eighteen months is the transition age, when words are used to express ideas and are adopted as substitutes for gestures. By the end of 2 years, the normal child asks for food, toilet and drink, verbalizes immediate experiences and poses questions such as "What's that?" At 3 years he asks rhetorical questions, and expresses desires, refusals and denials. He even formulates requests for help. Only gradually does he master the higher ranges of vibration frequency. Even at 3 years he is not able to imitate the frequencies involved in difficult consonants. Therefore, it is quite usual for him to continue with infantile malarticulation almost up to the age of 5 years.

Just as visual fixation and pursuit have a patterned motor expression, so auditory experience has a motorized component. Human ears may not prick; but there are numerous other neuromotor sets. At 18 months he swings rhythmically with his whole body in response to music. He hums spontaneously and sings syllables with wide ranges in tone, pitch and intensity of voice. At 3 years his rhythmic responses are less comprehensive but not less discriminating. He bends at the knees, sways, nods his head or taps his foot to keep time. He sings as he rocks in a chair. He recognizes a melody. He sings phrases of songs. He may reproduce the entire song. He begins to match simple tones. He enjoys group participation in rhythmic play. He gallops, jumps, walks and runs, keeping good time to music.

By all these diversified activities, the child strengthens his auditory rapport with his social environment. Speech is a complicated technique and emerges in an extremely intricate social context. A child with a hearing handicap is pitifully disadvantaged in his mastery both of the technique and of the social context of speech. He does retain one of his distance senses, sight, and thereby establishes contact with the persons who surround him. He begins to read their facial expressions. In time he interprets their gestures, but he is blind to the modulations of the speaking voice which accompany social interchange.

§3. SENSORINEURAL HEARING LOSS AND CENTRAL COMMUNICATION DISORDER

Early Symptoms

With the foregoing outline of the normal course of auditory development in mind, we are in a better position to understand the origin and nature of the behavioral symptoms which are distinctive of hearing impairments.

Impairment of the mechanics of the external or middle ear produces a conductive hearing loss, with decrease in the ability to hear across all frequency ranges. Air conduction is impaired, while bone conduction is intact. Sound is muffled but not distorted. When medical or surgical intervention is not curative, sound amplification with a hearing aid results in normal ability to discriminate language, except in unusual circumstances.

Sensorineural hearing loss due to impairment of the organ of Corti or, less commonly, to lesions of the eighth nerve poses an entirely different problem. This hearing loss is not symmetric but usually is greater at the higher frequencies. Loss of discrimination in the upper range renders the child unable to perceive or to imitate some consonants; loss in the middle range annuls vowels, semivowels and other consonants. The child hears some of everything going on about him, but it is distorted; the necessary acoustic detail is missing, and discrimination and language comprehension are lost. The resultant handicap depends not only on the degree of loss but on the frequencies at which loss occurs. It is a sobering experience for anyone to sit in a soundproof room and try to recognize words as frequencies are screened out progressively. Only then can the world of a child with a high-frequency sensorineural hearing loss be appreciated fully. Mere amplification of all sound does not remedy the situation for him. In the vast majority of instances there is residual hearing; modern hearing aids can amplify sounds differentially across frequencies sufficiently to restore some balance and permit reasonable discrimination of the spoken word. However, when there is a loss of 70 decibels or more at all frequencies, sound amplification adequate for the development of good speech rarely can be accomplished. The term *deaf*, as contrasted with *hearing impaired*, now is reserved for this relatively small percentage of individuals.

The behavior of children with severe sensorineural hearing loss across all frequencies is equivalent in many respects to the behavior seen in sensory aphasia. Traditionally the term *aphasia* has been applied to adults who lose speech secondary to some type of cerebral injury. Because of resistance to the concept of congenital aphasia, *central communication disorder* or *central auditory imperception* is used to describe those children who have no sensorineural hearing loss but nevertheless behave as though they were profoundly deaf. The terms are appropriate because the difficulty lies in the processing, patterning and interpretation of the incoming sensory information within the brain. Sound often is so confusing that complete inhibition of response to all auditory stimuli results.

This type of auditory imperception may be an isolated phenomenon. In infants and preschool children, evidences of other impaired central nervous system function usually are easily detectable—disorganized behavior, neuromotor abnormalities, decreased response to visual and tactile cues, seizures or varying degrees of intellectual impairment. Because both sensorineural and central communication hearing impairments can have common etiologic antecedents and common associated deficits, differential diagnosis may be difficult; however, it is very important for training and education.

There are some differences between the behavior of a child with sensorineural hearing loss and one with a central communication disorder. In the first few months, the "aphasic" infant may not show any deviations; after this age the two pictures are so similar that a single description suffices. In the first few weeks after birth, the psychologic growth of an impaired infant is not much affected, but in a few months he begins to show a developmental deficit. He may smile, laugh and vocalize, but his vocalizations are reduced in range and amount. Even his laughter may diminish; however, it suffers less at first because it is less dependent upon auditory and social stimuli. His vocalizations tend to become brief and monotonal. He does not indulge in the long stretches of experimental sound play in which the intact infant seems to delight. In sound play, the normal infant in time talks to himself, just as he looks at himself in mirror play. He does not indulge merely in sound production; he practices sound perception. As he matures, he modulates his vocalization to perceive the effect of the modulation.

The impaired infant cannot indulge in such profitable solioquy; he becomes more mute with time. Since he has no echo equipment for duplicating his own sounds, he has no means of imitating those of others. Nor does he have a social motive for improvising sounds. Therefore, absence of spontaneous sound improvisation is an early symptom of auditory handicap.

Likewise, reduced social rapport and diminished vocal intercommunication are premonitory signs of subnormal audition in infancy. Increased visual alertness and responsiveness to facial and pantomimic gesture may compensate for the auditory lack, and sometimes mask it, particularly in an expressive, reactive child. In itself, extraordinary visual attentiveness is a suggestive symptom. Multiplying signs of social remoteness also may be detected.

Symptoms of auditory disability vary, not only with the gravity of the defect but also with the temperament and treatment of the child who carries the handicap. However, retardational effects begin to appear, even in the field of adaptive behavior, prior to his first birthday. The infant sees the passing show of life as a silent cinema, discontinuous, devoid of sound effects and spoken script. The lack of sound accompaniments attenuates the reality of things; there is less meaning in a clock which does not tick, a spoon that does not click, a ball that bounces without a thud or a laugh that is inaudible. Hearing was intended to make the remote near. Auditory handicap tends instead to push the child into remoteness. Therefore, it has a subtly retarding effect on practical as well as social intelligence even before the usual period for articulate speech.

The failure of speech development accentuates the apparent retardation. There is a disproportionate reliance on concrete gesture. Words as signals and symbols are not in his power. The well-known declaration "all gone" which normally voices the idea of termination and of disappearance at 18 months is utterly beyond his scope. During the transition period between 1 and 3 years, when primitive gestures give way to words, the impaired child is peculiarly beset. He has not lost something that he once had; he is perpetually foiled in getting something which he ought to have, something which is almost indispensible for the very process of development.

Auditory imperception threatens the personality even more than it does the intellect of the child. The threat is due to the weakening of lines of communication; when social intercourse is thwarted, symptomatic behavior problems arise. Frustrations lead to tantrums, yelling and head banging. Irritability is common. When, as so often happens, parents and physician fail to recognize the problem, confusion becomes confounded; tensions are set up; ill-conceived discipline and training are resorted to; strange rebellions and obstinacies are provoked. This infant—toddler period breeds characteristic symptoms, some of which are due to the defect in the mechanics of development, while others are due to faulty management. The negative and "rebellious" symptoms are easily misinterpreted. A child may stamp his feet for three reasons psychologically quite different from each other: he may be vexed with others because they do not understand him; he may be vexed with himself for his failure to make himself understood; he simply may wish to call someone to him. An actual incident will illustrate. A boy is engrossed in play at nursery school. When it is time to go outdoors, the teacher brings his coat. He looks up and suddenly begins to stamp his feet, and screams a loud monotonous shriek in vigorous protest. The teacher is taken aback, for the child is intelligent and usually obedient. He has missed his cue; it is not time to go home. When he is shown the play yard, he understands at once and his shriek terminates abruptly.

When these impaired children seem stubborn and unreasonable, it is because they have ideas of their own. They must have more of their own than of any other kind, when insufficient pains are taken to communicate to them the ideas of others. (The mother who said impatiently, "He is too lazy to talk," was unreasonable too.) If such children seem suspicious, it is not so much because of fearfulness as because of an uncomprehending alertness as to what *might* happen. When they know what is going to happen, they become acquiescent and even good-naturedly cooperative. This is well illustrated in the conduct of a boy who at the age of $2\frac{1}{2}$ years was referred as a behavior problem, with irritability and tantrums as the chief complaint. The parents had fallen into the habit of managing him forcibly when he seemed resistant. They removed his coat by tugging, over his protest; they dragged him upstairs when he refused to walk. During the examination he seemed very intent on carrying out his own ideas, rather than heeding the examiner's directions. He worked with concentration when interested, but became resistant when transitions had to be made. He found that he could make a fine noise by stamping on the experimental staircase. He proved to be profoundly deaf. His parents, not recognizing the condition, had resorted to severe disciplinary methods which only aggravated the tantrums and rebelliousness. His behavior *symptoms* were taken to be the problem. *Deafness* was the real problem.

These incidents properly fall under the heading of symptoms, because this kind of behavior is typical of the way in which the impaired preschool child reacts to the ever-present barriers of noncommunication. His reaction is exacerbated if the parents insist upon some uncomprehended verbal form of communication at the expense of a comprehended gesture. The only way in which the barriers can be lowered is to foster gesture and dramatization at every opportunity, until the foundations for communication are laid firmly. A critical study of behavioral symptoms by means of a developmental assessment will reveal cases which otherwise remain concealed and misunderstood.

Diagnosis

Congenital sensorineural hearing loss is often familial. If a parent or older sibling is affected, a new infant usually is brought for evaluation early in life and a diagnosis established. Particular attention must be given in other instances following meningitis or encephalitis, blood group incompatabilities and prenatal infections such as rubella or cytomegalic inclusion disease. However, all infants should be screened in the course of routine care and developmental evaluation. No child has ever stepped up and said, "I am deaf," or "My hearing is blurred." A child so handicapped assumes it is part of the order of the universe. Much less does an *infant* make a subjective report of his condition.

When expert audiologic consultation is not available, and sometimes when it is, precise diagnosis depends on that most comprehensive and integrated index of the child's well-being, his behavior. Hearing impairment can be suspected, inferred and finally established on the basis of behavioral symptoms such as we have outlined already. Table 14-1 lists various symptoms and clues which may be used to derive a diagnosis and to help differentiate between sensorineural loss and central auditory imperception. These diagnostic signs are subdivided into five developmentally related categories, and the separate items arranged in an approximate genetic order. The items are not of equal importance, and they do not all appear in a single individual. Some are characteristic of the first year, and others of the second and third years. No item should be ignored if there is the least suspicion of auditory handicap. When a mother brings her child to the doctor and hesitatingly suggests that she isn't quite sure that the child hears, begin to assume that he does not hear.

The behavioral response of the normal infant depends on his maturity. Prior to 24 weeks of age, he responds to a variety of perceived sounds by altering his activity—immobilizing or becoming more active, smiling or crying. By 28–32 weeks of age, he turns promptly and consistently to sounds of low intensity over a range of frequencies exemplified by quiet voice, sibilant sounds, crumpled tissue paper, rattle and hand bell. An infant's failure requires repetition of the screening test and then further investigation. Inconsistent or fragmentary responses to some sounds do

Table 14-1. SIGNS SUGGESTIVE OF IMPAIRED HEARING IN
INFANTS AND YOUNG CHILDREN

I. Hearing and Comprehension of Speech
    General indifference to sound
    Lack of response to spoken word
    Response to noises as opposed to voice

II. Vocalizations and Sound Production
    Monotonal quality ⎫ Normal quality in central
    Indistinct   ⎭   communication disorder
    Lessened laughter
    Meager experimental sound play and squealing*
    Vocal play for vibratory sensation
    Head banging, foot stamping for vibratory sensation
    Yelling, screeching to express pleasure, annoyance or need

III. Visual Attention and Reciprocal Comprehension
    Augmented visual vigilance and attentiveness ⊹
    Alertness to gesture and movement ⊹
    Marked imitativeness in play
    Vehemence of gestures

IV. Social Rapport and Adaptations
    Subnormal rapport in vocal nursery games
    Intensified preoccupation with things rather than persons
    Inquiring, sometimes confused or thwarted facial expression
    Puzzled and unhappy episodes in social situations
    Suspicious alertness, alternating with cooperation
    Markedly reactive to praise and affection

V. Emotional Behavior
    Tantrums to call attention to self or need
    Tensions, tantrums, resistances due to lack of comprehension
    Frequent obstinacies, teasing tendencies
    Irritability at not making self understood
    Explosions due to self-vexation
    Impulsive and avalanche initiatives

---

*Quality of jargon normal in central disorders
⊹Likely to ignore visual and tactile cues and have disorganized
  behavior in central disorders

---

not indicate that he will have the ability to hear and interpret the human voice. The most common reason for failure of the screening test at this age is mental deficiency. When developmental assessment indicates this is not the cause for less mature responses than prompt sound localization, expert audiologic evaluation is indicated. In special hands, psychogalvanic skin resistance conditioned reflex testing or EEG evoked potentials can demonstrate the level of response to pure tones. By 18 or 24 months, if there has been delay in diagnosis, the child can be conditioned by play audiometry to give an overt behavioral response such as dropping a cube in a cup, and a reasonable pure tone audiogram obtained. Consistent positive or negative responses are relatively easy to interpret; however, equivocal results continue to present problems, and the behavior of the child then must be the guide to management.

    At all ages, a cautious approach to audiometry must be used and the examination started at threshold intensities. If normal responses are obtained across frequencies at 10 decibels, the child does not have a sensorineural defect. A child with central auditory impairment tends to inhibit responses to disturbing sounds, and 90 decibels can be irritating and even painful. If the examination is begun at 90 decibels, *all* responses may be inhibited; then it may not be possible to demonstrate the normal response to 10 decibels until after a relatively long period of auditory training. The fact that the child does not respond to 90 decibels provides information, but it is a different kind of information, useful only if normal responses at threshold levels have been shown.

Errors in diagnosis and delays in referral may result because the child with a high-tone sensorineural loss may hear the slam of a door, run to the window to see a truck or look for the airplane overhead. Even snatches of mumbled but articulate speech are not inconsistent with this diagnosis. The child with a central communication disorder can present even more puzzling fragments of behavior. He turns sometimes when a rattle is shaken gently behind him yet ignores the clash of cymbals equally close; he runs to see what is happening as his mother starts to unwrap a package in the next room; he fetches a wet washcloth when she tells his sister of her headache. When mental deficiency has been ruled out, the observed peculiarities of conduct often are interpreted as a psychiatric disorder. "Emotional blocking" is a favorite explanation when there is residual or selective frequency hearing, or beginning integration of sound patterns within the brain, and strife has arisen between parent and child because of imputed willfulness. The child hears some sounds; therefore he cannot have hearing impairment—so the argument runs.

It is the lack of responsiveness to the spoken word which constitutes the handicap, and the essence of that handicap is obstruction of communication. There is a safe rule which would prevent harmful delays of diagnosis and remediation: when a child acts as though he were deaf to the human voice, *treat him as though he has a hearing impairment.* To manage a child so handicapped as though he can hear, or ought to hear, leads to grave mistakes.

Management

The cardinal objective in management of a child with hearing impairment is the conservation of all possible communication. *Socialization* to preserve the optimal growth of personality is a major goal.

Sensorineural Hearing Loss

Ideally a diagnosis of congenital hearing loss should be made by the age of 6 months, when the infant reveals his sensory defect by reduced vocalization and subnormal auditory social rapport. To compensate for his defect he watches vigilantly, but only his caretakers can fill the void of incompleted interpersonal relations. Through gestures and dramatized intimacies, contacts can be built up, and the remoteness of the child can be forestalled. The mother should initiate auditory training by pantomime, with abundant talking close to the infant's ear; this begins some of the necessary auditory feedback while his precise status is being evaluated.

The normal infant at 36–40 weeks begins to develop speech. He uses particular sounds in referring to specific objects or classes of objects. This is the ideal time for an infant with sensorineural hearing loss to receive his hearing aid. It is the age when he is most receptive and when the normal progressions for the development of speech are fostered most easily. The infant whose world expands and presents him with new experiences and new delights not only wears his hearing aid—he demands it, because it helps him. The best prognosis for normal development of speech and education in a regular classroom results when auditory training starts this early. The older the child when a hearing aid is fitted, the more difficult the adjustment and the greater the likelihood of complete rejection. Children with fairly good potential in audition sometimes become functionally deaf because they have not had an opportunity in early life to exercise their residual hearing. Conversely, infants with mild to moderate impairment whose mothers have recognized the problem early and have supplied sound amplification with their own voice, in combination with gesture and pantomime, have developed normal speech without a hearing aid. However, the fate of infants should not be left to such lucky events. Even a mild hearing loss which would cause little difficulty for an adult can have a profound retarding effect for a child who has no prior experience on which to build. Continued reassessment is needed, and participation in special nursery school programs generally is necessary before graduation to a regular classroom is possible. This graduation is possible for the majority of cases diagnosed and treated from infancy.

When the sensorineural handicap is so severe that use of a hearing aid cannot prevent serious retardation in development of language, special methods of education are needed. The objective for these children is not speech but *social intercommunication.* This type of management will tend to relax tensions and to prevent the conflicts between adult and child which too often impede the early progress of the deaf. The child will be fortified in his natural desire to understand and to defer to cultural demands. His trust in life will be strengthened as he becomes more closely identified with the social group—the cardinal need in the mental health of the deaf child. It is a significant developmental fact that young deaf children naturally watch the expression of the whole face rather than the mouth for their cues. Lip reading comes later, and formal instruction should wait until socialization is well established. Day school programs are gradually, and correctly, coming to replace residential schools for the deaf.

Central Communication Disorder

Children with central auditory imperception frequently have associated disorganization of other aspects of their behavior. Evidence of normal levels of response to auditory stimuli can be demonstrated, and often it is impossible to be certain that such children cannot interpret what they hear until an age of 18 months or later. The approach to treatment is more controversial. Some maintain that sound amplification is appropriate only if limited to specific situations in auditory training sessions. There is logic to this view since normal perception of sounds at threshold is present. Auditory stimuli already are confusing, so little benefit can be expected from bringing closer the rattling of the garbage cans down the street. These children tend to reject their hearing aids, and the breakage rate is high. It behooves us to listen to what they are trying so wisely to tell us. The primary objective again is social intercommunication. Fortunately, compensation occurs for most of these children, even when they are not recognized or handled wisely. They begin to understand and then reproduce speech, and eventually handle language and speech adequately enough to enter regular school. This is not always the case; for such children the diagnostic differentiation is a difficult process, and the residual handicaps may be great.

The mental health of the parents also requires consideration. They cling to the hope that hearing can be restored by medical or magical means; they plead for a fenestration operation, having read a popular article on the treatment of otosclerosis in adults; spines are "adjusted," hearing aids purchased without discrimination, airplane rides suggested and invariably the adenoids are removed, usually with little or no effect on hearing. The layman entertains an exaggerated idea of the facility of the profoundly deaf in lip-reading and in speaking, with training; to the parents of a deaf child it spells hope that their child can pass as a hearing person. Slightly more realistic parents will concede the need for a hearing device, but then expect there will be no handicap! The truth is, when there is not enough residual hearing on which to build speech there will always be a handicap. The aim of a well-adjusted parent should be to help his severely handicapped child to become a competent, contented deaf person, able to communicate with others easily, rather than a poor imitation of a hearing person, laboring always to conceal his handicap. Outlook for the later life of a hearing-impaired child is discussed in the final section of Chapter 15.

§4. ILLUSTRATIVE CASES

In good hands and with the early fitting of hearing aids, the first four of the following children today most likely would be making satisfactory progress in community programs, even in regular school. The case reports would conclude differently. Facilities for Case 5 still are not easy to find.

Profound Congenital Deafness

Case 1 had a second cousin who was born deaf, and a normal older sibling. She herself had never responded to any sound, not even a loud clap of thunder. She had four developmental examinations:

    16 months—general maturity level 12—15 months
    21 months—general maturity level 18—21 months
    28 months—general maturity level 30+ months
    40 months—general maturity level 42 months

She showed an early mild symptomatic retardation, which was gradually overcome, and an above average developmental rate was attained. She experienced very little difficulty in establishing lines of communication with her family. As early as 16 months she was beginning to point to what she wanted and to respond to simple gestures. By 40 months she indicated with beautifully executed and understandable pantomime that she no longer used a baby's crib, but was a big girl and slept in a big bed. She did have considerable emotional difficulty due to her hearing loss, expressed first in tantrums when she did not understand or could not be understood, later by great anxiety and suspiciousness about new situations, when they could not be explained to her. Much of this was due to the parents' early maladjustments which resulted in submitting the child to many medical examinations and procedures, including adenoidectomy. Speech training was begun against our advice during this suspicious phase at $3\frac{1}{2}$ years, and her reaction to it can be summed up by her vocabulary at the end of 6 months: "bye" and "home."

She later went to a special school for the deaf, making excellent academic progress, good progress in lip-reading, and slow progress in speech production.

Familial Sensorineural Hearing Loss

Case 2 is of interest because of the family history and situation. The father was deaf, one of 12 children of whom 3 were deaf. He had "no voice" and never learned to speak, although he attended an excellent school for the deaf for years. He was employed and supported his family. The mother also was deaf; she was one of 5 children, 2 of whom were deaf. She lip-read and spoke, but used a familiar person to interpret her speech to strangers and strangers' speech to her. The examiner could, however, understand single words of the mother's speech, which was limited to 1–3 word sentences and generously larded with gestures and nods. The parents believed their boy could hear but did not speak because he could not learn speech from deaf parents.

At 30 months he was reported to be very noisy, sometimes heard a loud voice or bell, but understood nothing said to him, and had no words. He had nursery school experience with hearing children but proved difficult to manage, fought, grabbed, became angry and was very fearful of strangers. In the examination he was anxious to please and looked eagerly for cues, approval and permission. General maturity level was 24–27 months. The diagnosis was familial hearing loss in a low-average boy.

Unsuspected Hearing Loss, following Meningococcic Meningitis

Case 3 was a normal baby who had meningococcic meningitis at 6 months of age, with a supposedly complete recovery. A note by the referring physician *at 33 months* read "Does not talk. Points, hears and obeys commands. Impression: environmental factors." The mother was inept and impatient. The child was violently noisy and assertive, antagonistic to the examination at first, and suspicious throughout. She heard the bell but not voices, and she ignored all purely verbal situations. Her general maturity level was 30–36 months. The diagnosis was postmeningitic hearing loss in a girl with average intelligence.

The mother had no suspicion that her child could not hear. She accepted the new diagnosis immediately as though a light had dawned and made everything about the child comprehensible to her. She even expressed remorse at her previous lack of patience and understanding.

Hearing Loss from Maternal Rubella with Family Maladjustment

Case 4's mother had rubella in the third month of pregnancy. The birth and early development were normal, but the boy was a feeding problem, and the parents emotional. At *33 months*, in requesting examination of their boy, the parents wrote: "At 18 months used an occasional word but never seemed to speak. Still does not talk and has forgotten the few words he knew. A poor eater. His hearing is apparently normal." He was an attractive boy, alert to visual cues, and sailed through the examination at a 30-month level wherever he could get his cues by eye. He turned away from verbal situations. He heard his father's voice (father concealed), listened, looked puzzled and shrugged his shoulders. He did not recognize it or locate it as a normal child does.

At 42 months he watched lips for cues and reproduced some sounds, obediently but without meaning. General maturity level was a full 42 months. The parents were forever testing his hearing, the mother heckled him and the father bellowed heavy commands at him. They felt the stigma of his hearing deficit very keenly and were evading realities. The boy had a hearing loss due to maternal rubella; he was normally intelligent. The problem was the family adjustment, and the effect it would have on this handicapped boy.

Mental Deficiency with Impaired Hearing

Case 5 had a paternal uncle who was mentally defective. She made slow developmental progress in infancy, did not display visual attention until she was 8 months old and it was then noted that she did not seem to hear. *At 47 weeks,* general maturity level was 32 weeks. Vocalizations were meager, with no response to sound. *At 15 months,* she heard loud noises and the radio. General maturity level was 40 weeks with atypical patterns. *At 32 months,* general maturity level was a defective 18 months. The parents accepted a diagnosis of mental deficiency with hearing loss. They had never been satisfied that hearing loss alone could account for her slow development, although they had received a good deal of assurance from various physicians that this was the case.

Central Communication Disorders

The following cases include some verbatim recordings of language interchange during the course of developmental examination between examiner and children with a central communication disorder. Some introductory comments on their language and the parents' complaints will be helpful.

In the milder forms, parents complain with an uncertain and apologetic air that the child's words are never his own; he can say what has been said to him, but he cannot formulate his own sentences. He does not know how to ask a question, but always uses a declaratory form even when he obviously means to ask a question. Or he does not know how to answer a question, but can only repeat it. Or, again, he may not comprehend what an answer is, but repeats his question over and over, with increasing insistence and concern, until his question is repeated instead of answered; then and only then is he satisfied. He may experience an inordinate difficulty in achieving the transposition of "you" and "I," calling himself "you" and his mother "I" for months on end. He may be able to make spontaneous remarks of good content and quality, but comes up against an impasse if his remark must be responsive. The normal child stumbles a little over these language mechanisms in the course of his development, but he stumbles so slightly and for such a brief period that parents hardly notice the error. The $3\frac{1}{2}$ to 5 year-old child with a mild central communication disorder easily can give such rote information as his name, address and sex, can count and recite nursery rhymes. He can, in other words, return any answer that he has in stock as a pat answer. However, he cannot cope with the simplest question when he must devise his own reply. Parents are at first irritated by the monotony and repetitiousness of the child's conversation; they finally become alarmed at the child's apparent stupidity.

For the child with a severe handicap, the learned language responses are almost completely stereotyped. He cannot play with words, paraphrase or ring the changes. Language is a stiff and clumsy instrument which he wields only with the greatest difficulty. In such a child the outlook for normal use of language is less promising. The speech he acquires does not have the tonal monotony of the deaf child, but speech is so limited as to make him almost inarticulate.

It should be stated that in no instance in the following conversations is failure to respond correctly due to a withholding of response by the child; all the questions asked are fair questions, easily answered by the normal child of comparable age.

Case 6

CHILD, $3\frac{1}{2}$ YEARS (HOSPITALIZED)
Spontaneous remarks to the nurse: "I want my cup." "I want my blanket on me."
"Put it on my bed."

EXAMINER

(shows picture book)
"Do you want to play?" . . . . "Yeh." (smiles)
"What's that?" . . . . (confidently) "That's a _____ that's a _____ ."
"What's the girl doing?" . . . . "She's doin' _____ she's doin' _____ ."
"What's that?" (dog) . . . . "That's a _____ that's a _____ that's a _____ ."
"What does he say?" . . . . "He says _____ ."

Case 6 (Cont'd)

EXAMINER	CHILD, 3½ YEARS
"He says bow-wow."	"Yeh!"
"What does this girl have?"	"She's got a ____ a ____ a ____."
"It's a spoon."	"Yeh!"
"What happened to her dinner?"	"It spilled."
"What's this?" (dog again)	"It's a ____ a ____ a ____ I don't know maybe."
"What's your name?"	"John Doe."
"Say 8537."	"8537."

Note that this child verbalized his wants without difficulty. Speech was clear; he was alert, interested and eager to play. He could not name an object but seemed to recognize the name when it was supplied to him. Each time a question was put to him, he seemed confident of his ability to answer, and surprised when the word was not forthcoming. He repeated digits with ease, and the old learned response to the question of his name rolled out without hesitation. His adaptive behavior was normal for his age, and he was not retarded; however, he was "aphasic." The condition for which he was hospitalized (osteogenesis imperfecta with fracture) did not yield any ready explanation for the "aphasia."

Case 7

EXAMINER	CHILD, 3½ YEARS
(showing picture card and pointing)	"A dog, a house, shoe ____ clock."
(showing Binet picture card)	
"What do you see?"	"What do you see?"
"What do *you* see?"	"What do *you* see?"
"What *do* you see?"	"What *do* you see?"
"What do you *see*?"	"____ You see ____ girl."
"What else?"	"What else?"
"What else?"	"What else?"
"What else?" (insistently)	"What else ____ a house."
"What else?"	"What else?" etc.
(no visual stimulus)	
"What runs?"	"What runs?"
"Does a doggie run?"	"Does a doggie run?"
"And a car?"	"And a car?"
"What sleeps?"	"What sleeps?"
"What scratches?"	"Scratches?"
"What bites?"	"What bites?" etc.
"What's your name?"	"Say your name is Johnnie Jones."
"Are you a little boy or a little girl?"	"Little girl. 25 Third Street."

This boy was referred for study because of his language difficulties and because of the question of serious mental deficiency. The parents stated, "He does not *use* speech, not to express his wants, not to relate his experiences, nor even in the most rudimentary conversation. He never answers questions. He understands speech and will carry out requests. He never greets anyone or responds orally to a greeting. He repeats sentences that he has heard, with dramatic emphasis. The relevance of his speech varies from nil to complete. He is completely unsocial." He showed very deviant behavior, particularly in the development of his social relationships and feelings toward others. Adaptive behavior in the examination situation was at age, but ordinarily he operated at a much lower level.

Note that he could name pictures spontaneously, but that he merely repeated and repeated a question, varying his inflection to match the examiner's. Occasionally, after much persistence, a pertinent response was elicited. Like the previous boy, he could give his name, but note the form of his reply: it was what someone else had said to him. He gave his sex incorrectly because he was merely repeating the question, and then by rote he gave his address although it was not called for. His only spontaneous remarks were of a repetitive nature, obviously reproductions of questions and answers he had once heard.

Case 8

EXAMINER	CHILD, 6 YEARS
"Why do we have houses?"	"I don't know what you say, houses, because I haven't a house."
"Why do we have books?"	"Cause, cause, cause I have a couple of books."
"What do we do with our eyes?"	"See the eyes."
"What do we do with our ears?"	"See the ears."
"What runs?"	(looks puzzled)
"Does a car run?"	"Yes."
"What cries?"	"A baby cries."
"What scratches?"	"No, two."
"What sleeps?"	"One two sleeps."
"What swims?"	"Two swims."
"Can you swim?"	(nods) "I pick my feet up."
"What burns?"	"Two five two burns, birds."
(examiner coughs)	"I got a bad cold, too."
"Put the ball on the chair."	(does so)
"Put the ball *under* the chair."	(looks about the room in perplexity, then puts it on the chair)

This girl was a friendly, cooperative child, anxious to please. Her hearing had been questioned over and over again because she apparently did not understand much of what was said to her; her mentality had been questioned repeatedly because her responses to questions and verbal instructions were hopelessly inadequate. Yet her hearing was normal by audiometric examination, and in nonlanguage tests she responded well within the normal range for her age. She was receiving special instruction in the hope of helping her to develop her faulty conceptual powers. The child's early history may well be of etiologic significance. She was born at term weighing 6 lbs 9 oz, after a difficult 52-hour labor. Delivery was spontaneous, but it was a breech presentation. The child was cyanotic, required resuscitation and did not suck. Difficulty with swallowing and chewing persisted until she was over 4 years of age.

15

Visual Disorders

Human visual perception ranks with speech in complexity and passes through comparable developmental phases. Moreover, seeing is not a separate isolable function; it is profoundly integrated with the total action system of the child—his posture, his manual skills and coordination, his intelligence and even his personality. For this reason, even minor defects in visual function, whether sensory or motor, have importance for both the pediatrician and the ocular specialist.

The grave defects of blindness and near-blindness strikingly reveal the significance of visual perception to child development.

§1. DEVELOPMENTAL ASPECTS OF VISION IN INFANCY

Vision is the most sophisticated and objective of all the senses. It gives the most detailed report of the outside world, simultaneously registering position, distance, size, color and form. But vision does not function in complete isolation; developmentally and psychologically it is closely correlated with other sensory activities, particularly touch and kinesthesia.

Vision is more precocious than audition in its development, but both looking and listening are criteria of cortical intactness in the newborn period. Although he resists excessive illumination by blinking, the infant soon uses his waking time for accumulation of visual experience and the exercise of ocular functions. Indeed, so fundamental is the sense of vision that it is the traditional criterion of wakefulness as opposed to sleep. An infant does not really wake up until he begins to look; when he ceases to look he goes to sleep. In the early months looking is half of living.

From the very beginning there is a motor component in the infant's visual behavior. The eyes do not function as mere receptors which catch rays of light; they are searchlight antennae which are in constant adaptive movement. The kinesthetic impressions registered by these eye movements are very important, as are the retinal impressions themselves, because the retinal impressions in isolation would not supply the complete data which are necessary for comprehension of the configuration of physical objects. The motor data furnished by the eye muscles soon are supplemented by comparable data supplied through pre-hension, manipulation and locomotion. Visual impressions supply the foci and cues for attentional fixations, but the infant's knowledge of the physical world is built up through his dynamic adaptations. The seeing child becomes by slow de-grees to the concepts of vertical, horizontal, circle, square and oblique. It takes time for the retinal maculae to attain full physiologic development and for the child to acquire the minutiae of experience which establish the precision, dimen-sions and stereoscopic qualities of his perception. The retina receives impressions, and muscles, fundamental and accessory, achieve adjustments to position, distance, size and form; the cortex organizes the experience.

§2. THE DEVELOPMENTAL IMPACT OF VISUAL DEFECT

Visual perceptions are really visual—motor perceptions; even in the normal infant they are products of long and gradual growth. The blind infant cannot attain even the most rudimentary spatial orientations until he can bring his muscular system to bear upon the problems of position, distance, size and form. But for him they always will be different problems, because he cannot use sight and motor responses in mutual self-correcting combination and reciprocal reinforcement.

One sense cannot substitute for another, or compensate adequately for another; it is very doubtful whether there is any significant increase in acuity of the senses which remain intact. The senses were meant to function synergistically, two or more modalities blending; even the primary tactual sense normally does not function in pure form. If this close reciprocal relationship between vision, touch and hearing is not recognized, it is impossible to appreciate the gravity of the handicap under which the blind or near-blind infant labors.

The blind child is so dependent upon touch that it is difficult for him to project his mental constructs beyond the periphery of his reach. As an infant he has more difficulty than the seeing child in attaining a perception of his physical self; it is involved ambiguously with garments, blankets and furniture. He does not have the assistance of sight to make the fundamental distinction between his anatomic self and all these appurtenances.

Like the normal child, he can come to an appreciation of distance and intervening space only by translating his body from one point to another. He begins to acquire a dim sense of remote objectives and of distance covered if he is permitted to creep and to walk. As so often happens, if his locomotion is restricted or denied, his spatial orientation remains benighted. Mastery of the finer details of distance and spatial relationships likewise is dependent upon ample exploration through active touch. His finger tips must make journeys to explore outlines and conformations. Here again, it is easy to underestimate the depth of the blind child's deficiency. If he does not know what an elephant is, it is idle to suppose that in his preschool years he will learn by presenting him with a miniature model. It is fatuous to hope that the blind child ever will attain equally penetrating and rich mastery of detail, as the seeing child does.

Retention of hearing also does not compensate the blind child fully, because any interpretation of what is heard normally depends so much upon what is seen. Hearing is a distance sense for the seeing child, but for the blind child hearing is an extremely subjective sense. Sounds do not acquire objectivity, localization, and distance meanings except through long and tedious training. The child also must have profound difficulties in building up images appropriate to the voices he hears, and in associating these voices with persons like himself. When the blind child acquires the spoken word, he has the same difficulty. Whether he speaks the word himself or whether he hears it spoken by others, it is difficult for him to give it an objective, detached status.

In discussing the handicap of the hearing-impaired child in Chapter 14, we used the metaphor of the silent motion picture film. We also may adapt this metaphor to the blind child. For him, the sound film is a succession of jumbled sound effects and a running commentary of words; he lacks all experience of the pictorial patterns and the pageantry of gesture and movement which constitute the essence of the film for the hearing-impaired and the normal child.

Blindness, therefore, constitutes more than a mere absence or impairment of a single sense. If it dates from birth or early infancy, it may dislocate drastically the entire mental life of the child. For these reasons, the retention of even a very slight amount of vision in a visually defective infant has a favorable effect on his behavioral organization. Any therapeutic or surgical procedure in infancy which can bestow even a modicum of sight is paramount above other measures. Unfortunately, any primary or secondary damage to the visual receptors is extremely likely to involve other structures of the brain and may produce mental deficiency. Therefore, the restoration of some vision does not always insure a favorable developmental outlook, even when accomplished early.

§3. DIAGNOSIS OF VISUAL DEFECT

The diagnosis of severe visual defect in infancy is relatively simple in an otherwise unimpaired infant; there is imperviousness to a flashlight, absence of protective blinking, and incapacity to follow a moving object with responsive head or eye movements. These constitute sufficient evidence of complete or partial blindness. An estimation of the degree of residual sight is a more difficult matter. However, the gravity of any sensory defect cannot be appraised purely in terms of sensory acuity or sensorimotor inefficiency. What is required is critical diagnostic appraisal of the total effect upon the developmental organization of the child. This total effect can be estimated best on the basis of the developmental assessment. An interpretive diagnosis of behavior must then determine the procedures of care and management.

Diagnosis of strabismus is important; its significance as a neurologic symptom already has been mentioned. In normal infant development, the eyes usually are well coordinated for conjugate movements by the age of 12 weeks. Persisting or recurrent strabismus beyond this age cannot be dismissed as negligible. Since infants have wide nasal bridges and pseudoepicanthal folds, the pupils often appear misaligned and strabismus may seem to be present. However, only if reflected highlights are eccentrically placed in the pupils does strabismus exist. If it causes diplopia, the image from the deviant eye is suppressed, *amblyopia ex anopsia* gradually results and if treatment is not instituted early, normal binocular vision never develops. Visual cortical degeneration has been demonstrated in animals, and probably occurs in humans also. The causes of strabismus are varied; every infant should be referred to an opthalmologist as soon as it is suspected. If surgery is indicated, vision can be preserved by patching the good eye to force the impaired one to function. Glasses or miotics will correct refractive or accommodative errors, and the squint may disappear. Even an infant under a year will wear glasses if they really improve his vision.

If what the infant does indicates that he sees, no weight should be put on the ophthalmoscopic appearance. Young infants, particularly very blond ones, normally have very pale optic discs. When retrolental fibroplasia was common, infants frequently were examined under anesthesia and visual abilities stated by the appearance of the eyes, although the behavior belied the opinion that blindness was present. Behavior is the most sensitive index of function.

Some severely mentally defective infants show a pseudoblindness in early infancy. In these cases, eye movements have an uncontrolled character in the early weeks of life, but become more coordinated toward the close of the first year. Even protective visual blinking may be late in appearing. However, the child's ability to look increases with age; his lack of response to visual stimuli is due to the mental deficiency. A differential diagnosis between such deficiency and true blindness must rely on a critical appraisal of the total behavior picture and the developmental history.

The appraisal of the developmental capacities of a blind child is a challenging task. The examiner should not assume that the ordinary methods of developmental diagnosis are inapplicable; many of the situations can be adapted to the handicap. Other situations can be improvised by following cues of the child's spontaneous behavior. Postural, prehensory, language and personal–social behavior patterns which require little visual discrimination can be observed and elicited. All successful performance which approximates the child's age should be weighed very favorably as a maturity sign. The interview should bring to light the maximum manifestations of adaptive behavior at home.

The blind child has a progressive ability to meet the basic tests of life, if he is otherwise normal. Some of the child's failures and difficulties must be ascribed to his handicap, but too much allowance should not be made for the retarding effect of the blindness *per se*. If he has normal potentialities, he will demonstrate them in his vigor, in the purposefulness, relevance and integration of his behavior and in his ability to establish a working rapport with parent and examiner. If his behavior is fragmentary and poorly organized or if it is excessively self-absorbed and undirected, the outlook is not promising, even though the child is active and is responsive to a few well-learned situations. However, the factors which determine the developmental fate of a blind infant may be so varied and numerous that prognosis always should be cautious and conservatively hopeful without fostering undue optimism. Even in combination with extreme prematurity, blindness does not necessarily produce serious retardation.

§4. EARLY MANAGEMENT OF VISUAL DEFECT

If the blind infant is overprotected because of misguided sympathy, he fails to have an active babyhood; if left alone he tends to be indifferent to the external world and his development is impeded through sheer environmental impoverishment. He may become anemic, physically underdeveloped, poorly nourished and flabby in musculature; he may acquire "nervous habits." These habits are well called *blindisms*, although some of them also occur in institutional syndromes of children who have not suffered visual deprivation. The most common blindisms consist of eye rubbing, finger flicking before the eyes, sniffing and smelling, arm twirling, body swaying and repetitive vocal tics and tricks. These blindisms are symptoms and substitute activities. They can be prevented only if we succeed in understanding the needs of the blind child for more adequate self-expression. In the infant and preschool years special accommodations must be made so that he may enjoy positive developmental experiences.

The blind baby needs special care, yet the cardinal rule for parents should be "Treat the blind baby as if he were a seeing child." This is a safe rule with reservations which common sense will supply. Strength, self-reliance and happiness must be encouraged. The blind infant should not be permitted to lie on his back for months. Perhaps as early as 16 weeks, he is ready to respond to propped sitting. The test at least should be made to determine his potentialities; taking further cues from his maturity progressions, he should be encouraged to grope, reach, grasp and manipulate. He should learn to walk, even though he gets bumps; he should romp and explore and play with toys; he should be as active in body and as investigative in mind as a seeing child. He should learn to dress and undress, comb his hair, take care of his person and possessions, keep himself clean and acquire agreeable habits of deportment. He should not be made overly conscious of his handicap, but rather of his obligation to take his place in the family circle. These are the primary lessons in the formation of his character, and they can be learned in a good home.

Sometimes an effort is made to provide educational opportunities in a special nursery or in a kindergarten department of a school for the blind. Such segregated nurseries and institutional provisions seem to complicate rather than simplify the problems of psychologic development. Institutional life multiplies the difficulties of adjustment both to the physical and the social world. The institutionalized child is confronted with other blind children equally unadjusted. An institution either becomes too stereotyped or introduces too many uncontrollable variables, to say nothing of the confusion of noise which inevitably arises when too many children are brought into close association. A normal nursery school is preferable and may be needed as a therapeutic test if the child has been overprotected.

Confusion is the very thing which should be avoided in the early education of the blind. Ideally there should be a deliberate simplification of the world of sounds for the young blind. There should be fixed orientations with respect to rooms, playground, doors and furniture. The dim world of the partially seeing should be earmarked by certain fixed sounds such as the chime of a clock and the ring of a doorbell; it should be eyemarked by conspicuous identification disks and by spotlights which draw attention to locations.

When a group of blind preschool children are gathered together, there are bound to be several among them who are aggressive and hyperactive. They will hurl blocks at random, some of which will strike heads. A blind child cannot learn the course of a projectile from such experiences. He makes no association between throwing a toy and being hit by a toy. These recurring mishaps are lawless, uncomprehended and emotionally disturbing. Well-defined and simplified educational paths must be laid out, and the protection of intimate individual guidance is needed. When an adult is at hand to safeguard, the blind baby can be encouraged to creep and the toddler to walk. Self-confidence can be imparted by progressive stages, with not too much reliance on the hard knocks of experience.

Such individual guidance is realized best in the family home. If the blind baby is deprived of parental care, foster home placement is much preferable to institutionalization. The needs of the preschool blind child are so vital that there is room for the development of a new kind of home teaching service. This service conducted by state and private agencies still is confined mainly to adults and to children of school age. Expert educational guidance can be provided both for foster and family homes through home visitors trained to understand the peculiar needs of the infant and preschool blind.

The early years of a blind child's life are most in danger of neglect and of misguided treatment. Every case presents individual problems which demand the counsel of the physician. A knowledge of the developmental characteristics of sensory defects will enable him to render valuable service. The following case histories indicate some of the problems that may be encountered.

Illustrative Cases

Case 1 was born 13 weeks prematurely, with a birth weight of 2 lbs. Although slightly cyanotic, and afflicted with atelectasis and cervical adenitis during the neonatal period, she made excellent physical progress, and weighed 15 lb 10 oz at the age of 35 weeks, approximating a weight norm of 24 weeks and height norm of 20 weeks. This was consistent with a corrected chronologic age of *22 weeks*. A developmental examination at that time showed a behavior picture approximating the 20-week maturity level, in spite of almost complete blindness. Flashlight inspection through the constricted pupils of both eyes revealed a whitish membranous sheet posterior to each lens: bilateral retrolental fibroplasia. The infant showed slight sensitivity to strong light, indicating a small residuum of vision. In the supine position, she extended her arms laterally, pumped with both feet, rolled to the side, squealed with pleasurable vocalization. She brought her hands to midline when the examiner pressed a rattle against her chest. Seated in the supportive examining chair, she exploited the tabletop actively with scratching, had an incipient groping and corralling approach to a cube and grasped the cube on contact. She noticed her mother's voice and quieted when talked to. The prognosis was favorable because of energy, integration and satisfactory personal–social adjustments.

Reexamination at 16 months (corrected chronologic age *56 weeks*) confirmed the favorable prognosis. Sensitivity to light apparently was lost. Irides were previously slaty blue, and now a dirty brown. Behavior was near a 56-week maturity level. She stood momentarily alone, withdrew a cube from a cup, released a ball in to-and-fro play, cast objects, comprehended several words and vocalized with incipient jargon. She showed spirited verve, emotional reactiveness combined with control and a perceptive parent–child rapport. Her outlook was excellent if adequate socializing experience could be provided throughout the next five years. This case demonstrates that a combination of extreme prematurity, blindness and neonatal complications does not necessarily produce retardation.

Case 2 was referred for observation at the age of *48 weeks* because of extreme blindness. Examination revealed pigmentary degeneration of the retinae and bilateral optic atrophy. An electroencephalogram showed absence of occipital alpha waves as the only abnormality in the record. The developmental examination indicated retardation within the 28-week zone of maturity. Muscle tone was good. There was fair vigor. Optimal behaviors included: props self on forearms in prone, gets up on knees and elbows, rolls over to supine, grasps cube with radial palm, transfers cube, vocalizes "da." The context of these behaviors was relatively good, but the behavior picture was not sufficiently decisive to warrant a favorable prognosis.

Reexamined at *18 months,* the child still presented an attractive appearance ("large beautiful eyes"). However, "blindisms" were more marked. She dug her fists vigorously into her eye sockets. Postural control was seriously retarded. She sat alone only briefly. She groped undiscriminatingly for a toy. Her vocabulary was limited to one word. Her behavior was fragmentary and poorly integrated. At the age of *2 years,* her exploitation of test objects was sketchy and infantile, consisting of mouthing, transfer, blowing and tapping. Despite slight gains in vocalizations and vocabulary, the maturity ratings nowhere rose above the 12-month level.

The final examination at the age of *30 months* showed minimal progress in the interim. Behavior continued to be infantile and increasingly stereotyped. Two more words had been added to her meager vocabulary. Developmental outlook was now extremely poor. In this case, the blindness is of unknown etiology. The developmental career suggests that the degenerative process was not limited to the optic nerve, and eventuated in progressive mental deficiency.

Case 3 was born with bilateral cataracṭs, but had some faint light perception in infancy. She played actively and showed great eagerness for visual experience. She would grope for a toy, grasping it on tactile cue, and locating its position by an auditory cue, when the object made a sound as it was placed on the table. Having grasped the object, she brought it very close to her eyes, examining it in a monkeylike manner. Her investigatory press was so strong that she fussed in the absence of toys. At the age of 1 year, she picked up a pellet on tactile cue, using a pincers type of thumb opposition. It is noteworthy that she had developed such a high degree of fine prehension, even in the absence of detailed visual experience. She made an excellent showing on the developmental schedules at the age of 18 months just prior to the needling of her cataracts. Vision was improved by the operation and by glasses. She made excellent progress, maintaining the alert expression and happy disposition which she manifested as a baby, and rating a near-average maturity level at the age of 4 years. She represents the type of child who benefits greatly from the specialized instruction offered by school-age sight-saving classes.

Case 4 was a boy born with complete bilateral anophthalmia, a very rare congenital anomaly—particularly striking in this instance because in all other respects he proved to be remarkably normal. Birth, neonatal and health history were uneventful. There were no complications during pregnancy, although the possibility of an unrecognized virus infection could not be excluded. Physically, this child made an agreeable impression, enhanced by magnetic personality traits. Cranium and facial features were well formed, but the eye sockets were sunken, the eyelids diminutive and closed and the eye lashes scanty. Puncta and lachrymal glands functioned. Palpation of the orbits indicated an underlying soft, amorphous mass. X-ray indicated that the optic foramina were closed and the optic nerves presumably wanting.

Systematic developmental examinations at 16, 28, 40 and 52 weeks and 18 and 24 months showed consistently normal behavioral development throughout this period. At the age of *16 weeks,* he held the rattle actively, brought it to his mouth, engaged in mutual fingering in spontaneous play, maintained good head station in the seated position, scratched the tabletop, vocalized with squealing and well-defined laughter, heeded the examiner's voice and interrupted activity to listen to sound. Head rotation was restricted, and the head tended to plunge with exaggerated abruptness. This latter atypical behavior and the impassiveness of countenance were attributable to the visual defect, indicating that facial expressions require learning; exploitation was vigorous, and in form and context the behavior patterns approximated those of a seeing child of similar age. A favorable prognosis was made on the basis of spirit, emotional characteristics and the integrity of the total behavior picture.

Similar approximations to normality were demonstrated in the subsequent examinations. At *28 weeks* he banged and transferred a cube; at *40 weeks* he plucked a pellet pincerwise; at *52 weeks* he cruised from chair to chair, and released a ball with a slight cast; at *18 months* he walked well and combined two words responsively; at *24 months* he had a vocabulary of 30 words and combined 3 words spontaneously; at *27 months* he participated in nursery school play and made excellent personal–social adjustments. Although the culture makes increasing demands on discriminative vision, much of his behavior under adequate safeguards was essentially normal in basic pattern and purpose. For example, while trying to climb into a chair he exclaimed, "I can do it!"

This case is highly significant from the standpoint of developmental diagnosis. Nature performed an unwonted experiment for our instruction: in the embryonic period, she limited a lesion neatly to the receptor organs of vision, and left all the rest intact. It represents a test tube demonstration of the fundamental role of maturation in the patterning of human behavior. Our culture is highly dependent on visual cues. The culture cannot, through its seeing agents, impart these signs to a blind child. He is deprived of all ordinary opportunities of imitation. Nevertheless, he conforms to an impressive extent to the culture, because through intrinsic growth processes he is able to bring forth patterns of behavior which proceed into desirable channels—if his parents provide experiences favorable for their development. This does not happen when normal growth potentialities are wanting, destroyed or damaged. Too often the complications of deafness and blindness are not limited neatly to the sensory functions; other structures and functions are affected, the growth potentialities thereby reduced, and the child proves to be seriously defective. Often the mental deficiency is ascribed mistakenly to the sensory defect alone. A case such as this indicates how normally behavior can develop under favorable circumstances.

§5. VISUAL CORTICAL DYSFUNCTION

There is a group of children whose handicaps are due to cerebral impairment, involving chiefly the visual areas. More than strabismus results; a serious visual defect is the presenting symptom. These patients often are referred for diagnosis as blind or near-blind infants.

Very early in life, irregular, roving or nystagmic eye movements are noted, together with failure of fixation and apparent blindness. As the weeks pass, vision tends to improve slightly, though it still is obviously very poor; the irregular eye movements persist for months. The outstanding findings on opthalmologic examination are strabismus, uncoordinated eye movements and pallor of the optic discs. Behavioral examination discloses that vision is very defective but not altogether absent; the infant cocks his head to see, the eyes rove and he sees but fleetingly, "out of the corner of his eye." Often he will perceive only a moving object.

The visual defect tends to involve macular vision more seriously than peripheral vision. These two kinds of vision have separate and distinct cortical representation;

thus, injury to the visual cortex representing the maculae may leave peripheral vision undamaged. However, in most cases peripheral vision also is fuzzy and fleeting; the infant cannot be said to really see or look, but only to catch fugitive, blurred glimpses of his environment. In the early weeks, he hardly responds to these glimpses at all, but by the age of 6 months he begins to try to use his defective visual equipment as best he can.

At the same time, the infant almost invariably will show evidences of associated impairment of motor function. These evidences may be only minimal, but it is very important that they be recognized. Any combination of visual and manual disabilities may distort and reduce adaptive behavior to a marked degree.

No two injuries are precisely the same; thus, clinical manifestations are varied. Any degree of associated motor involvement is possible; the visual handicap varies in severity, from total blindness to such a mild defect that it is overlooked in infancy and early childhood, particularly if the motor handicap is sufficiently marked to become the focus of attention. In other instances, poor vision is not suspected but a visual mannerism such as eye rolling or head wagging is so obtrusive as to cause concern. Personality and intellectual deficits are not uncommon. Each case requires careful individual evaluation in terms of the total child, his disabilities and limitations, and his assets and compensating forces.

A great many of these children eventually learn to use what little vision they have with considerable effectiveness; however, the precise degree of effective vision cannot be predicted in infancy. Most of them can walk about without guidance, though they may be unsure of thresholds and curbs; they see well enough to play well with toys, aided by clever guessing and filling in. In the early years, books and pictures are beyond their visual abilities as a rule, though many will pretend to read and will supply random names for the pictures they cannot see. Some compensate almost completely by school age.

Treatment directed toward the conservation of sight is indicated. If a child is tending to establish monocular vision, vision in the nonfunctioning eye should be preserved by covering the good eye with an eyepatch. He will tolerate the patch if he has any vision at all in the nonfunctioning eye, though he may need considerable help. An ingenious and conscientious mother will find that even a small infant will wear the patch if he is riding in his carriage or if she will give him extra attention and stimulation at this time. Operative correction of the strabismus should depend entirely on the opthalmologist's judgment. Corrective lenses should be applied for any coexisting error of refraction, but the parent should be warned that the visual defect is central and not in the eyes themselves; that glasses will not help this part of the problem. At school age, sight conservation classes may be indicated.

The parents also need orientation and education. They must learn to think of their child not in terms of his eyes but in terms of his total makeup, including his associated handicaps and assets. Prognosis for development depends on the normality of these assets and the intelligence of parental management.

Illustrative Cases

Case 5 had a normal delivery but was cyanotic for the first 12 hours of life. Irregular eye movements and failure of visual responses were noted early. In time, vision improved slightly, but the parents became concerned about the baby's poor developmental progress.

At *44 weeks* of age the infant had marked strabismus with wandering of the eyes. She cocked her head in attempting to fixate, saw very poorly and groped for objects. Her sitting posture was abnormal—unsteady with bowed back. The arms were tremulous with small athetotic finger movements. She held two objects and transferred awkwardly from hand to hand. General maturity level was 32–36 weeks.

At *15 months* of age she crept and pulled to her feet. Her exploitation was stereotyped, her prehensory approach tentative and overdeliberate. On one occasion she attempted to build a tower of two cubes. She had three–four single words and a limited soft jargon. General maturity level approximated 13 months. She had numerous visual mannerisms such as pulling and poking at her eyelids and the bridge of her nose. The abnormal eye movements were no longer present, but she was using only monocular peripheral vision. Examination of the eyes under anaesthesia at this time revealed some pallor of the discs, with probable defect in the central area supplied by the papillomacular bundle.

At *27 months* of age she was walking alone. Her gait was somewhat stiff and rigid, a little too erect. She did not grope her way, but was unsure of thresholds, and often dropped to her knees and crept through a doorway. Hand movements were uncertain, and she overreached and fumbled. She had about 10 words. General maturity level was 18–21 months. The ultimate developmental outlook still was uncertain. The visual handicap remained moderately severe, while the motor signs of cerebral insult were becoming decreasingly significant. This child may prove to be mildly defective, or she may organize further and show improvement.

Case 6, born at term, required resuscitation and showed cyanosis and feeding difficulties in the neonatal period. She was referred for examination because "the eyes roll in a purposeless way, less marked now than formerly. Does not recognize her mother."

At *26 weeks* of age she was a small infant with a small head and obviously poor vision. There was strabismus and occasional saccadic movements of the eyes. Tone was greatly excessive, and the reflexes on trigger. Her adaptive behavior was confined almost entirely to stereotyped hand regard, and apparently she did not perceive proffered toys. There was no grasp, the hand remaining open when an object was pressed against the palm. Head control was very poor. She chuckled and cooed. She was reported to have made great progress in the month preceding examination, but she showed a developmental level of only 12–16 weeks. The opthalmologist reported that the central areas of the fundi of both eyes showed a granular atrophic lesion of the choroid and retina, together with pallor of the nerve heads.

At *42 weeks* of age, strabismus was marked, and vision just barely adequate for grasp and exploitation. She could sit alone briefly, creep and pull to her feet. Hand regard was still present, and there was considerable fine motor incoordination. Hypertonia and hyperreflexia persisted. However, general maturity level was close to 36 weeks. The outlook seemed much improved.

At *15 months* of age she walked alone with a toddling gait. The manual disability was very slight. However, strabismus was very marked, and she used only the right eye. A slight left facial weakness and some general blanking out of facial expression were apparent. Her performance was normal in quality, the general maturity level 13–14 months. She was wearing an eyepatch over the right eye about 1 hour a day, tolerating it with social help. She was sufficiently "wise" to go into a corner to try to pull it off.

At 2 years of age the position of the left eye was corrected surgically with 90% cosmetic improvement. At *26 months* of age her gait was entirely normal, if a little cautious, and she used her hands well. Vision was adequate for walking about and manipulation of objects, but inadequate for picture identification or demonstrations with blocks and formboard. General maturity level was 21–24 months. The developmental outlook was relatively favorable; there remained a considerable visual defect which will have to be taken into account in planning for her education. Her development far surpassed anything that could have been predicted on the first examination at 26 weeks of age. Most remarkable was the recession of the motor signs of cerebral damage.

Case 7 was born 2 months before term following premature separation of the placenta. The infant did well, but at the (corrected) age of 5 months the mother was concerned because he frequently rolled his eyes downward and inward as though looking at the end of his nose, and appeared to lapse into a "dream state." The referring physician considered the behavior sufficiently abnormal to suspect a disturbance in vision.

At the (corrected) age of *25 weeks* he was a passive, chubby, inactive infant with poor head control and poor vision. The arms were held flexed and withdrawn, with athetotic movements of the fingers; the legs and toes were held extended. The reflexes were hyperactive. There was no prehensory approach, simply vague passive regard. He displayed frequent possible seizure episodes, looking down his nose with marked strabismus and general immobilization. Behavior was very atypical; no patterns above the 16-week level were seen. Feeding difficulties, choking and gagging were reported as prominent.

At the (corrected) age of *40 weeks* he did not respond to toys at all unless they were moved and shaken, when approach would suddenly break through his passive immobility. Grasp was poor, and objects seized were immediately dropped. He could sit alone very momentarily. Adaptive behavior was depressed to the 24–28 week level, while language behavior was nearer 36 weeks. A report from the opthalmologist stated "probable optic atrophy."

At the (corrected) age of *17 months* he could take a few uncertain steps alone. When the right hand was held to assist his walking, the left arm reflexly assumed a typical hemiplegic posture. He used the right eye only, cocked his head and strabismus was marked. The hands frequently assumed athetotic postures. General maturity level was 52–56 weeks. Eyepatch treatment was begun at this time.

At the (corrected) age of *30 months,* motor signs were almost imperceptible, though he still choked on solid food and the hands were perhaps a little clumsy. Vision remained very poor and was not quite good enough to enable him to respond to many of the examination situations. He could not see any demonstrations not involving movement (as drawing). General maturity level was above 24 months, but language was lagging, with a vocabulary of only three–four words. He was wearing an eyepatch 1–2 hours daily.

At the (corrected) age of *4 years* he had a free, easy stride, but his hand movements were not quite precise. Feeding difficulties were finally resolved. His attention was fairly well sustained, and language development had accelerated; he had a fairly good vocabulary and used sentences. Vision was very poor; he did much covering of his visual inadequacies with random replies and evasive remarks, though he occasionally admitted, "I can't" or "I don't know." Actually, he was so adept at concealing his visual handicaps under ordinary conditions that the mother said "He seems to see all right at home. Perhaps I overestimate, but I don't think his vision is so bad." Adaptive maturity level was 3 years, language development $3\frac{1}{2}$ years. Operative correction of the marked strabismus was planned in the near future.

This boy undoubtedly sustained cerebral insult with mild motor and marked visual involvement. It was difficult to estimate his maturity with any assurance that one was doing the boy full justice, but language development was in the normal range. The visual handicap was serious and will create special problems in adjustment and education.

Case 8 was born 3 weeks postmaturely, weighing 7 lb 1 oz. The delivery was instrumental, the infant was cyanotic and she twitched for the first 24 hours of life. She had a single convulsion at 11 months of age.

She was referred for examination at *18 months* of age because she could not stand or walk. She had spastic monoplegia of the right upper extremity with associated signs of further mild, diffuse motor involvement. She used her left hand poorly, tapping, pushing and poking at objects without coordinated manipulation. She walked when one hand was held, overstepping with the right foot; she could not creep or pull to her feet. Reflexes were hyperactive, the right more so than the left. Her regard was vague and vision defective. She tended to fixate with the left eye, the right eye wobbling uncertainly. She had a rich jargon and 15–20 words. Gross motor development was atypical, fine motor at 40 weeks, adaptive at 10–13 months, and language fully average at 18–21 months.

Her progress was remarkably good, and on her last examination at $5\frac{1}{2}$ *years* her gait was normal except for overcautiousness on stairs. She used her left hand almost exclusively, bringing in her spastic right hand to stabilize the unsteady movements of the left. Vision was poor; she picked up the pennies, one by one, leaving two unseen on the table. She verbalized drawing a man and was satisfied with her product, but the drawing was totally unrecognizable. She identified large pictures, not too accurately. She guessed, fumbled and groped; she made excuses, "It's hard to do," "That's the way I do it," "What's the matter with this thing?" At the same time, she handled all the language and conceptual tests appropriate to her age with ease. She had been wearing glasses for 2 years with very little if any improvement in vision.

This child had a selective cerebral dysfunction, but the visual impairment, which was disregarded for the first 18 months, became her most serious handicap. She was ready for school entrance, but will require special educational measures adapted to her manual and visual disabilities.

§6. THE LATER LIFE OF BLIND AND HEARING-IMPAIRED CHILDREN

The fate of the infant suffering from sensory defect depends largely upon associated factors. For this reason, the more precise the early diagnosis the more implications it has for prognosis. The vocational outlook for the handicapped must necessarily enter into the physician's judgment and advice.

First and foremost, it is essential to achieve a differential diagnosis between mental deficiency with sensory defect and sensory defect with potentials for normal development. If this differentiation is not attempted, there is danger of excessive preoccupation with the defect itself, and this leads to the same errors of misunderstanding and management which arise in connection with cases of infantile psychosis (Chapter 16). Therapeutic tests, including long periods of observation under educational programs, may be necessary to establish a final diagnosis. If mental deficiency proves to be present, elaborate training measures directed only toward the specific defect are of doubtful wisdom.

In the relatively normal child, personality factors and social conditions, both extra- and intrafamilial, will prove of ultimate importance, particularly with the hearing-impaired, who are subject to emotional deviations which tend to separate them from hearing persons, and to segregate them with their own kind in adult years. The vocational outlook is good in numerous occupations which place chief reliance on vision as opposed to hearing. Early recognition, sound amplification and wise management may allow almost complete compensation in all but the most severe cases.

The adult blind present fewer problems of social adjustment. Personality factors are less likely to complicate this adjustment. The normal intelligence of the individual, supplemented by the protection of the seeing-eye dog, makes for relatively normal adjustments to community life. Detailed planning of life arrangements, as well as vocational placement, is important. Here, even more than with other forms of handicap, intelligent social work is of great value. The physician often is the first person to set into motion the assistance of social and community agencies.

16

Autistic, Psychotic and Other Disturbed Behavior

From a very early age, the normal infant is socially responsive to people. By 12 weeks, he smiles and coos back when stimulated by movement and the sound of a human voice. Nothing stirs the heart of the misanthrope more than a 16-week baby whose eyes crinkle and lips curl spontaneously in an appealing smile as he initiates social play. Invariably, the smile the 20-week-old gives his mirror image evokes answering laughter from a group of watching students. So absorbed is the infant with people at these tender ages that it may be difficult to divert his attention to test objects during a developmental evaluation. This phase passes in large measure; as he matures, his social perceptions become selective, discriminating and complex.

When the give and take of *social interaction* does not unfold, or is lost, the child's behavior seems to arise from within himself. It appears unrelated to environmental stimuli and is accompanied by a variety of repetitive bizarre mannerisms; there may be aggressive, destructive and self-destructive acts. Nowhere does more confusion exist than in this group of children, who currently are diagnosed as suffering from infantile psychoses, variously termed autism, childhood schizophrenia, atypical ego development or a heterogeneous group of other designations, frequently thought of as psychogenic psychiatric disorders, and so treated.

§1. HISTORIC CONSIDERATIONS

Although there were earlier references to childhood schizophrenia, modern interest in the subject of infantile psychosis stems from Bender's annotation on childhood schizophrenia in 1942[5] and Kanner's description of early infantile autism in 1943.[36] Kanner used the term to define what he believed to be a specific clinical entity with three cardinal characteristics. The pathognomonic feature was extreme aloneness and the child's inability to relate himself in the ordinary way to people,

320

from the beginning of life. The second characteristic was an anxiously obsessive desire for the preservation of sameness, leading to a restricted repertoire of spontaneous activity. The third facet was failure to use language for purposes of communication. Because of the presence of unusual feats of memory qr isolated performance skills at or above age level, all the children were believed to have normal or near-normal intelligence; their subsequent course belies this assumption. Kanner also reported an unusually high percentage of parents who were intelligent, cold and obsessive professionals, but he did raise the question of whether the child's behavior had caused the parents to withdraw. Nine points considered as criteria for the diagnosis of schizophrenic syndromes in childhood were presented by Creak in 1961.[15] In essence, they include the same behaviors described by Kanner, with perhaps more emphasis on backgrounds of serious retardation and theoretical formulations to explain the symptoms. Diagnosis has been confounded by a subsequent proliferation of loose and idiosyncratic definitions of terms, making comparisons of different samples difficult.

The genetic background of infantile psychosis differs strikingly from that of adult schizophrenics. Parents of the patients studied by both Kanner and Eisenberg at Johns Hopkins,[22] and by Rutter at the Maudsley in London,[65] had a low incidence of psychiatric disorders; when present, they were more often neurotic than psychotic. Similarly, siblings of autistic children rarely are abnormal. Clinical pictures of schizophrenia comparable to the adult disease, in children who have been essentially healthy, seldom develop before 8 years of age; they are seen with increasing frequency towards adolescence. Consensus is growing that the term *childhood schizophrenia* should be reserved for such previously healthy children, and *infantile psychosis* or *autism* employed for those in whom the picture described above has been present from birth or early life.

Children with overt organic syndromes are referred to psychiatric services for differential diagnosis infrequently, particularly in the first 2 or 3 years of life. The majority of children with bizarre behavior are seen in psychiatric facilities at later ages. If one has a population of young pediatric patients who exhibit psychotic behavior, one might expect to find a heterogeneous group of associated diseases and syndromes. On the other hand, elimination of all patients with other specifically classified disorders might leave an apparently discrete condition. Such a selection process could explain why debate continues about criteria for diagnosis, organic versus psychogenic etiology and treatment and prognosis.

§2. "PSEUDOSYMPTOMATIC RETARDATION"

The diagnosis of infantile psychosis probably is overemployed rather than underemployed by child psychiatrists and child guidance workers. Attribution by parents and professionals of a psychogenic etiology to bizarre behavior long antedated the recent interest in the topic that has burgeoned in the psychiatric literature. The following description appeared in 1941 in the first edition of this volume, as well as in later printings, prior to Kanner's description.[36] Only the word "amentia" has been changed.

The fact that behavioral development is subject to at least temporary environmental depression is known both to the laity and to the profession. Very naturally, therefore, parents of defective children eagerly look for extrinsic causes which might account for the observed retardation. The parents wishfully hope that these causes operate as an obstruction which can be removed by treatment, or which will spontaneously disappear and release the impeded potentialities of development. In relating the history of the case the parents usually adduce some plausible causative factor such as long hospitalization, forcible feeding, severe eczema with prolonged restraint, a dominating nurse, an illness or trauma.

In recounting the history of the case the parents add extenuating claims: "He does some things so well." "He understands so much." "It is as though he were thwarted and as though something were holding him back." "He has an excellent disposition." "He has more abilities than he likes to use." "One time he said a sentence very plainly." "He seems unhappy."

In these cases there are residues of behavior, or demeanor and of attention which resemble the normal so much as to lend a certain plausibility to the interpretation which the parents themselves advance. Often the behavior of the child is very bizarre and paradoxically enough the very strangeness of the behavior invites a diagnosis which may overlook the underlying mental deficiency. When the behavior assumes bizarre patterns there is a temptation to look for environmental origins and to place a psychiatric construction on the symptoms. For example, the child may show extreme fixations on one toy, or on one pastime such as pouring sand through a pipe, opening and closing doors. This particular behavior becomes a misleading focus of attention in the interpretation of the case. The behavior may even be invested with symbolic significance to the relative neglect of a multitude of symptoms which definitely point to fundamental mental defect.

Extreme stereotypies of behavior are a frequent characteristic in this group of cases. The stereotypy is in the nature of a cauliflowering overgrowth. There may be an excessive amount of rocking, or mouthing, of jargoning, of chewing, clicking, respiratory and other mannerisms. Mutism, negativism, seclusiveness figure in different syndromes. The negativism may express itself in heedlessness to sound or *obliviousness to persons.* It is frequently found in association with hyperactivity. If the child were apathetic his obliviousness might be more readily recognized as a form of inattention characteristic of severe mental deficiency. But the activity and the bizarre exaggeration are frequently associated with an attractive countenance and a faraway, wistful expression which builds up an impression of dormant or obscured normality. There is a certain abstractedness in the demeanor which is suggestive of unreleased potentialities.

If the physician yields uncritically to this impression he may describe the condition as one of symptomatic retardation. The parents are encouraged to believe that the child will find himself in time. A special course of training is resorted to, an intensive and expensive psychotherapeutic program is inaugurated. Parents go to heroic lengths to reeducate the child and to remove the obstructions which they believe are retarding or deflecting the child's development.

This description and the illustrative cases which accompanied it are duplicated in case reports of autistic and psychotic children which have appeared subsequently. Gesell and Amatruda labeled these children as having *pseudosymptomatic retardation,* because the bizarre nature of the behavior fostered an attribution of a psychogenic etiology which obscured the true nature of the organic disease. The term *pseudopsychogenic* probably would have been more precise. Our subsequent experience, as well as that of others, has confirmed their opinion that the vast majority of these children have mental deficiency of varying degrees.

§3. STUDIES OF "AUTISM" AND "INFANTILE PSYCHOSIS" IN EARLY LIFE

In a children's hospital, the entire spectrum of developmental disorders is seen, whether the patients are admitted specifically for evaluation of those disorders or whether they are coincidental to other acute or chronic diseases. One of the cardinal characteristics of autism and infantile psychosis is that they be present from birth or the first few years of life; therefore, observation of infants and young children during this period is more helpful than retrospectively gathered information in establishing the antecedents of behavior seen at later ages. The pediatric developmental service to which the children described in this section were referred routinely accepted patients under 24 months of age. Older preschool children were evaluated on a selective basis if they had severe motor or sensory handicaps or were diagnostic problems in other respects. Consequently, children between 2 and 5 years of age with bizarre responses rarely were referred if it was possible to establish the presence of normal intellectual potential elsewhere; children over 5 were seen for the first time only in unusual circumstances. A special investigation was undertaken of those very young children in whom a diagnosis of autism was made on the basis of their clinical symptoms. A preliminary report of the initial findings was made in 1961 and the full results are presented in the following pages.[39]

Diagnostic Criteria

The first diagnostic criterion was the presence of *persistent failure to regard people as persons*– the extreme aloneness of Kanner. The diagnosis was not made if the child clearly was aware of people but deliberately withdrew from them in fear or rejection. Presence or absence of eye contact is a concept which figures frequently in the literature in descriptions of psychotic children, and is used erroneously as a measure of social awareness. Although autistic children reach out with their hands, their regard is directed to eyeglasses, hair or moustaches; unaccompanied by normal social interaction, this kind of eye contact is inappropriate behavior.

The second diagnostic criterion, a desire for the preservation of sameness, had two facets: insistence on the part of the child that the environment remain constant, and the endless repetition of changeless behavior. Slavish devotion to routines emerges only when a child is old enough to be mobile and exercise some control over external events. An infant indicates his desire for constancy to the observer by crying at change; usually only the stereotyped patterning can be observed in the youngest patients. Interruption of the repetitive behavior can result in rage reactions in either age group. Bizarre repetitive mannerisms also are seen commonly in association with mental deficiency, particularly when the deficiency is severe. The vast majority of such defective children have social responsiveness that is very immature, but it is nevertheless appropriate to their developmental age. A diagnosis of autism or psychosis was not made merely because social rapport was infantile in character.

The third diagnostic criterion of Kanner was failure to use language for purposes of communication. The language characteristics of the population studied, because of their very young age, require special comment, but this is reserved for the discussion of results in the following section.

Many of the children in whom a diagnosis of infantile psychosis is made are considered untestable; however, those with normal or near-normal intellectual potential present no problem in evaluation. The children are capable of appropriate use of the test objects, even though exploitation often may be interrupted by frequent wandering off to engage in bizarre manipulations. In other children, because of residual islets of normal or near-normal behavior, the examiner frequently makes one of two errors. He may decide that intelligence is normal but unable to be expressed fully, or he may persist in trying to elicit behavior at the child's chronologic age. The chaotic, fragmentary and uninterpretable responses thus obtained fall into proper perspective if the examiner drops down to the functional level of the child; he may even need to drop down to early infancy to demonstrate the actual level of potential. Parenthetically, similar residual islets of normal abilities can be demonstrated in mentally defective children who do not manifest autistic behavior.

A different diagnostic problem may arise in the first 6 months of life. Absence of the characteristic social rapport and interest in people is striking when normal adaptive interest in test materials is preserved. When mental deficiency is present, the autistic nature of the behavior may be obscured in the first few months by the general inattentiveness and amorphous character of the exploitation; the process may become clear only when the infant is older.

Initial Evaluation of the Patients

Among the first 1900 patients seen in the developmental service, a diagnosis of the symptom complex of "autism" was made in 64, or 3.4%. This rather high incidence is related to the fact that about 85% of the total population was under 24 months of age. Since the original purpose of the investigation was to determine the relationship of the behavioral constellation to paranatal complications and their resultant continuum of organic brain disease, the 14 patients with phenylketonuria were excluded from further comparisons. The association of a psychotic behavior picture with PKU is well known; it was present in 14 of the 17 patients with the disease in the total population. The remaining 50 of the original 64 patients, with a median age of 18 months, were compared to the next 50 children in the case file who were abnormal, i.e., had some type of central nervous system dysfunction, but did not show symptoms of autism, and to the next 50 who were without neuropsychiatric disorder and who had been examined primarily for teaching or other purposes, such as adoption.

Both abnormal groups differed significantly from the normal comparison group, but did not differ significantly from each other in any of the variables examined—sociocultural factors, antecedent complications, motor and intellectual deficits or associated disorders. In the autism patients and in the abnormal comparison group without autism, there was a high incidence of those antecedent complications of pregnancy associated with the continuum of reproductive casualty. Table 16-1 indicates that one-fifth of the autism patients were of low birth weight, and over half had toxemia and/or bleeding during pregnancy, as well as neonatal complications. Rates were similar in the abnormal comparison group, and except for birth weight, significantly lower in the normal comparison group. In the normal group, the rates of low birth weight, and also those of paranatal complications, are higher than the ones usually found in the general population, because the sample was weighted heavily with adoption candidates.

Table 16-2 indicates the incidence of other abnormalities in the autism patients

Table 16-1. Prenatal and Paranatal Complications in Autism Patients, Abnormal Comparison Patients Without Autism and Normal Comparison Group (50 Patients in Each Group)

	Per Cent with Abnormality		
Abnormal Condition	Autism Patients	Comparison Groups	
		Abnormal	Normal
Low Birth Weight	21	24	14
Toxemia and/or Bleeding	56	39	15
Neonatal Complications	57	60	27
# Lacking Some Data	3	1	4

Table 16-2. Organic Disorders In 50 Autism Patients and 50 Abnormal Comparison Patients Without Autism*

	Per Cent with Disorder	
Disorder	Autism Patients	Abnormal Comparison
Developmental Quotient		
below 50	46	38
below 60	64	52
Convulsive Disorders	74	64
Strabismus	52	36
Cerebral Palsy	18⎫52	38⎫64
Other Specific Diseases	34⎭	26⎭
Developmental Quotient above 75	20	34

*All patients had at least one abnormality indicative of central nervous system involvement.

and the abnormal comparison group without autism, who by definition had organic disease of the central nervous system. Except for their lack of social interaction, the autistic patients did not differ significantly in any respect. Only 10 of the autism patients had initial DQs above 75; in half, the initial DQ was less than 50. In itself, such mental deficiency during infancy is evidence of organic disease of the brain; sociocultural retardation could not explain the degree of mental defect found in this young population raised in family home settings. Three-fourths of the autism children had some type of seizure episodes prior to or during the initial examination, and half had strabismus. Half had "cerebral palsy" or some other specific disorder—Dandy-Walker syndrome with obstructive hydrocephalus, Schilder's acute disseminated sclerosis, Hurler's disease, trisomy 21, papilloma of the choroid plexus, congenital hyperthyroidism, varicella encephalitis, meningitis with secondary hydrocephalus, hypoglycemia, craniostenosis, congenital rubella with hearing loss, hypsarhythmia and probable cases of congenital lues, a familial metabolic defect, or Cornelia de Lange syndrome. The specific disorders found in the abnormal comparison patients were virtual duplicates.

Language development clearly was related to the adaptive maturity level of the children as well as to their chronologic age. Table 16-3 shows that for the vast majority of the patients language behavior was similar to their adaptive level of function, regardless of age or DQ. Since 80% had adaptive behavior of less than 18 months and half of less than 40 weeks, using language for communication would not be expected; the eventual speech could not be predicted precisely, but its development could be expected to parallel the adaptive development in the vast proportion. However, two children functioning between 2 and 3 years of age already demonstrated central communication disorders; they could hear, but only occasionally did they comprehend what was said to them. No child functioning over 18 months had language appropriate to the chronologic age.

Table 16-4 shows that language development in the abnormal patients without autism also paralleled their adaptive behavior. The trend for those with DQs above

Table 16-3. Initial Language Development in Autism Patients

		LANGUAGE IN RELATION TO LEVEL OF ADAPTIVE BEHAVIOR		
INITIAL ADAPTIVE DQ	#	Similar	Lower	Speech Absent
DQ over 75				
Less than 18 mos. old	8	6	2	-
18 mos. or older	2	-	1	1
DQ 75 or less				
Function less than 18 mos.	33	30	3	-
Function 18 mos. or more	7	4	1	2
Total	50	40	7	3

75 to have more normal language development might prove significant with larger sample sizes; however, the overall similarity of the two patient groups is far more striking than the differences.

Convulsions can cause confusion, especially in young children, and must be taken into account in diagnosis. Psychomotor seizure activity, during which the patient is out of contact with his environment (Chapter 13), can mimic autistic behavior. Usually a seizure disorder is clearly paroxysmal, and changes in the level of awareness can be seen during the examination, or a definite history of such variability obtained. In such situations, a diagnosis of psychosis is incorrect; autism is not an intermittent phenomenon, with abrupt changes from normal social responsiveness. However, on occasion the seizure state is virtually continuous and it is impossible to make a distinction.

Case 1 in Figure 16-2, our youngest patient, probably illustrates this unusual situation. He was a fraternal twin, and the pregnancy was complicated by toxemia and first trimester bleeding; birth weight was 6 lb 2 oz. There was a history of frequent episodes of myoclonic jerking. We were persuaded to see him at the tender age of *11 weeks* because his total disregard for the hospital personnel had raised the question of blindness. He was intensely interested in the examination materials, and his exploitation of them showed acceleration, with adaptive function at 14 weeks.

Table 16-4. Initial Language Development in Abnormal Comparison Patients Without Autism

		LANGUAGE IN RELATION TO LEVEL OF ADAPTIVE BEHAVIOR		
INITIAL ADAPTIVE DQ	#	Similar	Lower	Speech Absent
DQ over 75				
Less than 18 mos. old	12	11	1	-
18 mos. or older	5	3	2	-
DQ 75 or less				
Function less than 18 mos.	27	24	3	-
Function 18 mos. or more	6	2	2	2
Total	50	40	8	2

There was some increase in muscle tone, but no other neuromotor abnormalities; gross and fine motor behavior also were at the 14-week level. During the examination he had frequent episodes of turning his head to one side, immobilizing and failing to respond to visual obstruction. There was no evidence of any social interaction, and total disregard of the examiners. With his otherwise well-integrated behavior, it was difficult to postulate a constant seizure state, although seizure episodes were present. He was diagnosed as having autistic symptoms and a normal intellectual potential.

He was discharged without anticonvulsant medication and readmitted to the hospital a few weeks later, totally unresponsive to his environment. The contrast in his behavior was so marked that a psychomotor status epilepticus was considered, and our recommendation to treat him with phenobarbital was followed. Much to our surprise, at *27 weeks* of age he was sociable, friendly and alert, though with severe athetoid quadriplegia; in spite of his motor problems, adaptive behavior was still within the normal range, at 23 weeks.

His subsequent course was far from benign. He was admitted to his local hospital innumerable times for severe respiratory infections, episodes of cardiac arrest, grand mal seizures and Dilantin toxicity. In spite of this and his severe motor problems, he persisted with intense energy, and at *24 months* cooperated in an examination for an hour or more, identified pictures and tried valiantly to perform. His seizures were never fully controlled, and he failed to grow; he looked like a toy doll in a picture taken with his normal sister. He developed rickets associated with renal disease and continued to deteriorate.

When he was last seen, at *54 months* of age, he had had a total of 22 hospitalizations. He was friendly at an infantile level, but had lost his interest and vigor. Gross motor behavior was at a 20-week level, his athetosis still was severe and all that remained of his original potential was some language comprehension at the 12–15-month level.

In retrospect, doubt persists about the nature of his total lack of social interaction in the face of sustained organized interest in objects at 11 weeks of age. His history illustrates how uncontrolled seizures can have devastating effects on the course of development.

Case 2. In another case, we made the error of ignoring the parental history. This 14-month infant was reported to be very loving, responsive and jolly, *at times*. She was said to have two words, know some objects by name, engage in nursery games and understand a few simple commands. The parents said that she used her feet more than her hands and "didn't look at things." During the examination the infant was totally oblivious of the examiners, and adaptive behavior was less than a third of normal, at 18 weeks. She was hypotonic, and motor behavior was only 28 weeks. Clearly, she was not a normal 14-month-old, but was she having seizures when we saw her? Would we have changed her future course if we had been wise enough at that time to consider this possibility and treat her, especially in view of the reported language behavior near her age? This child was lost to followup, but we know that she continued to be deviant, because we received a request for information from a private school for "exceptional" children.

Case 3 (Case 31 in Figure 16-2) was normal until 21 months of age when a prolonged grand mal seizure produced gross ataxia, loss of speech and complete disregard for people, but preservation of normal adaptive behavior. The abnormal symptoms persisted for 2 or 3 months. Speech and motor control returned, and she clearly was interacting with people, but was hyperactive and disorganized. Subsequently she suffered at least three more major convulsive seizures; at 55 months she had deteriorated intellectually to a 15-month level, and had no motor impairment other than motor retardation. She had definite social rapport compatible with her very immature level of adaptive behavior and used only one word. Thus, the psychotic disorder can be transient in the sense that it may persist for only a few months.

These three children were exceptions. For the other psychotic children the story was one of a persistent pattern of autistic symptoms; superimposed seizure episodes were clearly paroxysmal in nature, and in 14 instances they were typical grand mal convulsions. We did recognize most of the children with episodic "autistic" behavior due to seizures; in them a diagnosis of convulsive disorder was made and they were not included in this sample of 50 as cases of infantile psychosis.

Although three-fourths of both the autistic and the abnormal comparison patients had private patient status, only one-third of the parents in either group had had some college education. This population did not conform to the original description of highly-educated professionals.

In summary, at the time of the initial examination of these 50 autistic children, there was evidence in all of organic disease of the central nervous system. None had just psychotic symptoms. The 5 children without distortions of neuromotor integration all had gross motor retardation as a result of their mental deficiency. The remaining 45, whether or not they were mentally defective, had neuromotor abnormalities ranging from minor signs to overt "cerebral palsy." Lesser degrees of specific neuromotor abnormalities are identifiable in infancy by developmental evaluation, before compensation occurs (Chapters 10 and 11); they are not demonstrable by a standard adult neurologic examination in later childhood. The motor and mental defects were associated with convulsive seizures and a variety of other specific disease processes. Further, the autistic symptoms were qualitatively the same, whether the child had mental deficiency or normal intelligence, or whether the process had been present from birth or appeared after a definite cerebral insult, such as encephalitis or seizures. The psychotic patients differed from the abnormal comparison children only by virtue of having the autistic symptom complex, in addition to their other central nervous system abnormalities. These are not unexpected findings in a population drawn from a pediatric developmental service dealing with the first 2 or 3 years of life.

Followup Information

A systematic followup of the 50 autistic patients was instituted because we had seen some half-dozen children who had lost their autistic aloneness, in periods which varied from the few months noted in Case 1 and Case 3 above, to 1½ years. Did all the children compensate? What were the factors indicative of a favorable prognosis? Was the high incidence of mental deficiency secondary to the autistic withdrawal, as many workers have postulated?

The followup period ranged from 3 to 10 years, with a mean of 5 years. The median age of the patients was 7 years. Five of the patients died: one had Schilder's acute disseminated sclerosis, one hemorrhaged uncontrollably following operation for a papilloma of the choroid plexus, one had trisomy 21, and one had mental deficiency with athetosis and convulsive seizures. The fifth, Case 14 in Figure 16-2, was seen on several occasions after his initial evaluation. In early life he had progressed normally and was socially responsive, but he began to deteriorate after the onset of myoclonic seizures at several months of age. The autistic symptoms appeared before intellectual deterioration began. He had a Dandy-Walker syndrome with grand mal seizures and progressive obstructive hydrocephalus, requiring a shunt operation. He went downhill steadily and died at 8½ years of age in a school for the mentally defective. He remained autistic, grossly defective and blind, and still was having many seizures of various types. Five children could not be located; one family refused to cooperate but stated that their child's function was still only about one-third of normal.

For 32 of the remaining 39 there was either a formal examination by an individual unacquainted with the initial findings, or a school report, from an ordinary public school or from a facility for the mentally defective. In the remaining seven children, written information supplemented by telephone communication was obtained from a speech and hearing clinic, a physician, a public health nurse or a detailed developmental questionnaire completed by the parents. None of the children had been in any treatment program directed toward their psychotic symptoms.

Figure 16-1 shows the relationship between the adaptive DQ and age at the time of the initial examination and the persistence of the autistic symptoms. The patients represented by the open symbols had lost their autism and were making appropriate social responses to people, and those indicated by the half-black symbols were compensating. The black symbols denote children who still manifested autistic aloneness. The figure illustrates two main points: First, a greater proportion of children under a year of age when first seen had DQs over 75; the younger the child, the higher the DQ tended to be. At first it was disconcerting to observe the discrepancy in DQ between those over and under 1 year of age, but the observation held for the abnormal comparison group without autism as well. The finding could be explained by the fact that, all too often, infants were referred for suspected mental deficiency who had neuromotor abnormalities but a normal intellectual potential. Second, the autistic behavior had disappeared in three-fourths

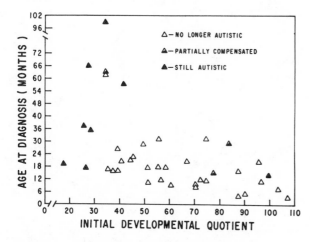

Fig. 16-1. Relationship of persistence of autism to age and developmental quotient at time of diagnosis.

of the patients. With few exceptions, it persisted if the child was over 3 years of age or the DQ was 35 or less when he was first seen. It disappeared in all those who were less than a year of age at their first examination. We do not have precise data on when these children began to establish normal social relationships. It was a gradual and variable process; some were relating appropriately by 2 years of age but not in earlier reevaluations; others were still autistic at 2 and 3 years of age, but not at 6 or 9 years. A pair of twins seen first at 5 years still were autistic at 9 years but not at 14. One child, who was 9 years old when we first saw him, was beginning to establish social contacts at 15 years of age.

Figure 16-2 shows the relationship between the initial and later adaptive DQs (or IQs). Only 6 of the 40 patients had subsequent quotients above 75, one of whom was functioning at about 50% of normal and having seizures when first seen at 22 months. The striking finding is that most of these children functioned less well at the time of followup than they did initially, in spite of the fact that they had lost their autistic behavior and had established social interactions. Some had known decelerating processes, such as trisomy 21 or Hurler's disease; others, represented by the black symbols, developed grand mal seizures. For a few, no specific disease process explained significant deterioration. Not all children admitted to state schools for the mentally defective deteriorated. However, the initial mental deficiency was not an artifact of psychotic withdrawal. At followup 60% of the children had DQs of 35 or less; one-fourth of these same children functioned at that low a level initially.

Table 16-5 demonstrates that language behavior at the time of followup again was related to the intellectual function of the child. The low IQ and low functional levels are adequate explanations for failure to speak. A high proportion of those

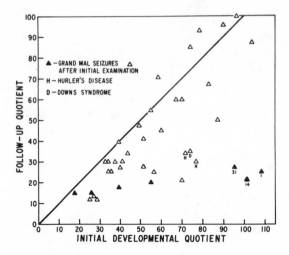

Fig. 16-2. Relationship between initial and followup developmental quotients in autistic patients.

severely mentally defective had language that was more retarded than their adaptive behavior, a common finding in a defective population; some of these possibly will never speak, especially if they are institutionalized. Six other children, all functioning above an 18-month level, had hearing impairment (Chapter 14). One was a sensorineural hearing loss secondary to congenital rubella; the other five had central communication disorders, or "aphasia." Deafness was suspected at one time, but they gradually began to comprehend and then use language, although with various idiosyncrasies. Echolalia and pronoun reversals were concomitant, as they are in normal children 21–30 months of age. One child could spell out some words with block letters at age 15, but still did not talk. The intellectual level of the child determined the usefulness of his language for communication purposes. Only three of these children with hearing impairment, the ones with the best intellectual

Table 16-5. Follow up Language Development in Autism Patients

		LANGUAGE IN RELATION TO LEVEL OF ADAPTIVE BEHAVIOR			
FOLLOW UP ADAPTIVE DQ	#	Similar	Lower	Impaired*	Speech Absent
DQ over 75	6	4	-	2	-
DQ 36-75					
Function less than 18 mos.	0	-	-	-	-
Function 18 mos. or more	10	5	2	2	1
DQ 35 or less					
Function less than 18 mos.	12	2	4	-	6
Function 18 mos. or more	12	2	4	2	4
Total	40	13	10	6	11

* 1 with sensorineural hearing loss, 5 with central communication disorder

function, had lost their autistic aloneness completely at followup. The incidence of specific communication disorders in this group of psychotic children would seem to be relatively high, but far from a universal characteristic. Clearly though, absence of speech at older ages correlates most highly with severe degrees of mental deficiency.

No systematic followup was conducted for the abnormal comparison group without autism. Information available for 15 patients indicates a subsequent course, quite parallel to that of the autism patients, which depended on their initial status and specific disease process.

§4. STUDIES OF OLDER CHILDREN

Our findings agree well with those of Rutter and his coworkers, who reexamined 63 children diagnosed as psychotic at the Maudsley Hospital in London; 57 of the children had autistic features.[66] Because their average age was 6 years when they first were seen, they probably represent a sample with more severe, certainly more persistent, psychotic symptoms than those exhibited by our population. Mean age at followup was 15½ years, and all the original patients were reexamined. There is a remarkable similarity between the characteristics of these children and ours.

Initially, just under half the children had IQs below 50 and about one in five tested above 80. About half of the children had no speech at 5 years of age, only eight of whom had measured IQs above 60. The psychotic behavioral manifestations could not be differentiated on the basis of IQ score, the presence or absence of speech, an onset from birth or later, the presence of a definite antecedent environmental stress such as hospitalization or the existence of signs considered definite or suggestive organic brain disease.

At the time of followup, the initial IQ obtained proved to be a good predictor of the later IQ, with a correlation of 0.80. The brighter children remained brighter, the dull tended to become duller, especially if they were institutionalized. Half the children still had IQ test scores below 50. In no case did the IQ rise appreciably in the nine children who no longer were autistic; in fact it tended to fall more often. Sixteen of the patients were considered to have definite signs of brain dysfunction, but the "stringent criteria" for this categorization are not stated; 15 of the 16 had grand mal epileptic seizures, 10 of whom developed their convulsions after the initial evaluation, about the time of adolescence. Another one-fourth were felt to have signs suggestive of brain damage, including disorders such as congenital lues and toxoplasmosis, but without physical abnormalities. Rutter treated mental deficiency separately from organic brain disease, and it is not possible to determine how much overlap existed between the 50% of children with initial IQs of less than 60 and the 50% considered to have other evidences of organic central nervous system impairment.

The initial IQ was found to be the best predictor of eventual outcome. A total of 10 children achieved a normal level of speech development, and 7 of the 32 who were mute at 5 years learned to speak. However, only 2 patients with an initial IQ less than 60 learned to speak, only one of whom used his speech to communicate. Failure to learn to speak was highly correlated with a low IQ; lack of speech was a poor prognostic sign only if mental deficiency also was present. Five children had definite receptive aphasia, and 14, lesser degrees of the same disorder; one-third of these children had been considered deaf at earlier ages. It is not entirely clear whether Rutter considered this aphasia to be evidence of organic brain dysfunction. In general, as language was acquired, it followed the normal developmental progressions. Finally, outcome and adjustment were not influenced by psychotherapy, but they were affected by whether or not the child received any appropriate educational experience.

Rutter agreed with our findings and concluded that infantile psychosis is not part of schizophrenia, and is unlikely to be a homogeneous disorder. Neither is it a special form of mental deficiency, since it can be associated with normal intelligence. Although there is high incidence of receptive and executive speech defects, he differentiated infantile psychosis from developmental aphasia, since most aphasic children use nonverbal communication and are not autistic. He concluded that infantile psychosis most likely will prove to have heterogeneous causes, leading to generalized impairment of brain function, with mental subnormality, aphasia, autism and other defects.

On the other hand, Kanner and Eisenberg believe that autism is a specific entity which is distinguishable from schizophrenia by the early age of onset, and from mental deficiency because of evidence of good intellectual potential. However, Eisenberg contradicts himself when he acknowledges at the end of his discussion of childhood psychosis that Rutter "suggests, and I believe correctly, that my earlier observations on the presence or absence of useful speech by age 5 as a predictor of outcome may have been 'largely due to the high correlation between absence of speech and low intelligence.' "[21] Kanner's recent report of the subsequent course of the 11 children he described originally indicates that only 1 of the 9 for whom he was able to obtain information had normal intelligence and had made a satisfactory adult adjustment; a second was functioning in a simple routine position and a third had died.[37] Kanner attributes the poor outcome in many of the rest to the fact that they were in state hospitals, but most of these individuals did not enter such institutions until after adolescence. In 6 children the history strongly suggests organic brain disease because of convulsions, delayed motor development, general slow development, an abnormal neonatal period and prematurity.

In the larger followup study of 63 patients at Johns Hopkins reported by Eisenberg and Kanner, no IQ scores were given, so precise quantitative comparisons are not possible.[22] At adolescence, 3 patients had made a "good" and 14 a "fair" adjustment, a total of 27%. It is not possible to determine from the report how many of the patients with a "poor" adjustment were capable of establishing social relationships compatible with their intellectual level of function. Outcome appeared to be related to the severity of the disorder rather than to the type or amount of therapy.

Rutter also characterized his outcome in the same broad general terms.[66] His results were perhaps somewhat better, if one assumes that the criteria for the categories were more or less comparable to those of Eisenberg and Kanner: good, 14%; fair, 25%; poor, 13%; very poor, 48%. None of the "good" and all but one of the "very poor" children were either untestable or had an initial IQ of less than 60. If one devises similar crude generalities for our 40 patients on the basis of their educational placement (or on DQ, for those at home and not in any program), 13% were "good," 10% "fair," 30% "poor" and 48% "very poor." To the latter group must be added the four additional children who died.

§5. DIFFERENCES, SIMILARITIES AND THE NATURE OF "AUTISM"

It is clear that the chief difference between our population and those of Kanner and Eisenberg and Rutter is the fact that ours was drawn from patients in a general pediatric service who were referred for developmental evaluation. The other two samples were seen in psychiatric services. None of Kanner and Eisenberg's patients had overt neuromotor abnormalities, but there may have been a few in Rutter's sample; it seems clear that children with cerebral palsy were rarely, if ever, included. Mention is not made of hydrocephalus, trisomy 21, Hurler's disease or any other of the conditions we found. It is unlikely that children with such overt abnormalities are referred to psychiatric facilities, even if their behavior is bizarre, although now there may be a trend toward making such referrals and having the patients accepted.

The second difference is the younger age of our children; three-fourths were less than 2 years old at the time of their initial evaluation. It would seem unreasonable to imply that the diagnosis was incorrect on this basis, since one of the cardinal criteria for infantile psychosis is that it be present from birth or early life. We were careful to point out that we made the diagnosis only in the presence of persistent failure to relate to people as persons. This type of behavior is distinctive and readily perceived when one is sufficiently familiar with the normal social responsiveness of very young children. The relatively high incidence of the disorder in our total population probably is related to the fact that the autistic aspects of behavior tend to disappear with increasing age. As already mentioned, neuromotor abnormalities are more readily demonstrable in early life by developmental assessment, before compensation occurs. The third difference would seem to be related to the severity of the autistic symptoms, or at least to their persistence. Only 10 of our patients had failed to establish social interactions by 6 years of age, the mean age in the other two populations.

In other respects, our sample was remarkably similar to Rutter's. There was a comparable incidence of mental deficiency and of grand mal convulsive seizures. There were patients in both samples with central communication disorders. Many of the other distortions of language behavior, similar in the two groups, were probably more apparent than real and related to the marked mental deficiency. The children were following the normal developmental progressions in language, but were markedly discrepant in terms of their chronologic age. The clinical estimate of outcome showed similar percentages in the good, fair, poor and very poor categories. The IQ is the basic factor in determining this eventual adjustment, and is emphasized by the fact that 60% of Rutter's patients with a "very poor" outcome were untestable at his initial evaluation of them, and 70% had no useful speech at age 5 years. At followup, virtually all our patients with absent speech unassociated with a specific hearing impairment had DQs of less than 35. Those whose age was comparable to the initial age in Rutter's sample were not untestable if the developmental examination was employed for their evaluation.

In spite of the absence of reported formal test scores, we suspect that the Johns Hopkins population was not too different, since almost three-fourths had a "poor" outcome and half of the sample had no speech at 5 years. Since mental deficiency is the most common cause of such marked retardation in language development, failure to speak by 5 would be similar to the prognostic criterion proposed by Brown, the inability to play meaningfully with toys.[10] Both are alternative ways of stating that the outlook is less favorable if mental deficiency also is present.

Since our original contact with these 50 children, we have observed another 75–100 very young children with autistic behavior. Their characteristics are no different from those of our original sample. Scientific parsimony would seem to dictate that "autism" or "infantile psychosis" is not a specific disease entity. It is a description of a *complex of behavior symptoms* which, in our experience, is associated with organic disease of the brain. The etiologies are as varied as are those which produce similar organic brain dysfunctions unaccompanied by these particular symptoms. In the vast majority, but by no means all the cases, there is an association with mental deficiency of varying degrees, and there is a high incidence of language disorders in addition to those related to the mental deficiency itself. There is also a very high incidence of typical and atypical convulsive disorders (Chapter 13), from which the psychotic behavior is distinguishable because of the paroxysmal nature of the former. The autistic symptoms sometimes last only a few months, and the vast majority of the children eventually lose their autistic behavior and establish social interactions; however, they are as mentally defective as before, or more so. The prognosis depends in large measure on the level of intellectual abilities.

The characteristics of autistic behavior are not differentiable on the basis of these other associated factors. No data are available as yet to indicate that involvement of a specific area of the brain is responsbile for the appearance of the symptom complex in some children with cerebral dysfunction and not in others with similar types of dysfunction. That there may be some metabolic derangement is suggested by the high frequency of the bizarre behavior in PKU patients, and the fact that these symptoms sometimes respond rather dramatically to dietary therapy.

We offer the hypothesis that autism represents a global aphasia, in which central nervous system dysfunction is so severe that the complexities of social stimulation cannot be integrated or interpreted by the child, with the result that social interaction only produces further interference with his central nervous system function. Integration improves with maturation, as it does in a variety of the other disorders discussed in this volume. Some credence is lent to the hypothesis that the child is unable to cope with the multiple impacts of social demands by the evolution of compensation reported to us by several parents. The infant responds first to his mirror image, which imposes no demands for behavior on him. (One of the children in the sample appeared to be blind until she was placed in front of the mirror, when she patted her image repeatedly and it was clear that she could see.) There follows a response to other infants, other children and finally parents and other adults. The terms "autism" and "infantile psychosis" should not be applied indiscriminately to all types of deviant and stereotyped behavior in the absence of the characteristic feature of persistent failure to regard people as persons. These terms have heuristic value in defining a population which might form a nucleus for research, particularly in relation to treatment methods.

§6. MANAGEMENT

The first responsibility of the physician is diagnosis, not only of the symptoms and the intellectual level but also of the associated disorders responsive to specific therapy. Treatment of convulsions is most important. While anticonvulsants do not modify the psychotic behavior, unless the seizures are masquerading as psychosis, they may be vital in preventing subsequent deterioration.

The available evidence indicates that outcome is not influenced by the amount and kind of psychotherapy, and psychotherapy as such does not seem warranted. This does not mean that general methods of behavior management and behavior modification programs should not be undertaken, in order to avoid compounding the situation by unwise procedures (Chapter 18).

The nature of the difficulties should be explained fully to the parents, with particular emphasis on the fact that they have not caused the abnormal behavior. They should not attempt to force social interactions on the child, but must be alert to any spontaneous overtures and make prompt responses when they occur. The parents will need continuing support, and various methods of providing this also are discussed in Chapter 18.

The most important long-range planning should be provision of educational experiences appropriate to the abilities of the child. These probably should start at a time when the child is mature enough to participate in a nursery school program. It should be a "normal" nursery in the sense that the other children have the same general level of abilities, but do not necessarily manifest psychotic behavior.

§7. ILLUSTRATIVE CASES

It is fitting to end this chapter with the two brief case reports and comments which Gesell and Amatruda presented in their original discussion of "pseudosymptomatic retardation."

Case 4 was physically a beautiful, appealing child. She sat alone at 7 months. At 10 months she had convulsions followed by possible encephalitis. Examination at *33 months* revealed a developmental level of 18 months. The parents felt that some emotional block was at the basis of the retardation and absence of speech, and had provided a special speech tutor who insisted that the child was "bright but highly negative."

The apparent obliviousness to persons fostered continuance of the theory that emotional inhibitions were operating. Excessive training zeal set up tensions and "nervous habits" in the child. These abated when more attention was paid to physical well-being instead of speech instruction. Reexamination at *4 years* showed an extremely slight advance in all five fields of behavior.

The parents were advised as follows: "If you can bring yourself to shaping your child's world to her needs and can do it cheerfully for her sake, your own distress will be reduced. If there is a remote chance that a change will occur, you will be increasing that chance more by these means than by constantly sustained efforts to teach her beyond her capacity to learn." Not until 2 years later was the diagnosis of mental deficiency accepted.

Case 5, a small, wiry, active child, was examined at the age of *42 months.* Like Case 4, he was completely oblivious of persons, but displayed flashes of attention, such as brief interest in a picture book. The mother firmly believed that "except for inattention to words, he is like a normal child."

The parents concentrated their solicitude on the heedlessness to the spoken word and the failure to talk. They wondered whether it was due to deafness, aphasia, endocrine disorder or possibly retardation. Their preoccupation with language factors threw the whole behavior picture out of focus for them, and they underestimated the seriousness of associated behavior, which included rather aimless running and vocalizing, snatches of hand regard, tongue sucking, clicking, rubbing of the abdomen, blowing, etc. This boy did not walk until the age of 27 months, but this was attributed (by the parents) to feeding difficulties. There was a history of vomiting, forced feeding and slow weight gains. It was suggested (again by the parents) that the forcible feeding methods had set up an emotional blocking.

A series of previous physical examinations had resulted in conflicting diagnoses of deafness and endocrine disorder. We ruled out both of these complications and then considered a third possibility, namely "a profound emotional blocking." This too was ruled out on the grounds that the observed emotional behavior was consistent only with a pervasive retardation affecting all fields of behavior. Emotional factors could scarcely account for the fact that this child did not walk until the age of 27 months. A diagnosis of mental deficiency was indicated.

The prognosis? He had learned to walk, he will in time learn to talk a little. Any progress he makes will be exceedingly slow, a matter of years. There will be no revolutionary emotional release or reorientation at adolescence. School, in the ordinary sense, will be quite beyond him. The parents finally accepted the diagnosis of mental deficiency, but only after a vast amount of miscarried effort and hope, much of which might have been spared.

The cases of *pseudosymptomatic retardation* have a way of making undue trouble for all concerned. Our case histories show that the parents of these children do a great deal of "shopping around." They try one expedient or one program after another. Meanwhile the child is growing older, and in retrospect it proves that the retardation was fundamental and inherent in the damaged nervous system. It is organic and not due to "emotional blocking" or to "environmental impediment," but is based upon a true mental deficiency. The intellectual impairment may be of any degree.

Part III

The Protection of Early Child Development

17

Developmental Screening*

This volume has presented a detailed discussion of normal and abnormal neuro-psychologic development to provide a background on which the clinician can build, in order to become skilled in differential developmental diagnosis. Although every child needs and deserves developmental supervision, the specialist's skills should be conserved for accurate diagnosis of difficult problems. The number of children in whom abnormal development is suspected is enormous, the need for service great and the supply of specialists limited.

Thus, there is a need for developmental screening to be carried out at a variety of levels—from parents through child care workers, public health nurses, general practitioners, pediatricians and other specialists who deal with children. A screening interview and examination indicate if the infant is demonstrating behavior appropriate for his age. If he is not, the particular areas involved and the extent of the deviation can be determined, and a decision made about the need for referral for more detailed evaluation, and the level of expertise required.

Screening procedures unfortunately still are being made by selection of several behavioral items at widely spaced ages, or single items at monthly intervals. The rationale seems to be that the physician is too busy to devote any significant amount of time to the details of development. The reader who has progressed through this volume will realize that this abbreviated an approach grossly oversimplifies the complex nature of development. It is somewhat analagous to saying "Give me a single test for metabolism, I don't have time for details." Two such abridged procedures were compared with complete examinations and proved to be so inadequate that their use should be abandoned entirely. A more recent widely used screening procedure which avoids these particular pitfalls, the Denver Developmental Screening Test, suffers from other defects, notably combining adaptive and fine motor behavior, the omission of several key concepts in adaptive behavior, and too wide as well as inappropriate age ranges for many items.[23] Moreover, it has not

* The Developmental Screening Inventory, as well as much of the other material in this chapter, first appeared as a supplement to Pediatrics,[48] and is reprinted with permission of the publisher.

been validated by adequate comparison with an infant examination which predicts later development.

Practical experience in the evaluation of development has been a minor part of pediatric training, and attention usually has been directed only towards a few landmarks of motor behavior. The use of an effective screening inventory would do much to raise the present level of developmental evaluation. Parents can provide the initial level of screening by answering a questionnaire appropriate to the child's age and providing supplementary information. In the two common American patterns of medical care, there then can be a second level of screening by general practitioners or by well-baby clinic nurses and other child care workers. In a teaching center, the medical student could, with use of an adequate inventory, acquire an acquaintance with development in the day-to-day care of his patients. The pediatric resident during his training can establish a firm knowledge of normal growth and development as the basis for detecting deviations.

For the practicing pediatrician, an adequate screening inventory can provide the shortcut he desires, making it possible for him to apply systematically the knowledge that he already has. This can be accomplished by surveying a child's behavior at frequent regular intervals. With the proper questions and observation of behavior, a few minutes at each visit will suffice to determine if the child is behaving at his age level. Adequate screening also will conserve the time of the small number of expert developmental consultants as well as permit such a consultant to function more effectively, because he is provided with a satisfactory history of the pregnancy, newborn period and course of development. The family physician will be in a better position to provide continuing support and counseling for parents during long-term care of a child with a significant deviation. Finally, an adequate screening inventory can be used in large-scale research; it would prove most useful in the evaluation of present programs of maternal and infant care.

§1. CRITERIA FOR AN ADEQUATE SCREENING IVENTORY

In evaluating development, one is concerned with both present and future function. The complete examination from which a screening inventory is derived must be an adequate predictor of later abnormality. First, then, it must have validity. This predictive value can be determined only by longitudinal studies, and such data must derive from followup correlations between the complete infant examinations and those done at later ages.

Second, since a screening inventory does not include all the behavior patterns evaluated by a complete examination, the results achieved by it must correlate with those of the full developmental evaluation. Ideally, no child called abnormal by the complete examination should be called normal on screening (underscreening), and there should be a minimum of normal infants called abnormal (overscreening). To determine if screening gives the same results as a complete developmental evaluation, one uses the history and observations obtained at an examination to complete the screening inventory. If the diagnostic classification from the inventory does not agree with that of the examination, the inventory is not likely to give satisfactory results under any other circumstances.

Third, for prediction as well as for present management, intellectual defect and motor disability must be distinguished by the inventory. Behavior must be evaluated separately in the different areas of functioning, since only adaptive and language behavior are related closely to later intellectual function. A sufficient number of items must be selected from the complete examination to permit evaluation of important developmental concepts in each area of behavior. The materials needed to accomplish the evaluation should be available readily.

Fourth, the inventory should yield reproducible results when used by different individuals observing the same examination; that is, it must be reliable. In order for this to be achieved, the behavior items in the inventory must be stated as precisely as possible, so that examiner, observers and the person giving the history know what is meant in each instance.

Fifth, the age intervals must be small enough so that correct diagnostic classification can be achieved even if the chronologic age of the infant lies between two inventory age levels. In the first year of life, changes occur so rapidly that items must by provided at 4-week intervals. Because they represent stages at which major integrations occur, the key ages of the developmental schedules provide the most information, but the infants may not always oblige by presenting themselves at these key ages.

Finally, supplementary information (Section 6) must be obtained from the parents about convulsive seizures, hearing, vision, the loss of previously acquired behavior and any concerns they have about the infant's progress. Developmental quotients derived from the screening inventory are the starting points for evaluation, but the supplementary information may indicate that more detailed examination is necessary, in spite of quantitative adequacy.

§2. CORRELATION BETWEEN THE
DEVELOPMENTAL SCREENING INVENTORY AND THE EXAMINATION

The Developmental Screening Inventory (DSI) in Section 4 consists of selected items from the developmental schedules, presented in full in Chapter 3, in each of the five fields of adaptive, gross motor, fine motor, language and personal–social behavior. The foldout section covers 4-week intervals from the ages of 4 to 56 weeks, and 15 and 18 months. It is followed in Section 5 by a supplementary inventory encompassing 21, 24, 30 and 36 months. Data indicating the predictive validity of developmental assessment already has been presented in Chapter 5. Present concern is with whether the screening inventory based on it will identify abnormal infants.

Two decades ago, we evaluated a questionnaire for infants 40 weeks of age in a sample of 901 infants. A question on standing was omitted, no supplementary information was obtained, and the scoring system for the responses to the questions made the assumption the infant was exactly 40 weeks old; in spite of these facts, the results were sufficiently encouraging to warrant further development of the procedure. When the results of a complete examination done by a physician were used to answer the questionnaire, all infants with intellectual deficiency or severe neuromotor problems were detected. Discrepancies occurred for infants whose chief motor problems were confined mostly to the lower extremities.

The present Developmental Screening Inventory covers an age range from 4 weeks to 18 months. The two youngest ages are included primarily to assist in the detection of *abnormal* infants 12 and 16 weeks old. When this DSI was evaluated initially, no supplementary information was included. The results of a full examination of 58 patients between the ages of 16 weeks and 18 months were used to answer the DSI. A secretary transcribed the information on the developmental schedules to the comparable items on the DSI, and a staff physician assigned maturity levels without knowing the age of the child. Age was supplied, developmental quotients calculated for each area of behavior and diagnoses made. The child was assigned to one of four diagnostic categories: (1) Abnormal neuromotor status and abnormal intellectual potential; (2) Abnormal neuromotor status with normal intellectual potential; (3) Questionable neuromotor status with normal intellectual potential; (4) Normal in both areas.

All but 1 of the 20 infants with abnormal neuromotor status, with or without intellectual defect, was identified as abnormal by this procedure. The one 36-week-old who was underscreened was having innumerable seizures and was grossly ataxic from Dilantin intoxication. In spite of this, it was possible to give him maturity levels close to his age in his seizure-free intervals, and his gross deviation in motor behavior was not apparent in the bare recording of his accomplishments. One 18-week infant called normal on the complete examination but assigned an abnormal neuromotor status on screening had a severe cardiac disorder and marked malnutrition. At the time of the examination it was felt that the extremely poor head control manifested was a result of the other diseases, and not due to involvement of the central nervous system, particularly since fine motor behavior was normal. These results indicate the importance of obtaining supplementary information.

These 58 patients had been screened by junior medical students, to determine what results would be obtained when the DSI was employed by individuals who had no experience in pediatrics and no training in the use of the instrument. The students merely were given the DSI and a screening kit, told to read the instructions and then proceed with their examination. All 20 infants called significantly abnormal by the full staff examination also were identified as abnormal by student use of the DSI. However, the students did assign more abnormal diagnostic classifications than did the staff to the remainder of 58 infants. Closer scrutiny indicated that this amount of overscreening was not necessarily inherent in the DSI, but was related more to the students' lack of experience, and sometimes lack of interest. It resulted to a considerable extent from failure to correct age for prematurity, calling an infant seriously abnormal because a DQ was only 90, or recording items as negative because more advanced behavior was present, and then misinterpreting these negatives; occasionally observations were sprinkled haphazardly over the forms without any attempt to record or interpret systematically.

Subsequently we tested the DSI to determine how effective it was if parents answered the questions. A questionnaire derived from the DSI was mailed to the parents of all 603 infants born in three small communities in a year's time. Seventy-five percent returned the questionnaire, and there was staff contact or information from the family physician for an additional 10%. Twenty-eight weeks was the age selected for this investigation, in order to identify deviants and plan for their care early; this age also is one at which the time required for the screening process is relatively short. The questionnaire covered the ages 20–32 weeks and included the supplementary information questions (Appendix A-6). Half the infants for whom parental responses indicated behavior at age then were screened by a nurse who had received some training in the use of the DSI, as were all infants for whom the parents' answers indicated there might be developmental delay or seizures. When the questionnaire or the subsequent screening suggested abnormality, the infants were brought for a full developmental evaluation by a physician, who also examined a sample of the apparently normal infants, without knowing the category to which the child belonged.

Eighty-seven infants were seen by the physician, and the results of the full developmental evaluation used to answer the DSI. Only 5 infants were diagnosed by the examination as Abnormal and had mental deficiency or a significant neuromotor handicap. Four of these were classified as Abnormal by the DSI; the fifth was identified because of a history of possible seizures, but classified by the DSI as having only minor neuromotor abnormalities. Seventeen of the 87 had a Questionable diagnosis, with minor abnormalities, with or without seizures. Two of the 17 infants were not identified by applying the observations of the full examination to the DSI because their disability was unilateral and they could perform at age; however, one of these infants did have a seizure history.

Evaluation of the parents' responses to the DSI questionnaire produced similar results. All 5 with major deviations also were classified as Abnormal by the parents. However, 1 of the 17 mothers whose infants had minor neuromotor abnormalities reported erroneously that the infant could do everything at and above his age; she was the only mother who did this. By contrast, 8–10% of mothers reported less mature behavior than the infants demonstrated in the examination; i.e., they overscreened.

A scoring system was developed for all possible combinations of responses to the items on the DSI questionnaire, in each area of behavior. The classification of an infant by the system as Normal, Questionable, or Abnormal took into account the infant's age and discrepancies within and between areas of behavior. With the exceptions already noted above, application of the scoring system to the DSI questionnaire responses identified the Abnormal and Questionable infants. This was true whether parental responses or the results of the physician's evaluation were used to answer the DSI questionnaire.

One difficulty which emerged in these tests of the DSI probably would apply at all ages. Screening will not necessarily provide knowledge about some neuromotor abnormalities or qualitative aspects of the child's behavior, both of which are major factors affecting diagnosis. Infants with unilateral minor neuromotor disabilities who are able to perform at age are not identified. A second problem may be the comparatively young age selected in the last study. Not all 28-week infants can be expected to bear their full weight when supported; for a few who cannot, some deficit may exist. Careful attention must be paid to all their behavior, and followup conducted in 4–8 weeks to be certain all these infants are bearing weight and do not have persistent defects.

The DSI also has been used, but not on a systematic basis, with parents who bring their infants for an evaluation. If parents are asked to report current behavior, the classifications derived from the DSI questionnaire completed at home have good correspondence with behavior observed in the examination, and abnormalities are identified. However, when parents are asked to provide a review of development from 16 weeks up to 18 or 24 months or longer, inconsistencies in the developmental progressions sometimes appear. In general, parents don't supply information in the review which would lead to calling an abnormal infant normal; rather, their answers indicate the need for more definitive examination to define the nature of the abnormality. When the parents provide this review of past development, the information also permits an estimate of the current levels of function.

The supplementary DSI for the ages 21–36 months has been evaluated opportunistically rather than systematically. It tends to underestimate the adaptive ability of children who have difficulty with drawing. This problem is counterbalanced if entirely normal language behavior is present. In contrast, delay in speech is not indicative of mental deficiency if adaptive behavior is normal and the child hears and understands what is said to him at his age level.

Careful and interested application of the DSI, with the supplementary information questions, leads to detection of all infants with significant abnormalities and discrimination between neuromotor and intellectual handicaps; it also identifies almost all with minor neuromotor impairment. Parents clearly have an interest in the developmental status of their children. The practicing physician should be expected to obtain better results than a medical student, nurse or other child care worker. Unquestionably, he is more concerned, since his patients, his reputation and even his economic interests are affected. In addition, he must take further definitive steps if he finds that DSI screening reveals abnormality.

§3. PRACTICAL USE OF THE DSI

The student who already has had practical experience in developmental evaluation, either under supervision or by assiduous self-instruction, can proceed without difficulty in the use of the DSI. He merely will survey fewer behavior patterns than he does in a complete examination.

For less highly trained examiners, instructions are provided on each individual Developmental Screening Inventory as well as in the following section of this chapter. They should be read in their *entirety* before attempting to use the DSI. Because of space limitations, the items on the DSI appear in very abbreviated form. Those items which we believe are too specific for the parents to observe are blocked out in the history column. In Appendix A-6 the remaining items are expanded in the form of questions, which are more precise; these expanded forms should be used in interviewing parents to obtain the best information. Ways in which these questions can be utilized by sending them to the parents prior to the examination of the child are discussed in Chapter 4 and Appendix A-6. Additional information is included in the instructions accompanying the DSI, under the heading of "Specific Behavior Patterns." A complete description of all of the items on each developmental schedule from which the DSI is derived is found in the glossary sections of Chapter 3; reference to these glossaries will be of inestimable help to those who do not read the entire volume.

The Screening Inventory permits classification of children into three groups in each area of behavior: N (Normal or Advanced); Q (Questionable); A (Abnormal). The supplementary information in Section 6 must be obtained even for those infants clearly acting at or above their chronologic ages, to be certain they do not have other problems. However, the DSI and the supplementary questions alone will not yield a definitive diagnosis for infants in the Questionable or Abnormal categories. The procedure provides the basis for deciding if serial observations are indicated or if immediate referral for a complete diagnostic evaluation is necessary. For many infants, screening will indicate that intellectual potential is normal and only minor neuromotor abnormalities are present (the Questionable category). These infants will need to be followed, but compensation is to be expected for most of them and there is no immediate need for treatment or referral for diagnostic consultation.

§4. THE DEVELOPMENTAL SCREENING INVENTORY (DSI) FROM 4 WEEKS TO 18 MONTHS*

Development proceeds in an orderly predictable manner, with the same variability in behavior for normal infants found in all biologic measurements. By asking some

*Copies of the DSI may be obtained from the editors. In quantity, they may be purchased at cost.

This inventory is a screening procedure, and a definitive diagnosis should not be made on the basis of a single screening by itself. Some infants identified as deviant by it will require prompt referral to a consultant or a center for a complete diagnostic evaluation. Other deviant infants will require serial observations to determine if such referral is necessary.

questions of parents, observing the infant's behavior, and recording this information systematically, an estimate of the level of function in various areas of behavior can be made which correlates very highly with the maturity age assigned on the basis of a complete Developmental and Neurologic Evaluation, from which the items are adapted.

This screening inventory will be of value for serial observations in well-baby supervision, as well as for diagnostic problems referred for evaluation. READ THE ENTIRE INVENTORY BEFORE ATTEMPTING TO USE IT.

DO NOT BE ALARMED BY THE LARGE NUMBER OF QUESTIONS. They cover the age range from 1 to 18 months and any *one* infant can *usually* be evaluated by 2 or 3 consecutive age levels at most. We have tried to phrase the items as clearly as possible; specific explanations for some are listed in the instructions. It will help to understand them if you *look at the adjacent age levels,* e.g., lift vs. hold at 8 and 12 weeks in Gross Motor Behavior; offer the parents both alternatives. ASK THE QUESTIONS AS THEY ARE STATED. (Appendix A-6).

START by asking questions appropriate to the chronologic age of the child. If the answers are negative, drop to a lower age level; then work back up. It is best to cover ONE AREA OF BEHAVIOR AT A TIME rather than one age level at a time. Remember that the infant may be slow in one area and normal in other areas. Keep asking questions above the child's chronologic age until no more positive answers are obtained. When you start your interview, TELL THE PARENTS SOME QUESTIONS ASKED WILL BE ABOVE THE CHILD'S LEVEL OF ABILITIES.

Record the parents' answers [H = History Col.] and your observations [O = Observed Col.] on each visit, to the left of each item. For behavior which depends on your observations only, the history column is blocked out. Record responses + [Present], − [Absent], or × [Unknown]. If an infant is seen every 4 weeks, there may be some overlap in behavior; confusion can be avoided by recording in different colors. Failure to progress normally will be obvious if significant overlap between visits persists.

Blocks are provided at the upper left and lower right of the form for recording the age level at which the child is functioning and the diagnoses. In each of the five areas of behavior, assign maturity levels in weeks, or months, based on your clinical judgment of the age levels your recorded history and observations describe best. You can interpolate between the adjacent age columns, e.g., 35 weeks, since a 32-week infant adds 36-week behavior gradually over the next 4 weeks. DO NOT FORGET TO TAKE THE PARENTS' HISTORY INTO ACCOUNT. This is particularly true in language behavior, which may not be exhibited during the examination. We have found parents' reports to be very accurate when clearcut specific questions are asked.

Assign a diagnostic category in each area on the basis of your age levels. With just these items, expect to be able to divide the infants into three diagnostic categories: [A] definitely abnormal, [Q] borderline or questionably abnormal, and [N] normal or advanced. Do not expect to make a precise diagnosis. REMEMBER THAT THERE IS NORMAL VARIATION AROUND THE AVERAGE OF 100

AND THAT THE AGE PLACEMENT OF AN ITEM IS THAT AT WHICH ROUGHLY 50% OF INFANTS ACHIEVE SUCCESS. If an infant has a history of normal language behavior, at least at 36 weeks and beyond, it is dangerous to make a diagnosis of mental deficiency, even though adaptive behavior is retarded. Be suspicious of the presence of abortive grand mal convulsive seizures.

Age in weeks must be *counted on the calendar;* there are 13 4-week periods per year. Don't forget to SUBTRACT THE WEEKS OF PREMATURITY from the chronologic age.

Conduct of the Developmental Screening Examination

TEST OBJECTS. In the actual examination the test objects are very specific, but they can be approximated and should consist of the following, which can be purchased in most supermarkets or from sources listed in Appendix A-1.

a round embroidery hoop 4 inches in diameter with a string about 8 inches long no more than 1/16-inch diameter

an aluminum cup 3.5 inches in diameter

a plastic bottle in use in most pharmacies, 2 inches high and 1 inch in diameter

round cinnamon candies used in cake decoration [for the 8-mm pellet, or "crumb"]

a child's picture book

a large crayon and paper

ten 1-inch wooden cubes [those readily available are usually 1-1/4 inches]; the surface should not have embossed designs

"small toy" usually refers to the 1-inch cube, but the plastic bottle also qualifies and is more appropriate at 40—48 weeks in connection with the crumb [pellet]

Even these objects are not essential. On the hospital wards, tongue blades, a stethoscope, or a small flashlight can be used early; the small paper medicine cups or the pop-apart plastic beads or other toys that the infants frequently have can substitute for the cubes. For the pellet [crumb] a piece of paper rolled into a *small* ball is fine. The tape used to tie toys across the cribs is rather large but it can substitute for string. At the older ages some child on the ward usually has a book, and a medicine glass can be used for a bottle. A large notebook or a file folder can serve as a table if no tray is handy. The mother, or a nurse or attendant, can support the young infant in a sitting position.

GENERAL COMMENTS ON CONDUCTING THE EXAMINATION. Note that at the age of 20 weeks and below the Adaptive Behavior items are observed when the baby is *lying on his back* in *supine.* At 24 weeks and over he is expected to do similar things when in a *sitting* position; initially he will need to be held supported or tied into a high chair so that his hands will be free to manipulate the test objects.

ALL INFANTS SHOULD BE EVALUATED IN SUPINE, SITTING, PRONE, AND STANDING, except that above 32 weeks a normal infant need not be placed on his back. Start in the supine position routinely up to 20 weeks of age and up to 32 weeks if the infant happens to be in that position; after 32 weeks start the examination in sitting. If a younger infant happens to be in his mother's lap, he may not want to lie down and the examination can be started in sitting.

The infant must cooperate if information useful in assessing behavior is to be obtained, and his degree of cooperation is often directly related to the manner of the examiner. If you talk to the infant before and during the examination in a friendly manner and do not push him to perform, good rapport usually is established. The examination often is more successful if it does not follow immediately some painful or upsetting procedure you have performed, but even in such situations presenting the toys usually will secure his cooperation. OFFER SOME TOY OTHER THAN A TEST OBJECT BEFORE HANDLING THE INFANT. WHEN HE TAKES IT HE USUALLY HAS ACCEPTED YOU AND WILL LET YOU PICK HIM UP.

PRESENTATION OF TEST OBJECTS.

Supine. Start with the object in the midline at the infant's feet and bring it up toward eye level. Hold it about 12–15 inches from the infant for visual responses and within reach if he is mature enough to grasp.

Sitting. Tap the object at the edge of the table in the midline with clear up and down motions of the arm. When the infant has fixated on the object, slide it *within reach* with a smooth horizonal motion; do not jerk your arm up and down on the way in. When presenting ring and string, put string down in reach, tap *ring* up and down, and put ring on table, but out of reach.

MOST BEHAVIOR IN INFANCY IS SEEN DURING SPONTANEOUS PLAY AND NOT ELICITED ON COMMAND. Present one cube, then the second, add the third, add the rest of the cubes and then the cup, and observe what he does. ALWAYS GIVE THE INFANT AN OPPORTUNITY FOR SHOWING THE MOST ADVANCED BEHAVIOR FIRST: e.g., spontaneous behavior when given an object; verbal request and/or pointing before demonstration, as in putting cube into cup; reach and grasp before visual following or placing in the hand, at younger ages.

REMOVE THE OBJECT(S) at the end of each situation or group of related situations before presenting the next one, but HAVE THE NEXT OBJECT READY before trying to take away what the infant is holding. IF HE OBJECTS STRONGLY, PRESENT THE NEXT ONE BEFORE TRYING FURTHER. This procedure usually works. DO NOT USE FORCE.

Talk to the infant, or better, describe what he is doing while you are doing the examination.

Specific Behavior Patterns

POSTURES IN SUPINE

4 weeks: *asymmetric* or tonic-neck-reflex (t-n-r)—the fencing stance with head

[4] WEEKS OR LESS — ASYMMETRIC [TO]NIC-NECK-REFLEX

4 Weeks or less	8 Weeks	12 Weeks	R
H O	**H O**	**H O**	
regard toy only when it is brought in front of eyes	Delayed regard of toy you hold in midline over chest	Prompt regard of toy dangled in midline at chest level	
[c]an follow dangled toy only to midline, not past it	Follow dangled toy past midline	Follow toy, or Ex's hand, in 180° continuous arc, side to side	
[d]rop toy put in hand at once	*Retain* briefly toy put in hand	Glance at toy when put into hand	
[h]ead sag forward if held *sitting*	Head bob erect if held *sitting*	Head bob forward if held *sitting*	
[a]symmetric tonic-neck-reflex postures predominate	No head droop if suspended prone	Symmetric posture head, body seen	
[c]lear nose from bed in prone	*Lift* head to 45° in prone [on abdomen] recurrently	*Hold* head up 45° when in prone [on abdomen] sustainedly	
[b]oth hands held tightly fisted		Hold hands open or close loosely	
[h]and clench as toy touched to it	. . . .	Hold toy put in hand with active grasp	
[i]mpassive face	Alert expression	Coo and chuckle	
[v]ague indirect regard	Direct definite regard	"Talk" back just if you nod head and talk to him	
[m]ake small throaty noises	Make single vowels—"ah, eh, uh"		
[r]egard examiner's face and decrease activity	Smile back just if you nod head and talk to him	Look at examiner predominantly	
[i]ndefinite stare at surroundings	Eyes follow moving person around	Hold up and look at own hand	
		Pull at clothes	

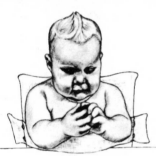

28 Weeks
Transfer Objects

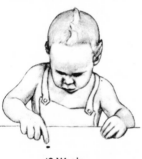

40 Weeks
Index Finger Poking

40 WEEKS — [P]ICKS UP CRUMBS & THREADS [PLAY]S NURSERY TRICKS

40 Weeks	44 Weeks	48 Weeks	C
H O	**H O**	**H O**	
[p]lay inside cup with toy you put there, touch and manipulate it	Take toy out of box or cup	Play with one toy after another of a group in same way, in sequence [e.g., drop to floor, move to another spot on table]	
[h]old small toy and try to or pick up crumb at same time	Put small toy inside cup or box if shown, but not let go of it	Exploit crumb only, ignore bottle	
[p]oke with index finger at things	Poke at crumb inside bottle		
[s]it erect and steady indefinitely	Stand at furniture without leaning against it, lift one foot up and down	Hold furniture and walk around it	
[g]o, not fall, forward to prone		Walk if both hands held at shoulder height for balance	
[c]rawl [creep] on hands and knees			
[p]ull self to standing			
[p]ut small toy down, take hands off	. . . .	Pluck crumb easily with thumb and index finger, not resting arm or hand on tabletop	
[p]luck crumb up promptly, usually with thumb and index finger			
[s]ay and mean "ma-ma" and "da-da"	. . . .	. . . .	
[h]ave one other "word"			
[p]lay nursery trick just if asked			
[p]lay nursery trick only if you do it first; doesn't understand meaning of words [does above]	Hold out toy to you, but not let go of it	Take toys off table to another surface [e.g., floor] deliberately in play	
	Reach for image of toy in mirror		

	H	O	**20 Weeks**	H	O	**24 Weeks**	H
Wave arms, move body at sight of toy; dangled if on back, or put on table if held in sitting			Bring both hands up towards toy, on back or if supported *sitting*			Reach and pick up or take toy with both hands	
Regard [look at] toy in hand			Grasp toy only if held near hand [approximately one inch away]			Reach for toy dropped within reach	
Take toy to mouth when on back			Look after toy dropped in sight			Put toy in mouth when held supported in *sitting*	
Head steady, set forward, *sitting*			Head erect, steady, held *sitting*			Grasp foot when lying on back [in supine]	
Symmetric postures predominate			No head lag when held by hands and pulled to *sitting*			Roll to abdomen, get both arms out from under chest	
Hold head 90°, look directly ahead in prone [on abdomen]			Push whole chest off bed, prone				
Scratch, finger, clutch at clothes			Scratch on tabletop, or on bed in prone [toy in sight not essential]			Pick up small toy and hold in center of palm with all fingers	
Bring hands together in midline and play with own fingers							
Laugh out loud			Squeal like a little pig, voice up high			Grunt and growl [deep sounds]	
Excite, breathe heavily, in play						Initiate "conversation" with toys or people	
Initiate smile just when people come up and stand beside him			Smile at self if *close* to mirror			Know strangers from family	
Recognize bottle just on sight			Put both hands on bottle when feeding			Smile and talk to self if put *close* to mirror	

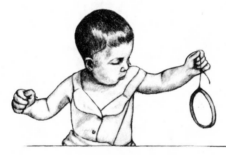

52 Weeks
Dangles Toy by Its String

56 Weeks

15 Months
Builds Tower of Two

15 Months

	H	O	**56 Weeks**	H	O	**15 Months**	H
Try piling one small toy on 2nd just presses it or it falls off			Put toy into cup or box just if you point and ask him to			Pile 1 small toy on 2nd [tower 2]	
Put toy in cup or box if you show him first each time			Imitate scribble with crayon after you do it			Get 5-6 [of 10] small toys in cup or box; doesn't put all 10 in	
Dangle toy by string, deliberate						Stroke crayon *in air* imitatively after you draw vertical stroke	
Walk with only one hand held			Forget to hold on, stand alone momentarily			No longer creep or crawl	
			If standing up, take few steps alone, fall headlong			Get up in middle of floor and walk alone	
						Collapse and catch self when falls	
. . . .			Pick up two small toys in one hand at same time, deliberately			Drop crumb into bottle just if you point and ask him to	
						Help turn pages of book	
Say 2 "words" plus ma-ma and da-da			Say 3 or 4 "words"			4-6 words, including first names	
Let go of toy into your hand if you hold hand out for it			When asked to, look at object: ball, shoe, light, T-V set, etc.			"Talk" foreign language—jargon	
						Pat at pictures in book	
Help in dressing-push arm thru sleeve if you get it started			Use slight casting motion and play ball *with* you, throwing it towards you			Indicate wants by pointing or vocalizing [grunt, "uh-uh-uh"]	
Offer toy to own mirror image						When fed leaves dish on tray	

TIONS

28 WEEKS
SUPPORTED SITTING
NE HAND APPROACH
& GRASP

32 Weeks

	H	O	
Reach and pick up or take toy with one hand only			Pick up one small toy and then second one
Transfer toy easily, hand to hand			Hold these two prolongedly
Bang toy up and down when *sitting* supported	■		Secure toy by string if string contacted by hand
Lift head from bed if on back			Sit 1 minute erect unsteady on *hard surface*
Sit if put on *hard surface* leaning on hands			Stand, hands held shoulder height
Stand if chest held under arms			Pivot in circle, prone, using arms
Pick up small toy, hold to radial side palm with 2nd and 3rd finger			Try to pick up crumb by raking with thumb, 2nd and 3rd fingers, usually little arm movement
Put whole hand on crumb, rake it			
Say "Mum-mum-mum" especially crying			Make single consonant sounds, "da, ba, ga, ka"
Make same vowel sound in series: "ah-ah-ah, uh-uh-uh, oh-oh-oh"			
Feet to mouth when lying on back			Bite and chew toys, not just lick
Reach out and pat self if put *close* to mirror			Persist in reaching for toys out of reach

H = HISTORY

O = OBSERVATION

DIAGNOSTIC CATEGORIES:

N = Normal or Advanced

Q = Questionable

A = Abnormal

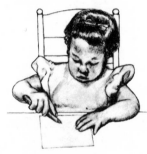

18 Months
Scribbles Spontaneously .

18 MONTHS
OOKS SELECTIVELY AT
D IDENTIFIES PICTURES

								DATE
								AGE
Dump crumb out of bottle—may show								**MATURITY LEVEL**
Scribble when you hand him crayon, i.e., spontaneously								
Imitate stroke *on paper* after you draw vertical stroke								**DIAGNOSIS**
Run stiff-legged								**MATURITY LEVEL**
Rarely fall when walking								
Climb into adult chair								**DIAGNOSIS**
Walk upstairs if you hold one hand								
Turn pages of book 2-3 at once								**MATURITY LEVEL**
Stack up 3 small toys [tower 3]								**DIAGNOSIS**
Point to picture, if ask: dog, baby								**MATURITY LEVEL**
Look back and forth as you point from 1 picture to other in book								**DIAGNOSIS**
Walk or crawl, pulling string toy								**MATURITY LEVEL**
Hug and love doll, stuffed animal								**DIAGNOSIS**
Use spoon to feed, spill good bit								

READ INSTRUCTIONS

DATE								AREA OF BEHAVIOR		
AGE									H	
MATURITY LEVEL								ADAPTIVE		
DIAGNOSIS										
MATURITY LEVEL								GROSS MOTOR		
DIAGNOSIS										
MATURITY LEVEL								FINE MOTOR		
DIAGNOSIS										
MATURITY LEVEL								LANGUAGE		
DIAGNOSIS										
MATURITY LEVEL								PERSONAL-SOCIAL		
DIAGNOSIS										

This inventory is a screening procedure, and a definitive diagnosis should not be made on the basis of a single screening by itself. Some infants identified as deviant by it will require prompt referral to a consultant or a center for a complete diagnostic evaluation. Other deviant infants will require serial observations to determine if such referral is necessary.

REFERENCE TEXT:

H. Knobloch and B. Pasamanick: Gesell and Amatruda's Developmental Diagnosis. Hagerstown, Md., Harper and Row, 1974. Chapters 3, 4, 17 and Appendices A4 and A7.

Instructional Films available from the Department of Photography and Cinema, The Ohio State University, Columbus, Ohio 43210.

1. Developmental Evaluation in Infancy.
2. The Gesell Developmental & Neurologic Examination at 16, 28, 40 and 52 Weeks.
3. Normal and Abnormal Neurologic Function in Infancy.

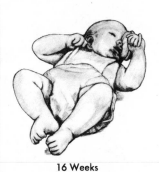

16 Weeks
Toy to Mouth In Supine

36 Weeks

Last Name

First Name

Case #:

Birth Date:

Birth Weight:

E.D.C.:

Days Prematurity Assigned:

AREA	H	O		H	
ADAPTIVE			Drop one of two toys picked up to take third one offered		
			Hit toy in hand at toy on table		
			Hold toy in one hand and play with attached string with other		
GROSS MOTOR			Sit 10 plus minutes steady on *hard surface*		
			Stand at furniture and not lean against it if put there		
FINE MOTOR			Pick up small toy in ends of fingers		
			Pick up crumb, thumb and index finger		
LANGUAGE			Say da-da, ba-ba, without meaning		
			Imitate cough, tongue click, etc.		
			Know own name		
PERSONAL-SOCIAL			Hold own bottle, pick up if dropped and finish it		
			Feed self cracker, do good job		

READ INSTRUCTIO

§ 5. DEVELOPMENTAL SCREENING INVENTORY SUPPLEMENT FOR AGES 21-36 MONTHS

K E Y   A G E S

INSTRUCTIONS

TOWER
F.Mot.: # built without Ex.
holding to help
Adapt.: Concept: Ex. holds to stop
from falling if awkward manually

TRAIN
▢▢▢▢ --Demonstrate out of
reach: say--one car, another,
push & say "choo-choo"
Imitates = pushes cube, or moves
hand & says "choo-choo"

COMBINE
2 different ideas--"What's
that" is one

DIRECTIONS
Order--put on table, on chair,
give to mother, to me

PRONOUN
Need not be in sentence; need
not be all 3 pronouns

TEST OBJECTS
Pencil, key, penny, ball

2+ = two or more

TOWER: Both Adapt. & Fine Mot.
items [See 21-24 Mos. Instr.]
COPY = make from model
IMITATE = after demonstr. If both
appear, always ask to copy first-
-is at higher level

CHIMNEY: ▢▢▢▯ [See 24 Mos.]
one, another, chimney for
smoke, point & push

HOUSE: ▯▢▯ Copy: point & say
downstairs, door, upstairs
Imitate: while building say--one
like this, one like this, then
as for copy

"DRAWING" = just a scribble; may
not understand what child says,
but credit if makes sounds,
partic. if points at same time
May indicate, not tell, for
Action, Use = close to age level

SEX: Are you a boy or girl?
Say sex of child first

PREPOSITIONAL COMMANDS [use chair]
Order: on, under, back of, front
of, beside

	H	O	21 Months	H	O	24 Months
A D A P T			Push train and say "choo-choo" [see instructions]			Align 2+ cubes for a train [demonstr.] [see instructions]
			Build tower of 5-6 [Ex. may help]			Imitate vertical stroke
						Imitate circular scribble
G R ' M O T			Walk upstairs, hold rail			Walk up & down stairs, may hold rail, wall
			Walk down, hand held			Run, stop no holding to wall, table, etc.
			Squat on haunches to play			Kick ball on request
F ' M O T			Tower 5-6 cubes, without help			Tower 6-7 cubes
						Turn pages singly in child's large book
L A N G			Combine 2-3 words [bye dad, go car]			3-word sentence; use pronoun: me, you, mine
			3 directions--no pointing or gesture			Test object: name 2
						4 directions--no pointing or gesture
P ' S O C			Use cup, put down when finished			Hat on, pull up pants
			Pull person to show them something			Domestic mimicry: sweep, dust, hammer
						Spoon right side up, feeding self

	H	O	30 Months	H	O	36 Months
A D A P T			Add chimney to train			Imitate 3-cube house
			Imitate horizontal stroke [& vertical]			Name own "drawing"
			Make any 2+ strokes to imitate a cross			Copy circle
						Imitate cross
G R ' M O T			Walk on tiptoe [dem.]			Pedal tricycle
			Jump: both feet off floor			Jump off bottom step
			Try to stand 1 foot not holding on			Stand 1 foot momentary balance
F ' M O T			Tower 8 cubes			Tower 9-10 cubes
			Fingers hold crayon [adult fashion]			
L A N G			Tell first & last name			Tell action in book
						Use plurals
			Test object: tell use [pencil, key, penny]			Tell sex
						2 preposit. commands [no point. or gesture]
P ' S O C			Refer to self by pronoun: I, me want			Feed self, spill little
			Help put toys away			Put on shoes
			Push wagon, carriage, back out if stuck			Understand take turns
						Unbutton buttons if accessible

turned to side, arm and leg extended on that same side, other hand fisted at occiput.

16 weeks: *symmetric*—head usually in midline or freely movable, arms both either in at chest or out.

12 weeks: head more apt to be asymmetric than body.

HEAD CONTROL IN SITTING (needs full trunk support)

4 weeks: head sags against the chest once it is brought forward.

8 weeks: it sags but can bob to an erect position.

12 weeks: head set forward between hunched shoulders; infant looks ahead, but head bobs down at times.

16 weeks: still hunched; does not bob forward unless turned away to side.

20 weeks: head is in line with the upper trunk, no longer hunched, and no bobbing.

PIVOT (to move about in a circle in one spot)

32 weeks: infant does this lying on his abdomen by crossing one arm over the other.

SITTING

28 weeks +: must be done on *hard surface,* not bed.

40 weeks: *goes* to prone—controlled, not falling; straight over, *not* to side first. Must be able to sit steadily before he can do this.

GRASP (reach out and take promptly in one motion; differs from approach with eventual prehension. Progresses from ulnar side of hand to radial digits.)

12 weeks: *hold an object actively;* obvious if he lifts it off bed. Otherwise knuckles whiten, which they do not do if toy rests passively in his hands.

20 weeks: can't reach out and pick up toy but shows he is trying by *scratching at the table when he sees it.* May scratch without toy being present.

SMALL TOY (CUBE) GRASP

24 weeks: has whole hand palmar grasp and all fingers press toy against center of palm.

28 weeks: is still in the palm, but is held at the radial side, primarily by the index and third fingers and is pressed against the thumb too.

36 weeks: there is a space between toy and palm and it is held with thumb and ends of index and third.

"CRUMB" (PELLET) GRASP

28 weeks: can pick up small toy but not crumb-sized object—can only land on this with his whole hand or try to get it with raking movement of whole arm.

Grasp of small objects then proceeds in same way as grasp of larger objects—towards the radial digits, with suppression of movements of whole arm and hand.

40 weeks: Pluck—grasp promptly between *ventral* surfaces of thumb and index finger.

MISCELLANEOUS

40 weeks: Put toy down—controlled removal of hand from object, not just dropping.

40 and 44 weeks: plays with cube in, or removes from cup, *when thy rest are left beside it* (may have to take a cube from his hand if he is holding two).

18 months: pulls toy on string after himself as walks or crawls around; not just pulling it towards himself.

LANGUAGE

4 weeks: sounds are made but have no definite form—are just noises in the throat.

36 weeks: he puts consonant sounds together without meaning: da-da, ba-ba.

A "word": a sound used consistently to mean something—a person, an object, a group of objects.

A nursery trick: wave "bye-bye," play "pat-a-cake," "peek-a-boo," "so-big," etc.

15 months: "Talking" a foreign language is "jargoning," i.e., making voice go up and down, pausing as though at end of a phrase, etc., in conversation, and expecting you to understand what he is saying. It is not "just baby babbling."

§6. SUPPLEMENTARY INFORMATION

1. Does your child turn to look at you when you talk in a normal voice?

2. Do you think he hears?

3. Has he ever had any convulsions or fits?

4. Does he ever stare off into space, and keep right on staring if you *put* your hand in front of his eyes and *hold* it there?

5. Does he ever start to cry for no apparent reason, and keep right on crying no matter what you do to try to comfort him?

6. Is there anything about your child that worries you?

7. Has he ever lost any behavior once achieved?

8. What age child do you think your child is acting like in:
   Controlling his body and hands?
   How his mind works?
   Making sounds or talking?
   Understanding what you say?

9. Does he use both of his hands and both of his feet equally well?

10. Is he taking any medication? What? How much per day?

18

Guidance and Management*

Health in children derives from a very wide variety of sources: in physical integrity and vigor, in the economic, social and emotional climate of the family and society in which they exist, in opportunities for education and learning, in the early recognition of problems and in the promptness and effectiveness of remediation. A significant handicap of any sort—physical, psychologic, environmental, or social—constitutes a strong deterrent to optimal mental health.

Whatever social legislation the future may hold, the inherent technologic trends in medicine will lead to a mobilization of its diagnostic and supervisory resources at the beginning of the life cycle. Pediatrics and obstetrics hold the most strategic position in the whole scheme of preventive and constructive medicine. Health protection begins with the beginnings of life and growth, and depends on comprehensive, continuous, and coordinated programs of care.

On a professional level, the neonatologist and obstetrician first of all must cooperate in fostering optimum conditions throughout pregnancy. The vast majority of developmental problems have their origin in the critical period of gestation. The neonatologist is extending his activities into the developing specialty of fetology. The next task is to insure survival of the newborn infant. The final and longest task is to safeguard his optimal growth. By this simple logic, development as well as disease falls within the province of clinical pediatrics, preventive medicine and public health.

In child development, diagnosis involves prognosis and prognosis involves treatment. The three are interdependent. Since development is a continuing process even for subnormal and handicapped children, child care professionals and parents must enter into a partnership to keep pace with the behavioral changes as they

---

*Permission has been granted by the publisher and editor to reprint the portion of the material in this chapter which first appeared in *Current Pediatric Therapy—3*, edited by Gellis and Kagan.[47]

occur. There are no absolutes in the task of parent—child guidance. The problems of care and management all must be reduced to the relativities of age and maturity. These relativities apply with equal force to subnormal, deviant, handicapped and normal children.

§1. NORMAL CHILDREN

The most acute solicitude of parents arises in the crises of illness and accident, but the most enduring and deepest concern of parents is with development. Prolonged illness, sensory and motor handicaps, severe malnutrition, prematurity of birth, convulsions, speech delay and numerous deviations of conduct often lead to acute parental anxieties about the child's future growth. However, even if there are no handicaps or complications, parents maintain profound interest in the progressions of their child's development. Development, in a biologic sense, is an inescapable problem for the child, and it is entirely natural for many so-called normal children to encounter difficulties along the pathway to maturity. It is normal for normal children to present developmental problems.

Parents are entitled to guidance in managing these normal difficulties. It serves no good purpose to tell a mother exactly how she should do a thing; it is more important to tell her how to approach and view the problem. The child is changing, so the problems change. However, if individual development is ignored, too much reliance on general rules will not fit the specific child; there will be a temptation to do too much through sheer training and discipline. In many aggravating behavior situations it would be better to do nothing at all than to pursue strenuously a mistaken course. Maturation is the key concept which must enter into all guidance. If the physician or other professional worker involved in child care is convinced of this concept, he will impart its implications.

Therefore, one cardinal precept of developmental guidance must be stated negatively: *Avoid doing too much.* Parents do not scold an infant for his failure and difficulties in early locomotion; they are not emotionally tense about them. The same objective attitude should be taken in all aspects of child management. The ways of natural growth and maturation are truly devious, but in the normal infant they are certain. Progressive neuromotor organization underlies all forms of behavior. We do not teach a child to crawl, creep, stand or walk; we give him opportunity. He does his own growing. Research has indicated that acceleration of some of these developmental processes may be possible, but it has not indicated if any value to the child will result. Potentially, there may be a cost in disorganization of total growth and development.

The success of child care depends not so much upon successful rule of thumb techniques as upon the underlying attitudes of parents and attendants. Here lies the most promising field for guidance. The adult—infant relationship is one of the most vital and most accessible factors in effecting a mental hygiene of infancy. Literally, the mind of the infant can be reached by altering faulty attitudes in the parents.

The physician need not step out of character when he consciously addresses himself to the adult—infant relationship as a dynamic reality; this is the essence of developmental guidance. However, it should be guidance rather than authoritative control; the common sense of parents should not be distorted by unwarranted introduction of untested theoretical concepts. Every parent has some philosophy of life which is expressed in methods of management, if not in articulate sentences. If the philosophy is democratic, there will be respect for the individuality of the infant and tolerance for the difficulties which he encounters in his development. Such a parent will arrive at the infant's point of view, and the infant's point of view is beyond doubt a developmental one!

§2. ABNORMAL CHILDREN

The early years of life are when physically and mentally handicapped children are most in danger of being neglected. The first 3 years are of special importance both for identifying these children and for initiating adequate medical and educational measures. Physician and parent alike are tempted to wait until the handicapped child is of school age. There is a vague optimism that he will outgrow his handicap, or there is actual resistance to acknowledging the handicap. The result is that the first formative years are lost. Sometimes the child actually is misunderstood and unwittingly mistreated. Both he and the parents make a false start, when it is supremely important to get a right start. In mild cases, the handicap surprisingly often is not even noticed. The failure to detect these children at an early age and direct the family to specialized services compounds the problems consequent to already experienced social inadequacy—in school, in the home and in peer relationships—and renders reorientation of the social and educational milieu more difficult.

In Chapter 17 on developmental screening, we pointed out that the physician is not necessarily the first professional person to detect something amiss, but he has the ultimate responsibility for making a diagnosis, estimating the seriousness of the handicap and initiating constructive attitudes in the family circle. The care of a handicapped child often proves to be a complicated problem which requires the cooperation of social worker, public health nurse, visiting teacher, home visitors and many others, as well as community, state or federal agencies.

Finding adequate facilities for the care of the physically and mentally handicapped, particularly the latter, is easier said than done. While community-based programs are improving, they still are fragmented, disorganized and inadequate. In the past they have been available primarily for children of school age. Increasingly they are being provided during the preschool period. Institutional care is necessary for a small portion of mentally defective children, even if adequate community facilities are available, but a host of social factors and insufficient funds have created disgraceful conditions in many state-supported institutions. Some private facilities may be better, but are beyond the means of most parents.

The chief responsibilities of a physician unaffiliated with a multidisciplinary developmental clinic are to be aware of the available facilities, direct the parents to them and work with the various agencies in developing a plan suited to the problems and potentials of the child. Allied professionals generally have more expertise than the physician in the social and educational aspects of management. In a developmental clinic, the role of the physician should not be that of a traffic director, nor should it be confined to the physical examination. He should develop and utilize his skills as a developmental diagnostician. In the last analysis, parents usually turn to the physician as the final arbiter when they have an abnormal child.

§3. IMPARTING A DIAGNOSIS

There are certain principles which should be followed in establishing and transmitting the diagnosis to the parents, whether this be done by a physician in his office, by a pediatric consultant or in a special evaluation clinic. Most of the points in the diagnostic procedure have been discussed throughout this volume, but they are summarized here to present a coherent picture.

If the parents are to be satisfied with the diagnosis and prognosis given them, and receptive to the necessary plans for management, they must know the basis on which the diagnosis is being made. The diagnostic process is thus an integral part of treatment. Parents usually are well aware that something is wrong, but even if it is obvious that a gross defect is present, the physician must not give the impression of making a "snap" diagnosis. Consequently, a careful history must be taken which includes the family history, pregnancy, labor and delivery, neonatal period, illnesses, seizures and the course of development. The parents also should be present at the developmental evaluation. This clarifies their feelings, systematizes their own observations, permits them to see behavior and symptoms which will be important in management and allows the physician to observe interactions between the child and the parents.

In the diagnostic evaluation, particular attention must be paid to the following points: Any conditions which are amenable to specific medical or surgical therapy must be detected and treated. Malformations of the central nervous system such as myelomeningocele or hydrocephalus should be corrected promptly. There is no correlation between the severity of the defect or the thickness of the cerebral cortex and the intellectual potential. Even if mental deficiency is demonstrated after the newborn period, care is facilitated if there is no open infected area or if the head has not grown to grotesque proportions.

Neuromotor and intellectual defects must be distinguished from each other in order to make the correct diagnosis. Such a differentiation can be made, but only by considering the intimate interrelations between neurologic integrity and maturational status, and not by attempting to fragment the infant into neurologic and psychometric portions. It is as harmful to label an intellectually potentially normal infant as mentally defective, because he has a motor handicap for which he may or may not compensate, as it is to tell the parents that a child with mental deficiency is just a little slow in motor development and will grow out of it. Associated handicaps also must be evaluated. Most commonly these are "cerebral palsy," sensory impairment or convulsive seizures. In the presence of uncontrolled convulsions, it is not possible to give a firm prognosis; prompt treatment is vitally important (Chapter 13).

Interpretation of the findings to the parents is as essential as the diagnostic evaluation, and time should be set aside for this immediately after the recording and synthesis of the findings. An unfortunate procedure in many multidisciplinary clinics is that so many different appointments are scheduled and spread over such a long period that it may be several months before anyone sits down to talk with the parents. Unnecessary anxiety and hardship for the parents results. Not every child needs to be seen by every specialist or have every procedure carried out, even if teamwork is needed for some children. It is just as important to know when multiple investigations are not necessary, as the following case illustrates.

A mother brought her 3-year old to a developmental clinic stating, "His smarts is all right, but he don't speak so good." After 26 hours of invested professional time, the team reached the following conclusion: normal intelligence with a speech defect. A developmental evaluation of an hour's duration, or even a screening procedure, would have confirmed the mother's opinion for her promptly and the child referred for speech therapy in another year.

Speaking with the parents about their child's prognosis requires both skill and sensitivity. This is particularly true in cases of mental deficiency, which bring with them the deepest frustration and disappointment which can occur in family life. The poignancy of this frustration needs no description; it is the ultimate negation of the expectations which normally center on a child. No one can impart a grave diagnosis properly who cannot imagine the nature of the sorrow involved.

During the postevaluation interview, physician and parents should be seated comfortably and any impression of haste eliminated. If a trial of treatment or further tests are indicated before coming to firm conclusions, the preliminary findings and the reasons for further steps should be explained. The physician should take 15–20 minutes to cover the points in a structured fashion; this will answer most of the parents' questions, even though he may have to go over some points several times.

The postevaluation interview can be conducted effectively in the following manner. Before giving his own opinions, the physician asks the parents three questions: "Is what your child did here today representative of what he does at home? What age child do you think your child is acting like now? What have you been told already?" Any ambiguities in the replies can be clarified and the distinction made between motor and intellectual behavior if the parents have not already done so. The physician then says he will try to answer four questions: "What is wrong? Why? What can we do about it? What can we expect in the future?" He gives his own evaluation of the child's level of function and tells the parents the child is not developing normally because the brain is not functioning normally. He uses the term "brain damage," but makes it clear that he means dysfunction and not an injury or lesion which can be seen or repaired. He then proceeds to discuss the ways in which brain dysfunction may manifest itself. Nothing is to be gained in shying away from terms which are emotionally loaded. If they have not already been used with the parents, they will be in the future. It is preferable to give a clear understanding of their meaning. Most parents prefer to know where they stand and what the physician thinks.

Although the child with organic brain disease usually has several rather than only one of the various manifestations, they are discussed conveniently by grouping them into six broad categories: (1) intellectual abilities, using the words "mental deficiency" (If the child does have mental deficiency, this area should be covered last; because of the grave import it carries, parents may fail to listen to the rest of the discussion. By the same token, if intellectual potential is normal and the difficulty lies elsewhere, it should be discussed first.); (2) neuromotor disabilities, including "cerebral palsy" and the lesser degrees of motor handicaps; (3) convulsive seizures; (4) sensory impairments, such as visual and auditory difficulties; (5) the integration and organization of behavior, including attention and the ability to establish social relations with people; (6) specific syndromes or diseases, important for genetic counseling or specific therapy.

There is no advantage in waiting for an auspicious time to "spring" a diagnosis. Parents generally are able to show an extraordinary capacity to confront reality if they are approached properly. There also is no advantage in waiting for the child to grow up. Infancy remains the best time for imparting a diagnosis of central nervous system dysfunction. When the physician has made a decisive diagnosis he should tell the parents without delay. In less-clearcut cases where he suspects serious retardation but has not made a conclusive diagnosis, the cumulative evidence of two or three comparative appraisals helps to bring about acceptance of the diagnosis. The parents also begin to watch and see for themselves. Such a progressive approach leads finally to a concrete discussion of prognosis. The time comes when the parents must consider realistically what the future holds in store. Again, candor is the best policy; it must not be ruthless, but it should be so revealing to the parents that they will understand what kind of training, supervision, safeguards and educational provisions will be necessary as the child grows older.

The resistance of parents to an adverse diagnosis is natural, but in the end they do not wish to be deceived and they will resent the inconclusiveness of any long delay. Ambiguous assurances and fostered optimism lead to expensive "shopping around"; parents should be advised against it. When a frank diagnosis finally is imparted, after a long period of futile hopefulness, most parents, no matter how bad they feel, react with grateful relief: "If we had only been told this in this way years ago!"

§4. MANAGEMENT IN MENTAL DEFICIENCY

Except in a few instances, mental deficiency cannot be cured, but long-term management is necessary. The primary problems in treatment usually are guidance of the family in their management and education of the child, and the provision of necessary special assistance for fostering development. Searching questions will be put by the parents: "Will he ever walk? When will he talk? Will I always have to take care of him? Won't he ever go to school? Will he be able to earn his own living?" These questions cannot be brushed aside; they are irrepressible. Adequate service consists in meeting them intelligently and in a helpful manner.

Above all, if the physician does not know what to expect because of the presence of modifying factors such as seizures or the possibility of deterioration, he must say he does not know and give his reasons. He should not hedge. Most often he will have to acknowledge ignorance when discussing why the mental deficiency or other abnormalities occurred.

Nothing is so beneficial to parent and child alike as acceptance of the current maturity age and rate of development. This overriding principle must be borne in mind in helping the parents. The child with mental deficiency usually follows the same developmental progressions that a normal child does, and in handling him the parents must ignore his chronologic age and treat him at his developmental age. He can be helped best to achieve his full potential by providing him with the opportunities appropriate to his level of function. Provision of maturity-appropriate toys, books and experiences in and outside the home will foster his development.

In discussing the future course of intellectual development, the physician should point out that the child will continue to learn, but at a rate slower than normal; the gap between how old he is and how old he is acting will become larger as he grows older; the development of more complex patterns of thought will continue, but it will reach a lower plateau than normal. Since the parents can divide the functional maturity age by the chronologic age appropriately, the physician gives them the approximate percentage of normal development that has been attained. In most cases, a mentally defective infant will continue to develop at approximately this same rate. The physician should be careful to point out he is not stating a precise intelligence quotient which will show no fluctuations in the future, but merely giving them a rough index of what level of behavior to expect at various later ages.

Parents feel guilty even if there is an adequate explanation for the deficiency, and it is essential to point out that they are not to blame, with particular emphasis on the point that the child's failure to develop is *not* the result of their failure to teach him how to do things, of not paying enough attention to him, or alternatively, of not letting him do things for himself. They will have to steer a middle course between trying to push the child beyond his capabilities and overprotecting him and hindering him from taking responsibility for things he can master. If the parents understand this, they will find it easier to exercise their own common sense.

In such a painful situation as mental deficiency, all kinds of esoteric treatment have been proposed. Families often spend thousands of dollars and disrupt the normal patterns of living in the hope that their child can be restored to a normal level of function. To date, none of the elaborate training procedures suggested has been demonstrated to be of value. Helpful books and pamphlets related to the management of children with mental subnormality are available from the U.S. Government Printing Office, and a list can be obtained from the Superintendent of Documents and given to the parents.

The main difference in the development of a mentally defective child is that he is capable of understanding things at a later chronologic age than does the normal, and repetition is required. However, qualitative changes in behavior usually are present. Even in the absence of neuromotor handicaps, there may be perceptual and perceptual–motor defects and other difficulties in integration which may result in disorganized behavior, hypoactivity, or hyperactivity. One of the major reasons for the development of destructive or stereotypic behavior is the mistaken concept that a mentally defective child, especially the severely impaired one, is incapable of responding to the ordinary rules of behavioral management. Any family must decide on the rules of conduct that they want in their home, and then help their defective child learn to abide by these rules, in the same way that they help their normal children to do so. The basic principle that behavior is governed by its consequences applies to all individuals. When it is possible to use it, reward works much better than punishment. If distressing or destructive behavior elicits a parental response, such behavior will increase. Unwittingly, the parents may foster the very behavior that makes it difficult to provide love and attention. The principle in changing the pattern is to make the rewarding consequences for the child contingent upon constructive behavior. This is the root of all behavior modification. However, it is not always simple to find rewarding activities within the limits of the child's capabilities if the impairment is severe; in certain instances, punishment or forcible intervention may be unavoidable. Preventing the development of abnormal responses is infinitely preferable and easier than treating them once they have arisen.

Emotional difficulties are at least as common for mentally deficient children as for intellectually normal children. When they have similar causes, unrelated to neurologic deficits or lesions, they require similar management. Unfortunately, insight psychotherapy, individually or in groups, has not been demonstrated to be effective for either normal or abnormal individuals. When it carries the implication that the parents' attitudes, management and lack of adequate stimulation are primarily responsible for the child's problems, such treatment can be detrimental.

Counseling directed toward parental support and development of the positive assets of the child, on a realistic goal-oriented basis, might be expected to result in greater and longer-lasting benefits. For this, the skills of a trained social worker, nurse or other child worker who can visit with the family as often as needed, are invaluable. Explaining to the parents that much of their child's misbehavior is triggered by organic disease that sets off unfortunate interactions with the environment often results in dramatic changes in the way they manage the child. The consequent improvement in the total milieu reverses the downward cycle that has been established. Frequently it will be necessary to begin anew at a level at which the child experiences almost invariable success. These successes then can be rewarded and gradually built upon to reverse the constant spiral of failure—punishment—further dysfunction—failure.

Disorganization and hyperactivity interfere further with developing consistency in management. They can be improved if the number of stimuli and choices for activity can be limited, and sudden shifts of focus avoided. Dextroamphetamine, methylphenidate or imipramine to tolerance, as measured by loss of appetite or irritability, may be helpful if other measures are ineffective. A good deal of the hyperactivity and disorganization associated with mental deficiency improves with age, as it usually does in children without impaired intellectual function.

Behavior modification also may be effective for the child who fails to establish any social relations and regards all people, including his parents, as inanimate objects. This is the behavior to which the descriptive term of *infantile autism* was given by Kanner[36] (Chapter 16). Although the child appears to be motivated entirely from within, developmental progress indicates that stimuli are being assimilated. The parents should talk to the child normally, even though he appears not to hear or pay attention, and should gradually increase social stimulation, without overwhelming him, as the child shows an increasing ability to integrate it. In the majority of instances, the symptoms of autism disappear as the child matures and he is reachable, even though his mental deficiency still is present.

The child is the patient, but the problems are peculiarly family ones, which involve brothers and sisters, and almost always concern the mental hygiene of father and mother. In many instances, the consequences of mental defect or other abnormality go so far beyond the child that they injure normal marital relationships or the functioning of siblings. One parent may blame the other, or both parents may harbor an altogether unwarranted sense of guilt. Sometimes emotions are projected against a hospital or a physician, with paranoid intensity.

It is the physician's responsibility to help the family to face reality as early and as steadily as possible. For all chronic conditions which contain aspects of life-long social dysfunction, numerous panaceas have been offered; the Doman-Delacato method of patterning and psychoanalysis are but two examples of the long list of untested therapies.[16] It is incumbent on all health care workers to develop competence in evaluating such therapies and protect parents who, in their understandable distress, are prepared to devote their lives to their handicapped child, to the exclusion of all else.

In the interval before the child is ready for education outside the home, much can be done to ease the burden of 24-hour care that the mother bears. The mother of normal children benefits from some time away from them. Even more is some relief advisable if the child is subnormal. This should be provided on a regular basis, even though it may be a limited one, and possible only to the extent of permitting the rest of the family to go out as a unit. Relief for the mother can be arranged by having the father contribute his turn at babysitting, or the home-making services of family care agencies may be utilized if they are available.

It is particularly important that the mother not devote herself to the abnormal child to the exclusion of the other children in the family. A balance must be struck between benefits to the subnormal child and unwarranted deprivation of the other children. The details of this balance, both financial and developmental, must be left to the parents. It should never be assumed that the presence of an abnormal child in the home automatically is deleterious to the growth and development of the normal ones. Aside from specific problems an individual case might present, the reactions of the children will depend on those of the parents. If they are ashamed and try to hide the child, their children will do likewise; if they accept the child and his problems, so will the children. Parents should answer questions truthfully when they are asked, in terms appropriate to the normal child's level of understanding. It is probably best to explain the abnormal child's problem in terms of illness and make analogies to other situations in which the reasons for the handicap might be more obvious. It is not necessarily harmful for children to learn early that everything in life is not perfect; they may then grow up with more humility and sympathy.

There are many community agencies which can provide help to the family, not the least of which are parent groups. Participation in parent and citizen groups for subnormal or handicapped children may be very helpful in the exchange of knowledge, provision of mutual support and amelioration of the feelings of isolation and guilt. Often mothers can develop a babysitting program, when no other facilities are available, and take turns having free time. Parent groups have been especially instrumental in changing attitudes and obtaining community services where none have existed previously; they will continue to be a potent resource for stimulating the development of care facilities. It is unfortunate that citizen groups frequently waste time and energy in providing direct care or in quarreling among themselves on semantic and financial grounds, instead of cooperating on long-range community goals. A society still can be judged by the care it offers its children.

Nursery schools for subnormal children serve the same function as they do for normal children. They provide opportunities for socialization with other children which might not be present at home, offer a variety of stimulating experiences and give the mother some time away from the child. In deciding when and for how long to send the child to a nursery school, the developmental level of the child again is of overriding importance. For example, five-day-a-week all-day nursery school is not recommended for an 18- or 24-month normal child. Similarly, it should not be recommended for 3- or 4-year children who function at half their chronologic age. It is better to suggest a more limited experience which can be increased as the child demonstrates enough maturity to cope with longer periods. These schools probably play a more important role with defective than with normal children, because many regular school systems have no facilities for coping with the mentally defective until they are 8 or 9 years old. Special techniques of management and education are necessary in the nursery school setting also.

Some communities are developing a home visiting program which provides advice and consultation to parents, usually those of preschool children. Such agencies can prove helpful to parents if they have adequate professional guidance. On occasion, the workers become overenthusiastic about what untested methods of training mean for a child with mental deficiency, particularly when they have no knowledge of the diagnosis that has been made. They may try to push the child beyond his capacities, and increase the parents' guilt by making them feel that they are depriving their child of needed help and therapy, if the child understandably resists such efforts. Trained professional supervision is necessary.

Long-range planning will vary with local and state facilities, with the financial status of the family, and with the abilities of the child. These facilities extend from private schools for "exceptional" children, through slow-learning classes in the public school system and community classes for those not able to function in an academic situation, to institutionalization in some cases. The child's emotional stability and personality are as important as his intellectual capabilities in determining his ability to adjust in a sheltered or competitive environment. Techniques in education of the child with mental deficiency are the same as those used in management—limiting stimuli and choices for activities, avoiding sudden shifts, patient repetition and reward for constructive behavior.

How detailed the discussion of long-range plans should be at the first diagnostic-prognostic interview depends on the age of the child and his abilities. If decisions are several years away, it is well to give the alternatives, mentioning the most likely possibility, but indicating that final plans should not be made until the child's progress and later functioning have been reevaluated. In the infant and the young child, the question of institutionalization rarely is raised at early discussions unless the parents ask questions about it. Ample evidence indicates that all children, particularly the more severely involved and younger ones, decline in their intellectual functioning and social behavior in a large institution where there is no program for structuring of activities or verbal stimulation. A recommendation for institutionalization should never be proposed and should be discouraged at birth and in the preschool period. Two exceptions exist: when a young child is totally oblivious of his surroundings *and* it is clear he will remain unresponsive to stimulation and will always require purely custodial care; or if the behavior is so uncontrollably destructive that there is interference with the total family adjustment. Foster home placement may be possible when emotional or social problems prevent keeping the child in the family. A temporary stay away from home also may allow reorganization; summer vacations at a camp are helpful. In all cases, care must be taken to ensure that the other children understand the reasons when placement outside the home is undertaken.

A few parents cannot accept a child even with only a mild degree of impairment and without any disorganization in his behavior. However, most will want to keep their child at home, even if it is not likely that he will benefit from the experience. The ultimate decision about future care still belongs to the parents, and this is particularly true about institutionalization. The physician must provide the information by which such a decision can be reached intelligently, and should give his support and encouragement if placement is indicated, but he must make it clear to the parents that the final decision is theirs.

Another aspect of total family planning centers on future offspring. The physician's or genetics counselor's responsibility is to provide the information about the risks for subsequent children, which are well known for conditions demonstrated to be hereditary, and unknown but probably slightly increased for other situations. The action to be taken on the basis of this information again is a decision the family must make.

Not every parent requires frequent conferences after the initial diagnostic evaluation by the specialist; in fact, most do not when it is conducted adequately, particularly when community resources are mobilized. However, at the end of the first diagnostic–prognostic session, all parents should be made to feel free to arrange for further discussions of points that have not been made clear or of any problems that may arise. Telephone conversations rather than office visits may sometimes be sufficient.

Finally, it is most important to specify when a formal reevaluation is indicated and by whom, whether it be in 6 months to determine progress or the results of treatment, or by an educational psychologist at later ages to decide on the best educational placement. Ongoing supervision of the child's total health care must be provided by a family physician. The expertise of the various members of a special evaluation clinic can be utilized by him. A social worker or nurse also can be extremely helpful in maintaining contact with the family as often as the individual situation demands.

§5. MANAGEMENT OF MOTOR AND SENSORY HANDICAPS

The management and psychology of the handicapped child was discussed in detail in Chapters 14 and 15 on hearing and visual impairments. Each type of handicap creates its distinctive problems.

In the case of children with motor impairment, a discriminating understanding is of special importance, because their true capacities cannot be measured by their motor abilities. A child may have a very restricted paralysis and yet be mentally deficient to an extreme degree, or he may have an extensive motor incapacity and yet be extremely intelligent and emotionally sensitive. When a competent diagnosis has been defined, practical questions of treatment arise at once.

The first years of life also are strategically the most important for handicapped children. Prompt medical, and sometimes surgical, care in infancy is the first essential if the child is to develop to his optimal capacity. A crippled child is not a sick child, and he can be treated like a well child even in infancy. He must not be overprotected; he can be propped in the sitting position if he cannot sit alone; he can be taken out in a carriage; he should be given experiences. A premium always should be placed upon mobility, so that the child can enjoy a sense of personal power. He should be allowed to hitch, roll and use an infant walker. When he outgrows the walker, a special homemade contrivance on wheels can be constructed.

The parents are entitled to feel that everything possible is being done to help the child; on the other hand they must be made to realize the limitations of physical therapy. Even if a child acquires the ability to walk, he may still be crippled. Moreover, he may never acquire walking at all. Yet he may benefit greatly from speech training. The ability to talk should be regarded as more important than the ability to walk.

In severe cases, parents should be warned that any training program will require years of patience and will at best yield slow results. Since the value of treatment depends upon the cooperation of the child, resistances which he offers must be respected. Most methods of therapy have been untested or are of no avail. In Chapter 10, we indicated that the most important aspects are the prevention of contractures, the provision of ambulation aids and the institution of social and educational experiences appropriate to the maturity level.

In all types of handicap, whether sensory or motor, the parents must understand the nature of the handicap and the purpose of the training and treatment measures. Their questions must be answered and the realities of the situation made clear. They must be helped to accept their child for what he is and to build the right attitude toward him. This attitude means acceptance of the child, a desire to help him and pride in his accomplishments. It does not permit overprotection or oversympathy; it never lets the child see the parents' disappointment; it meets the situation as a challenge.

19

Clinical Aspects of Child Adoption

The hazard of environmental retardation is especially serious for infants who are unwanted or abused or who for one reason or another are deprived of parental care. Many of them immediately become charges of the state. Such foster children face an uncertain future if they are maintained too long in a hospital, maternity home, institution or boarding home.

Child adoption is a social measure designed primarily to protect the welfare of such a child, by providing a home in which he will receive care and affection from parents as legally responsible for him as if he were born to them. The rights of the adoptive parents also must be protected, by insuring that the child is legally free for adoption and that the natural parents will have no further claim upon him. Termination of the rights of the natural parents is as important as establishing new parental ties. In order to safeguard all three parties involved in adoption, legal procedures must be supplemented by adequate social services. All adoptions should take place under the auspices of a duly authorized adoption agency, with review after a mandatory probationary period before the adoption becomes final.

§1. HISTORIC TRENDS IN ADOPTION PRACTICES

Adoption in one form or another has been practiced from time immemorial. Many of the early adoption agencies were and still are connected with various religious denominations, although state and local governmental agencies have become involved increasingly. In modern times, economic conditions and social attitudes have influenced profoundly the practices of adoption. During and immediately after the depression, there were many more infants available for adoption than there were families wishing to adopt. Emphasis was on placement only of "perfect" infants who matched the adopting parents in ethnic and religious backgrounds, physical characteristics and purportedly in intellectual potential. After World War II, with improvement in economic conditions, the number of families wanting to adopt outstripped even the boom in births. Emphasis then shifted to restrictions on the type of people considered suitable adoptive parents; they were almost exclusively white, legally married, church attenders, respected in the community and prosperous. Thus the "perfect" child also required a "perfect" home. Increased dissemination of contraceptive information and liberalized abortion laws have resulted in a sharp drop in the number of births. Women's liberation movements and changing life styles also have led to an increase in the number of unmarried women who keep their infants rather than releasing them for adoption, and these combined factors have led to a decrease in the number of healthy infants available for adoption.

In 1970 adoption was completed for about three-fourths of the available children. Only 12% of the adopted children were nonwhite, while two-thirds of those not adopted were. Further, almost all those adopted were less than 6 years old, and the overwhelming majority under 1 year. Thus, the greatest percentage of children not adopted were nonwhite, over 6 years of age, mentally or physically handicapped, or all three. Colloquially, this group is designated as "hard to adopt."[57]

Unquestionably, mentally or physically handicapped children fare better in a family of their own than in an institution or when shifted from one foster home to the next at frequent intervals. Just as clearly, there are parents who want to adopt such children. What is important is that the adoptive parents are acquainted fully with the problems they will face. When they are, there generally is no contraindication to adoption placement. The number of handicapped children placed in adoption undoubtedly would be increased if there were government funds available to help defray the additional financial burdens imposed by medical care costs.

Such situations are quite different from those in which parents who expect to have adopted a normal, healthy child discover that their adopted infant is abnormal. Such results can be disastrous, not only for the parents, but also for the child, whose welfare must be the prime consideration. Theoretically, it appears reasonable to assert that adoptive parents should take the same risks that other parents do in bearing their own children; in practice this does not occur, for two reasons. First, the chronic sorrow and feelings of being cheated are infinitely greater for adoptive parents, increasing the possibility of rejection of the child. Second, there clearly is an increased risk of abnormality in illegitimate children, for a host of medical and social reasons. In the first few months of life, it is nearly impossible to determine definitively whether an infant is normal; this is the chief contraindication to taking an infant for adoption from the newborn nursery, as well as the chief indication for a mandatory probationary period. No clear data indicate adverse effects from foster home placement, or even institutional placement, in the first 2 or 3 months of life. After this time, any deprivation which occurs is reversible, but the infant probably is affected to some degree. However, a healthy infant will respond favorably to a stimulating environment in large part.

Racial prejudice still is a prominent aspect of American life. We look askance at mixed marriages and raise our eyebrows when we see a nonwhite child with a white parent. Professional workers involved in making or evaluating the effects of transracial adoptions are not immune to these deep-seated feelings. While it is legitimate to inquire whether a black child in a white environment has difficult adjustments to make, rarely is the question posed about whether they are more difficult than those he must make in a totally black environment. Admittedly, there are no answers today to these questions. Fortunately, there is a healthy trend towards transracial adoptions. Invariably, this means the placement of a nonwhite child in a mixed or totally white home, and primarily in a middle-class home of above-average educational and socioeconomic level. The criterion for a transracial adoption should be the same as for any adoption—the opportunity for the child to grow in a stable environment that accepts him as an individual and fosters his developmental potential.

§2. AGENCY VERSUS INDEPENDENT ADOPTION

In the 1930s and 1940s, close to three-fourths of adoptions were arranged privately, while in 1970 the situation was reversed and less than one-fourth were carried out without the supervision of a licensed adoption agency. In many, but not all independent adoptions, relatives were the adopting parents. Long waiting lists, and the caution agencies use in their efforts to do the best for all parties, push some parents into the black or "grey" markets. Bureaucratic delays are enhanced by restrictive legislation and customs. Two-thirds of the states still require that adoptive parents have a religion, and further that it be the same as that of the prospective child. Less than a dozen prohibit or limit independent placement. Even under agency supervision mistakes occur, but they can be corrected and both child and adoptive parents protected.

The following cases illustrate what may happen when adoptions are not adequately regulated by social, medical and legal procedures:

1. A middle-aged woman feared divorce because of her childlessness. She adopted a baby in order to hold the affection of her husband. Jealousies arose instead, and the home broke up. A child who should have had a good home lost out.
2. An unmarried mother gave her child to an adoptive father who was so alcoholic that the child again became the ward of the state at 5 years of age.
3. A grandmother was given the illegitimate child of her daughter. It so happened that the grandmother was on parole from a state mental hospital and had to be returned to the hospital 6 weeks after the adoption.
4. An eccentric woman received an adoptive child but found she could not make him over; she tired of the experiment and rejected him.

5. An illegitimate baby boy was handed over by a maternity home and taken in adoption. He proved to be a premature infant in need of special hospital care and he also had a serious cardiac lesion. He had been placed in a home which could not accept a handicapped child.

6. A midwife arranged to hand over a newborn baby to a couple who eagerly wished to rush adoption through at once. A doctor who heard of the plans insisted on delay. In two weeks the Negro paternity of the infant became obvious. Placement in a family unwilling to adopt a black child would have been undesirable.

7. An unmarried woman gave her 2-day infant in adoption. He proved to be mentally defective and was unwanted by the prospective adoptive parents.

8. A woman had taken a 9-month baby into her home. She lavished affection upon him. For a baby, he looked quite normal, smiled, held up his head and apparently paid attention to his surroundings. But examination showed that he was definitely defective. At 12 months his function was at the 6-month level. The agency was advised against adoption placement, but something went amiss and a decree of adoption was granted. At 2 years of age he was still a "lap baby" and had a developmental level of 1 year. He was beautifully dressed in white lace-trimmed clothes. His mother still beamed upon him with a loving smile. She did not yet realize the problems she and her child would face.

In the first four cases, the welfare of the child was not protected adequately. In the last five instances, adoption could have taken place, but only if the adoptive parents were fully cognizant of the true nature of the situation and then wished to offer a home to such a child in need.

§3. THE PHYSICIAN'S RESPONSIBILITY

Every child adoption situation poses three questions:

1. What is the developmental and physical status of the child?
2. Why do the prospective parents wish to adopt a child? Will they provide a home which will protect and foster the child's development, no matter what his potential?
3. Are the natural parents of the child living? If living, why are they abandoning or surrendering the child?

Does the physician have any professional responsibilities to protect the standards and procedures of child adoption? Can he escape these responsibilities even if he would? He helps to bring infants into the world, those who need adoption as well as those who do not. He is regarded as something of a godfather to all children. The consequence is that he is asked frequently to find an infant for adoption, or conversely, he is asked to find a home for an infant who is abandoned or surrendered. These solicitations are likely to be highly charged with emotional tension. Sometimes they are surrounded with great secrecy, and heavy demands are made on the physician's judgment. So grave and complicated are the questions concerning adoption that the physician should hesitate to go too far in answering them. It is neither fair nor wise to expect him to assume the role of an expert in such an exacting field of child welfare. If he offers advice, if he takes any action whatever, he should be aware of the best modern practices in child adoption.

The physician does have essential contributions to make in the regulation of infant adoption. First and foremost, he should throw the weight of his authority behind officially accredited agencies, empowered by law to investigate, supervise and protect the status of the child. Stated negatively, the doctor should not, either as friend or as physician, undertake to initiate and sponsor an adoption. Indeed, it should be unlawful for anyone but a specifically licensed person to place a child in adoption. The physician should discourage all undercover, bootleg adoptions, and frown on the commercialized practices of those adoption agencies and maternity homes which operate on a profit basis. He should not let himself be drawn into privately arranged adoptions, even when they are undertaken in good faith. They are highly questionable ethically, wrong in method and the risk is too great.

Sound procedure also requires investigation of both sides of the adoption equation. In this, the physician's chief function is to render a careful judgment of the physical status and developmental outlook of any child whose adoption is under consideration. Here, developmental diagnosis assumes great social significance, and can reduce greatly the risks of adoption. The report of the physician defines precisely the status of the child and sometimes may give evidence of the child-rearing practices of the prospective parents. The physician also can contribute to an appraisal of the motives and emotional stability of the adoptive parents. Economic status is of less importance than parental attitudes and the wholesomeness of the parent—child relationship. Whether an unmarried person should rear an adopted child has been questioned, usually unnecessarily. In any event, the values of the physician should not enter into this decision.

To what extent the hereditary background of a foster infant should be weighed is a complex issue which often must remain unsolved. In a great many instances, the paternity of the child is unknown. Mental deficiency or poor performance in the mother is not a contraindication to adoption. Statistically, her mental deficiency is most likely to have been acquired rather than inherited; even if hereditary, it is not necessarily transmitted to the offspring in question. The child may well have a normal intellectual potential, even though it must be granted that he may be a carrier of a defect which could reappear in the succeeding generations. Candor requires that significant background factors should be known by the adoptive parents, but when the nature of these factors is interpreted duly, the parents probably will be ready to take a normal risk. There is some risk in all adoption, as indeed there is in the bearing of one's own children.

A probationary period of at least 1 year in the adoptive home should be waived only in very rare instances. It is a trial period which works no hardship, and is a natural supplement to investigation. It enables the physician to recheck his first developmental assessment; it gives all the responsible parties a chance to correct any error that may have been made; and it prevents impulsive errors by simply postponing the legal formalization of adoption. By such safeguards, society is overcoming the too-prevalent notion that adoption is simply a matter of placing an infant starving for love into the arms of parents yearning to bestow love.

The restrictions upon adoption should not be too severe, too rigid or too clumsy. We should think of adoption as a social resource which needs conservation. There are too many poor adoptions, not enough good ones, too many hasty ones and too many tardy ones, because of procrastination which keeps the children too long in boarding homes and congregate institutions.

§4. THE GROWTH CAREERS OF INSTITUTIONAL AND ADOPTED INFANTS

Accepted standards of child welfare now require that all dependent children should be under responsible medical supervision, at least while they are charges of the community. The function and significance of developmental diagnosis in this supervision of foster children can be illustrated best by a few actual cases. The following sketches also indicate how the symptoms of environmental retardation enter into the clinical control of infant adoptions. With the exception of Case 6, those selected are representative rather than exceptional. They exemplify the types of problems which arise both in connection with child adoption and in the supervision of young children placed in foster homes.

Normal infant; institutional retardation. Placed in foster home at 28 weeks; adoptable at 40 weeks

Case 1 was born out of wedlock. The mother was a young woman with a high school education. Birth was normal, and physical development satisfactory. The infant was reared in an institutional baby home. At the age of *24 weeks* she was referred for a developmental examination. The agency had planned to give her in adoption if she was normal.

She was a rather attractive infant with fairly well-defined emotional reactivity, who made a good general adjustment to the examination. However, her performance showed a wide range of scatter from 12 to 20 weeks, suggesting poor integration as well as retardation. There was a remarkable disparity between the level of her supine behavior and that of her sitting behavior.

Supine, she closed in on the rattle promptly and engaged in rattle play. She turned responsively to the ringing of the bell. Seated, she did not regard either cube or pellet, and gave only passive regard to the cup. She gave immediate attention to the examiner's incoming and outgoing hand. These attentional patterns were at a 12-week level, but the history of institutionalization and certain normal features in the behavior picture restrained a diagnosis of mental deficiency. A qualified favorable prognosis was made.

Immediate placement in a boarding home, rather than an adoption home, was recommended to determine the effect of a family environment. At the age of 28 weeks she was placed as a boarder with a foster mother who had three children of her own, ages 7, 10 and 15. These three children took great interest in the infant newcomer, who was returned for reexamination at the age of *40 weeks*.

This examination showed a marked improvement; much of the previous scatter had disappeared. The behavior was now well integrated at a maturity level of 36 weeks. She was healthy and happy. The prognosis now was favorable; the 12 weeks in the foster home had been so beneficial that adoption placement was recommended and accomplished in 1 month. The infant was reexamined at the age of *1 year*. Again she made a good adjustment to the examination, and demonstrated full average development.

In spite of a favorable personality makeup, this child showed symptomatic retardation as a result of 6 months of life in an institution. Three months in a family home was a therapeutic test which demonstrated her essential normality. Had she been referred for examination yet earlier in infancy, she might have been placed in adoption at a much younger age, to the advantage of all concerned. Had she never been subjected to institutional life, the symptomatic retardation never would have been a diagnostic problem.

Prolonged institutionalization, with retardation. Boarding home placement prior to adoption necessary

Case 2 was a small, dainty infant, who was born out of wedlock, birth weight 6 lb 4 oz, with a reported prematurity of 6–8 weeks. The birth history was normal. The child was reared in an institutional baby home, surrendered by the mother and made available for adoption. The report to the child welfare agency outlined the implications of our findings with respect to adoption.

At *17 weeks* this infant adjusted well to the examination. Head control was poor and she was barely able to lift her head in the prone position. She gave prompt attention to toys and made some prehensory effort. She contacted the cubes and grasped the rattle when it was close to her hand. She regarded the rattle in her hand and also engaged in hand regard. She smiled, was reported to laugh and selectively regarded the examiner and observers.

Her general maturity level was approximately 16 weeks, with gross motor behavior near 8 weeks. The supposed prematurity probably represented bleeding after conception. In view of her motor disabilities, we recommended at least one more examination before placement in adoption; however, because the prospect of adoptability was so favorable, we urged prompt boarding home placement. Delay in home placement would have meant prolonged institutionalization and continued deferral of a final adoption recommendation. Prompt home placement, it was hoped, would result in an equally favorable behavior picture at 24 weeks, when she could be recommended for adoption without further delay. The recommendation was not carried out, for a variety of those reasons which so frequently conspire against a child deprived of parental care. This child remained in her institutional home until the age of 15 months.

Examination at *24 weeks* yielded evidence of environmental retardation. Performance was at a 16- to 20-week level. There was delayed, feeble regard for the cube on the tabletop, excessive distractibility of attention to her own hand and to the examiner's hand and excessive regard for the examiner, typical of the institutional syndrome.

At *40 weeks* the syndrome had developed additional characteristic features. She made a poor adjustment to the examiner, with alternating, half-smiling, half-fussing and overfascinated regard. Placed in the crib, she rocked habitually.

At the age of 15 months she was finally placed in a boarding home, where she had an opportunity to play with other children and to find a secure place for herself in the affections of a family. After a period of shyness and withdrawal she made a good adjustment to the children and to the dog (hitherto she had not seen a dog!).

Examination at *18 months* showed the effects of family home life. Her behavior rated near the expected level, and placement in an adoptive home was recommended and carried out promptly.

At *21 months* she gave a high average performance. The mutual acceptance of child and home was evident. Continuation in this home with a view to ultimate adoption at the end of a probationary period of 1 year was recommended.

Legal adoption was completed for the child at the age of 2½ years. This child apparently was not handicapped to any significant extent, if at all, by her prolonged institutional experience. Under slightly different arrangements she might have been placed safely in adoption in early infancy, obviating the intermediate placement in a boarding home for therapeutic and observational purposes. There was no defensible reason for the extremely long residence in the institution.

Retardation and deviation in a faulty family home. Readjustment leading to a favorable adoption

Case 3 was an illegitimate child with a chequered career. After a short period in an institution he was placed in foster home A. Misguided management, combined with his sensitive disposition, caused him to develop atypical forms of behavior during the first year, and he acquired many unusual mannerisms. At the age of *48 weeks* his manipulation of toys consisted of a peculiarly limited patting with the palm or tapping with the index finger. In a similar way he tapped his lip and chin with his thumb. He showed serious retardation on developmental examination, but the behavior picture was so suggestive of environmental factors that the prognosis was qualified. Although the foster parents were anxious to adopt, we advised that the infant spend 6 months in foster home B, while measures were taken to assist the parents in foster home A.

This therepeutic test proved very productive. Reexamination at *56 weeks* of age showed considerable integration of behavior with disappearance of most of the mannerisms; however, retardation was still present.

Reexamination at the age of *18 months,* after 7 months in foster home B, showed further improvement. The boy was now normally assertive and emotionally more hardy. His maturity level of approximately 15 months indicated some developmental delay, but the quality of the behavior suggested potential normal development so strongly that return to his original foster home A was approved.

This restoration had fortunate results. With guidance, the foster mother acquired a better understanding of the child's emotional needs, and she improved her methods of care greatly. Even though 18 months is not the most favorable age for an adoptive placement, this boy made a good readjustment. At the age of *30 months,* developmental examination indicated a full average level of maturity, with attractive personality traits. Adoption was completed, happily for all concerned.

In this case, the combination of a sensitive child and faulty management produced symptoms similar to those which arise under distorting institutional conditions. An aggravated behavior problem might have been induced and adoption seriously prejudiced if this situation had been allowed to drift. Careful diagnosis and parent guidance by the physician, plus a therapeutic trial, placement in new surroundings and the assistance of a social agency, served to safeguard the normal potential of the child.

Normal infant with vital personality traits. Adverse home and institutional conditions.

Case 4 was a small, wiry, buttoned-eyed infant. She had four siblings, an affectionate father, but a psychotic mother. The children were severely neglected, untrained, cruelly treated at times and undernourished. She spent 7 months in this deleterious home environment and 5 subsequent months in a child care institution.

Developmental examination at the age of *12 months* gave no evidence of environmental retardation or deviation. Her performance was consistently and coherently at an average level. Blessed or born with an extraordinarily friendly and outgoing disposition, she had withstood the buffets of her natural home and become a favorite in the institution. Indeed, she was the pet.

Environment is an empty abstraction for clinical purposes, unless reduced to concrete terms which define the actual factors at work and include the susceptibilities and immunities of the child. The poor home had compensating features, and the forceful vigor of the child's characteristics withstood depressing effects. In the institution these same traits bent the environment to her own advantage. The institutional environment did not deflect her; she deflected its forces so that they converged favorably upon herself.

Environmental retardation in a mentally defective child

Case 5 was born out of wedlock and spent all of her first year in an institution. At the age of *6 weeks* she was small and scrawny, but apparently alert and visually perceptive. She made a relatively normal impression. However, at the age of *24 weeks* she presented an atypical behavior picture. She made an undiscriminating adjustment to the examination, and laughed in an automatic manner each time she saw the examiner. She did not perceive or exploit objects on the test table, but when supine engaged in regardful rattle play—a disparity of performance frequently associated with institutional retardation.

Reexamined at the age of *52 weeks,* her behavior proved to be seriously deviated and defective. Our clinical notes described her as a "wistful waif with deadpan expression." Animation was detectable only at rare and brief moments, for example, when she was lifted to a supported standing position. She responded to the translocation with a faint smile and a fleeting chuckle. The only vocalizations heard were soft clicking and sucking noises made with closed lips.

She was content to sit alone for indefinite periods, staring abstractedly and rocking intermittently. Nevertheless, it was possible to divert her attention momentarily to the pellet and bottle. Exploitation was confined to aimless pushing, poking and tapping. Rarely did she grasp an object; she tended to release propulsively before completing the grasp. If grasp was effected, it was maintained briefly with no increase of interest. Visual regard for test objects was highly variable; it might be delayed, precipitate, prolonged, fleeting or lacking altogether. There were snatches of motor behavior consonant with a 40-week level of maturity, but the functional organization of eye and hand were scarcely at a 16-week level. Her behavior was extremely defectively integrated.

Were we dealing with mental deficiency or with environmental deviation and retardation? Hypertelorism was present, and was counted as a developmental anomaly of unfavorable import. Diagnosis was suspended pending a therapeutic test in a foster home.

Reexamination was made at the age of *18 months,* after a period of 5 months in the foster home, where she received intensive individual attention. It took her 2 weeks to adjust to her new home, which she then accepted completely. At the age of 18 months she was the same solemn-faced eerie child. She still crept, as she did at 1 year, but could walk a few steps if placed in standing. Her adaptive behavior did not rise above the 40-week level, and achieved this level only in a fitful, fragmentary way. Her foster home experience had redirected the patterning of behavior into more conventional forms, and she now exploited toys more fully but still at an infantile level. In the absence of toys she reverted to table scratching and atypical fingering movements—manifestly an overdeveloped stereotypy. She articulated no words, but was said to imitate an "oh" sound. The attentional patterns remained bizarre and irrelevant, punctuated with frequent episodes of primitive hand play. The improvement under foster home conditions had been specious rather than fundamental. The therapeutic test did not need to be prolonged; her behavior was defective.

On retrospective analysis, this case proved to be misleading rather than complicated, and confusing rather than involved. It was atypical and yet it represented symptoms which were typical of environmental retardation and of mental deficiency. The case did not require differential diagnosis so much as multiple diagnosis. If in the interest of open-mindedness, we entertained the possibility of psychogenic depression, the case wore a plausible aspect of purely derivative retardation. However, the total evidence pointed conclusively to intrinsically deficient behavioral equipment, incapable of mature organic patterns of attention, and retarded even in the attainment of imperfect patterns. Fortunately, the patterns underwent palpable improvement in a noninstitutional environment; the overindividuation lost some of its excesses. We were left then with the simple but not amazing conclusion that a mentally deficient child can suffer environmental retardation and deviation. The tendency toward overindividuation in a defective infant under institutional restrictions exaggerates the abnormal behavior.

Extreme environmental retardation. Delayed recovery and ultimate adoption
Case 6 was highly exceptional rather than typical, but nevertheless instructive. It was distinguished by the sheer number and complexity of the complications which conspired to retard the course of early development—without, however, permanently impairing the latent normality. These various developmental factors were:

1. Premature birth
2. Congenital syphilis with a 4-plus Wassermann reaction in mother and child (followed by treatment)
3. Breech delivery, hyperactive reflexes, and slight spasticity, suggesting minimal cerebral damage
4. Microcephaly? (x-ray report)
5. Prolonged feeding difficulties
6. Severe upper respiratory infection, associated with acute suppurative otitis media, diarrhea, stomatitis, gingivitis and hemorrhagic nephritis
7. Isolation in hospital for 12 weeks
8. Institutional life for 15 months

The first developmental examination of this child was made at the age of *42 weeks* while she was still in a hospital, having just recovered from her severe illness. A serious degree of retardation was evident, even making allowances for prematurity. The general maturity level was at 20 weeks, but she sat momentarily with active balance. She regarded her own hands intently at the test table, scratched the surface and made poor and only occasionally successful prehensory approach on test objects. Both postural and adaptive behavior were so retarded that the behavior picture was considered defective, with a prognosis of possible improvement in a noninstitutional environment.

However, at the age of *65 weeks* she was still in an institution. The retardation remained severe. The infant was now able to pull herself to a standing position and to cruise holding the crib rail—her best performance at a 44-week level. But her exploitation of test objects was extremely meager and devoid of combining. Adaptive, language and personal—social behavior were scarcely above a 24-week level.

Mental deficiency was suggested strongly by this behavior picture, but at the age of *24 months,* after 9 months in a foster home, she showed considerable improvement. Her attention was more adaptive; she built a tower of three cubes; she scribbled vigorously; she placed a round block in the formboard; she had a vocabulary of seven words; she verbalized her toilet needs. Her performance had risen to an 18-month maturity level—a developmental increment of 12 months in 9 months of chronologic time, denoting a compensatory acceleration. Further improvement was predicted.

At the age of *34 months,* soon after placement in what was to be her adoptive home, the general maturity level had risen to 30 months. At the age of *4 years* she was an alert, attractive child, reaching almost a complete average performance on the developmental schedules—a remarkable realization of latent normality which had been impeded and deflected by numerous factors, both intrinsic and extrinsic.

No single feature of this case is exceptional; but the contemporaneousness, accumulation, and interaction of all the developmental hindrances depressed the level of behavioral output to an extraordinary degree. In retrospect it appears that the secondary factors served to conceal what was probably the most determining factor of all—a mild, slowly resolving cerebral injury. The transition from 30 weeks of institutionalization, to 12 weeks of hospital isolation, to 23 more weeks of institution exacerbated the depressive environmental effects. On the first examination, note was made that this infant was pathetically eager for attention; this item now takes on new meaning.

The total growth career suggests the validity of the concept of *reserve factors,* beyond immediate diagnostic scrutiny. They may come to the rescue when development is threatened or obstructed by hindrances such as were operating in this case.

Prompt adoption of a normal child in early infancy

Case 7, like so many adopted children, was born out of wedlock. Her birth and neonatal history was normal. From the hospital she was placed immediately in a boarding foster home. To paraphrase an old adage, blessed is the child whose developmental annals are brief. A developmental examination at *12 weeks* of age showed normal behavioral maturity. She was a healthy, attractive, well-cared-for infant, who made such a decisively good showing on the developmental schedules that direct placement in an adoptive home was recommended on the basis of this single and early examination.

The behavior picture was fully normal on subsequent examinations, at *28 weeks* and at *40 weeks.* She had been well placed, and adoption was completed in due time.

Early examination and other favorable circumstances permitted early adoption of this child, which has many advantages when adequately safeguarded. If there had been any significant complication in the medical history, or any evidence of even minimal cerebral injury, immediate placement in an adoptive home would have been inadvisable.

In conclusion, when the doctor is asked "Is it safe to adopt an infant?" he well may counter by asking "Safe for whom?"

It is safe for the *infant* if the motives, attitudes and expectations of the adoptive parents are healthy and reasonable.

It is safe for the *parents* if the baby conceals no defect or blemish which would disappoint their reasonable expectations.

It is safe for *society* if the adoption has been undertaken and completed in a realistic, planned manner, which safeguards simultaneously the welfare of the child, all the parents concerned, and any other children involved.

In making adoption recommendations, chief weight should be placed on the developmental examination; however, to repeat, the probationary period of 1 year should be insisted upon, to make possible the correction of any errors made by court, agency, foster parents or physician.

The whole procedure and philosophy of child adoption have suffered from misplaced sentiment and misplaced publicity. We need a more realistic and democratic approach to the neglected areas of this vast problem, especially for the large numbers of unadopted infants and preschool children who are lost from sight, because society has not organized adequate provisions for their identification through social service and developmental diagnosis.

20

Professional Training for Developmental Diagnosis

Every professional must know the history of his discipline and the history, structure, organization and dynamics of the society in which it operates. Without this information he is doomed to be a technician who must soon become obsolete, and possibly a hindrance to the growth and development of his discipline. This is just as true of the pediatrician, neurologist, psychiatrist and other child health workers as it is of any professional. This volume is not a text on medical sociology; however, pediatrics, child development and child health care are fundamental subjects in a health curriculum. The training of the pediatrician is discussed as a paradigm for all child care workers, since he is frequently the leader in one of the important aspects of the welfare of children.

Changes in the nature of pediatric problems place an increasing emphasis on the field of growth and development. How can this emphasis be implemented through medical schools and teaching hospitals? How can developmental pediatrics be brought more squarely into the scheme of pediatric education? This will necessitate basic theoretical instruction, concretely related to the clinical manifestations of normal and abnormal growth and development. This objective cannot be realized simply by adding a new subject, entitled "Growth and Development," to the curriculum. At both undergraduate and graduate levels, medical teaching must be correlated around fundamental themes.

For the pediatrician the fundamental center of correlation is the child as a unitary organism. To achieve this correlation, various fields of instruction can be focused more definitely on the life cycle of the child, using the normal progressions of this cycle as a basic frame of reference. It is this growth cycle which gives unity to the child and which integrates the three aspects of his development—anatomic, physiologic and behavioral. When the study of these aspects is pursued too independently, instruction tends to become disjointed. To be sure, the task of correlation falls in some measure on the student, but it is a complicated task; from

382

the beginning, the medical schools should assist him to acquire an integrated outlook on the whole field of child development, in both its normal and pathologic aspects. We need reorientation in medical instruction more than we need change of content.

There are few subjects in the field of pediatrics which cannot in some way be related to factors of age and developmental maturity. A developmental approach might bring an answer to the oft repeated question, "Why do we teach embryology at all?" Embryology becomes truly a basic medical science in any program of pediatric education which concentrates on the processes of child development. Moreover, we must adopt a point of view that gives equal weight to the postnatal as well as the prenatal aspects of human development. Broadly conceived, embryology includes physiologic functions as well as anatomic structures. There also is an embryology of behavior, and the whole organization of the child's development can be envisaged in terms of a dynamic developmental morphology.

The educational problem is to make these elusive developmental processes real to the student by using all possible concrete methods at our disposal. The teaching task is to take the whole subject out of the academic mist and impart a lively clinical appreciation of the stages and patterns of child development. This can be done only by contact with concrete, illustrative infants and children.

§1. DEVELOPMENTAL DIAGNOSIS IN A HEALTH CENTER

The term health center is used flexibly to denote a well-equipped school, hospital or clinic which maintains basic diagnostic departments, and is staffed with groups of specialists for referral diagnosis. Teaching hospitals which provide in-training and postgraduate courses and conferences would be included. Such centers at present are most highly developed in metropolitan areas, but with the growth of regional hospitals and health centers, comparable facilities will become more widely available.

In a diversified health center, developmental assessment attains the status of a diagnostic specialty. As such it has a separate locus, special examining rooms and appropriate equipment, described in Appendix C. It functions in a manner not unlike radiology, cardiology, opthalmology or any other diagnostic department. It uses its distinctive techniques to determine maturity status and developmental outlook, supplying data which are pertinent for diagnosis, therapy and guidance.

Such a department is in no sense a mere mental testing station. A mental age, an IQ or even a DQ has no value apart from clinical interpretation. In a health center, the findings of the developmental examination can be correlated closely with other clinical data. These findings are of special importance in complex cases requiring differential diagnosis and careful followup. With consecutive examinations, the significance of the developmental findings increases.

The physical arrangements for a division of developmental diagnosis at a health center should be planned to insure optimal responses on the part of the infant and young child. The surroundings should awaken a sense of confidence in the parents as well. The developmental unit offers a favorable setting for imparting the initial diagnosis and guidance; it also facilitates systematic followup supervision throughout the periodic contacts which are so essential in the care of cases of maldevelopment. It helps to counteract some of the prejudices which are associated with hospital and institutional surroundings. The problem of the handicapped child, in particular, often causes intense emotions on the part of the family, which may persist and express themselves in resistance to diagnosis and advice. A properly equipped unit has a reassuring and tranquilizing influence for the child and the parents. The unit serves equally well as a center for the examination and supervision of normal infants and young children.

§2. MEDICAL EDUCATION FOR DEVELOPMENTAL DIAGNOSIS

If developmental assessment is destined to become a major feature of clinical medicine, it is desirable to consider problems of professional training. Ideally, the training of physicians in this field should begin in the undergraduate years. Thereafter, it may be carried through to a high level of postgraduate specialization. The study of normal and abnormal child development can be carried on in close correlation, but knowledge of normality is basic and should be pursued systematically. Concrete, intimate instruction, both at undergraduate and at postgraduate levels, can be provided through the following procedures: self-instruction films and videotapes; observation (with discussion) of developmental examinations of normal infants of varying ages; observation and case studies of a wide diversity of developmental defects and deviations, examined in an active diagnostic service; and graduated participation and practice in the application of the diagnostic procedures.

Self-instruction films and videotapes delineate the characteristic behavior patterns of infants at advancing ages. The student examines these materials in precisely the same manner that he studies his histologic slides. He examines the patterns of behavior, and associates them with a given level of maturity. The basic films chart the normal progressions of behavior; he studies defects and deviations in the same manner. This method makes behavior as organic and as tangible as tissue, and child development is made less elusive.

Visual instruction must be supplemented by demonstration of the living, growing infant. For this purpose, a series of developmental examinations of normal babies at progressive ages should be arranged. Conferences should follow immediately; they lead to comparative, systematic discussions, because the diagnostic examinations of behavior are made with a standardized technique which exposes the lawful sequences of development.

The significance of normality is enhanced by similar examinations of retarded, atypical, disturbed, damaged and defective infants. Any pediatric service provides a plentiful array of these conditions of maldevelopment, and they are examined by the same standardized methods employed with normal infants. Many of these infants may have been examined at earlier ages. This doubles and deepens the developmental perspective. The child, in conference, is compared not only with the normal stages of maturity, but also with his previous self (often with previous cinema or videotape records to document the evidence). These comparative approaches give reality to development as a process.

Videotape is an important instructional tool. Immediately after the examination, the student can see himself and the child in action in order to improve his technique. During the examination, events sometimes move so rapidly that the time for comments by the instructor already has passed; with some students such comments merely unnerve them and interrupt their thought processes. Also, the student can do examinations on his own and review the videotape with the instructor later.

The extent to which each of these methods can be employed depends on the length and organization of the pediatric experience for the medical students and on whether or not house staff is assigned a regular rotation on the developmental service. When the student's exposure is casual and brief, one of the most effective methods of stimulating interest is to encourage use of the Developmental Screening Inventory (DSI) with all patients. After the student has done his own screening examination and committed himself to a diagnosis in writing, a full examination can be done with him and the diagnosis and its implications discussed. The same procedure can apply to the house staff, but they find it more difficult to free themselves from providing care for their patients; they are most likely to participate when they have an immediate diagnostic problem they wish to solve.

When a definite block of time, such as a month, is available, the methods outlined above can be employed more or less concurrently—beginning, of course, with the normal, but rapidly giving the student actual experience in carrying out examinations, and assigning him full responsibility for obtaining the history, discussing the findings with the parents and writing the report of the examination. Two or three students can be supervised by a single instructor; often the beginner can see more of the child's behavior when he is observing the examination of a fellow-student rather than being preoccupied by the sheer mechanics of what he is to do next. Through systematic presentation and concrete application, the study of developmental pediatrics can be raised to the status of a clinical subject.

§3. SPECIALIZATION IN DEVELOPMENTAL DIAGNOSIS

For the postgraduate physician, who already has served an internship and residency in pediatrics or neuropsychiatry, schools and hospitals should provide a specialty fellowship. After an induction period of observation and of laboratory study of the self-instruction materials, he is initiated into actual examinations of normal infants. As he develops skill and confidence, he is given increasing responsibility for the cases admitted on the diagnostic service. He soon discovers that the behavioral procedures are not as simple or as automatic as they may have appeared; he begins to respect them as diagnostic tools, which must be applied with finesse, and which become effective only as he can bring clinical experience to bear critically. In this way he arrives at a holistic outlook upon both everyday and unusual problems of child development. He thinks in terms of stages and patterns of maturity, of developmental trends and capacities. He envisages the infant and child as a growing organism, whose mechanisms of development permit understanding, diagnosis and supervisory guidance.

To acquire the essential longitudinal experience, 1–2 years full-time in a diagnostic and advisory service which deals with a wide range of normal and abnormal developmental conditions is necessary. Ideally, this specialized training should include periodic contacts with well-baby supervision, the examination of infants prior to adoption and foster home placement, of preschool children under nursery school auspices, and the differential diagnosis of a diverse array of mild and severe abnormalities, including mental deficiency, convulsive disorders, malformations, degenerative processes, cerebral injuries and other traumata, anoxia, infections and toxic lesions, endocrine dysfunctions, sensorimotor handicaps and environmental shocks and stresses.

§4. IMPLICATIONS

Enumeration of these conditions reminds us how gravely they may be neglected in the absence of facilities for developmental diagnosis and supervision. Whether the child be normal, handicapped or defective, the crucial medical and social problems call for a judgment of developmental status, outlook and guidance. Since it is the pediatrician or the family doctor who should be involved with these problems, it is he and his associates who must be prepared to make as definitive diagnoses and plans for treatment as possible.

Clinical and teaching personnel must be prepared adequately for responsibilities and leadership in the field of developmental pediatrics. To meet the mounting social demands, there must be reorientations in pediatric education. There is no other specialty equipped to take over this task of preventive and supervisory medicine. Allergist, cardiologist, orthopedist, neurologist and psychiatrist all have a role to play; but the pediatrician alone is conversant with the infant as a whole and concerned with the maintenance of a forward-moving sequence of development. The pediatrician is adept with babies, and by tradition he is interested in their total welfare.

The historic evolution of clinical pediatrics has very naturally brought about a preventive outlook for the period of infancy and early childhood. Psychiatry, on the other hand, has derived its ideas largely from the psychopathology of the adult, and from prescientific, untested and even detrimental concepts of psychodynamics and psychotherapy, with almost as many schools of thought as there are psychiatrists. Neurologists still are oriented to a great extent towards the isolated lesions that are superimposed on an organism which has matured.

There is arising a whole new school of neuropsychiatry, of which this volume hopefully is an example, that views mental and developmental disorders as a group of specific clinical entities or syndromes. The new approach considers interrelated genetic, physiologic and social variables to be exceedingly important in the diagnosis, treatment and rehabilitation of patients.

For the vast work in the mental hygiene of the early years, we must look to pediatric medicine. Pediatrics already is committed to a form of supervisory health protection which includes mental as well as physical welfare. Bodily growth and psychologic development cannot be divorced, and the methods of developmental diagnosis contain the essence of a psychiatry of infancy and early childhood.

To understand any child, whether normal or handicapped, we must understand his development. His ways of maturing are the sum and substance of his psychosomatic constitution. Only as we become aware of them can we plan adequate procedures of guidance and control. Here lies the significance of periodic examinations of infant behavior as an approach to the mental hygiene of early child development.

For most preventive efforts we must seek social action.

Appendices

Appendices

Appendix A

Examination Techniques

The basic methods of procedure for the developmental examination of behavior have been outlined fully in the body of the text. Appendix A is a brief manual of directions which assembles details of the examination for convenient reference in seven sections:

1. Examination Materials
2. Induction to the Examination
3. Examination Sequences
4. Examination Procedures
5. Record Forms, Recording and Appraisal
6. Questions for the Developmental Screening Inventory (DSI)
7. Table of Temporary Behavior Patterns

§1. EXAMINATION MATERIALS

The materials for the developmental examination are simple, and are pictured in Fig. 2-2. Some of the materials can be secured or improvised readily. However, care should be taken not to use objects which are markedly different from those prescribed in dimensions, texture and appearance, since weight and size do influence an infant's ability to handle them. The materials are being distributed on a nonprofit basis by the Psychological Corporation, 304 East 45 Street, New York, New York 10017. They may be purchased singly or in complete sets.

A list of the materials needed for carrying out the examination follows:

Ball, large: 4–6 inches in diameter
Ball, small: $2\frac{1}{2}$-inch diameter
Bell: 3 inches high with wooden handle and metal bowl $1\frac{1}{2}$ inches in diameter
Bottle, glass: $2\frac{1}{2}$ inches high, mouth 1-inch diameter

Catbells: 3 metal bells on shower curtain ring

Color forms and card: $8\frac{1}{2}$ by 11 inches with five forms and matching cut-outs, red. Circle, 2-inch diameter; square, 2-inch sides; triangle, $2\frac{5}{8}$-inch sides; semicircle, $3\frac{1}{4}$-inch diameter; cross, $2\frac{7}{8}$-inch length, $\frac{15}{16}$-inch wide arms

Crayons: Staonal #2 general marking crayon, 5 inches long, $\frac{1}{2}$-inch diameter

Cubes: ten red; 1-inch edges; squared corners; made of hard wood

Cup: aluminum, 12-ounce capacity, $3\frac{3}{4}$-inch top diameter, $2\frac{1}{4}$ inches high

Forms for drawing: set of 5-inch by 8-inch cards with form in heavy black outline. Circle, cross, square and triangle: 3-inch diameter, length or sides; rectangle with diagonals: 4 inches by $2\frac{3}{4}$ inches; diamond: $2\frac{1}{4}$ inches each side

Forms for tracing: $8\frac{1}{2}$-inch by 11-inch sheet. Double diamond: $2\frac{3}{8}$-inch outer sides, $\frac{3}{8}$-inch distance to inner sides. Double cross: $3\frac{3}{8}$-inch outer length, $1\frac{1}{2}$-inch wide outer arms, $\frac{3}{8}$-inch distance to inner figure

Formboard, three-hole: green, $\frac{1}{2}$-inch board, 6 inches by 14 inches. Three holes equidistant from each other and from edges: circle, $3\frac{1}{2}$ inches; triangle, $3\frac{3}{4}$ inches; square, $3\frac{1}{16}$ inches

Formboard blocks: white, $\frac{7}{8}$ inches thick. Circle: $3\frac{3}{8}$ inches; triangle: $3\frac{5}{8}$ inches; square: $2\frac{15}{16}$ inches

Picture book: Goosey Gander (a variety of nursery rhymes)

Picture card (a): dog, shoe, cup, house

Picture card (b): clock, basket, book, flag, leaf, star

Pellets: pink or white sugar, 6-mm diameter; flat on one side, convex on other

Performance box: green, $15\frac{3}{4}$ by $10\frac{1}{4}$ by $7\frac{1}{2}$ inches. Made of two layers of $\frac{3}{16}$-inch plywood, the inner layer shorter around the open end to serve as a stop for the drawer, which fits inside and holds the test materials (bottom of drawer matches $15\frac{3}{4}$ by $10\frac{1}{4}$ side of box). The open end of the box is $10\frac{1}{4}$ by $7\frac{1}{2}$ inches. With this placed to the observer's right, there is a metal carrying handle on the top ($15\frac{3}{4}$ by $7\frac{1}{2}$ inch side) and three holes on the $15\frac{3}{4}$ by $10\frac{1}{4}$ inch side facing the observer. From left to right, equidistant from the edges and each other, these are a vertical rectangle 3 by $1\frac{1}{8}$ inches, a $\frac{3}{4}$-inch circle, and a horizontal rectangle $1\frac{1}{4}$ by $\frac{3}{4}$ inches. The box is prevented from opening by inserting a metal pin through a hole drilled in the handle side of the box *and* through the drawer, attaching the pin to the outside of the drawer with a short chain to avoid its loss. See Figure 2-2.

Rattle: 6 inches long; bowl $2\frac{1}{4}$-inch diameter; slender $\frac{3}{8}$-inch diameter handle

Ring and string: wooden, red, 4-inch diameter; 10-inch string, 1-mm diameter

Test objects: pencil, key, penny, knife

Tricolored rings, or plaques on chain

Weighted blocks: set of five, $\frac{3}{4}$-inch edges, from 3 to 15 grams in weight

Picture books, cups, rattles, crayons and small plastic bottles can be purchased in local stores. Pellet substitutes must be firm as well as edible; cinnamon red-hots are satisfactory, but raisins and baby aspirin are contraindicated. Multicolored cubes and natural wood rings are available in quantity from the following sources (1973 prices given):

1-inch colored cubical blocks—$5.25/100
    Ideal School Supply Company
    11000 Lavergne Avenue
    Oaklawn, Illinois 60453
Hold-Tite 4-inch wooden embroidery hoops—$4.60/dozen
    Gibbs Manufacturing Company
    606 Sixth Street, N.E.
    Canton, Ohio 44702

Additional items which are part of the Stanford—Binet Test include[71] :

Aesthetic comparisons card
Geometric forms: card and matching forms
Incomplete man drawing
Missing parts card
Pictures, three cards

Special clinical equipment, described in Appendix C-2, includes the following items:

Clinical crib (Figure C-4)*
Tabletop for clinical crib*
Portable test table (Figure C-6)
Adjustable clinical table (Figure C-7)*
Infant examining chair (Figure C-5)*

The following items are obtainable on the open market:

Child's kindergarten table
Child's kindergarten chairs
Mirror (attach roller shade)

§2. INDUCTION TO THE EXAMINATION

Preliminaries and introductory procedures must be adapted to the general maturity characteristics of the child. The appropriate forms should be collated and the examining equipment and materials positioned properly for the expected maturity before starting the interview. Special suggestions and directions for making an easy, natural transition to the formal examination are given briefly below.

Note that the mother takes the active part in the induction. The examiner does

---

* The starred equipment is not essential if an ordinary examining table, portable test table and kindergarten table and chairs are provided.

not touch the child, but keeps his distance. This applies to all the age ranges. The mother removes shoes and stockings from an *infant* during the interview; other clothing is removed prior to the postural situations unless it interferes with the examination before this.

4–20 Weeks Maturity. At a favorable moment when the infant is quiet and contented, ask the mother to place him on his back on the crib platform or examining table. The examiner stands at the infant's left; the mother is invited to take a chair placed at the infant's right when it is clear that the infant is happy. The Supine Situations follow. Many 16- and 20-week olds may resent the supine position; the mother should be asked if her infant prefers the sitting position.

24–36 Weeks Maturity. At a favorable moment while you are interviewing the mother, when the infant is unapprehensive and playful, offer him an introductory toy, such as the tricolored rings or catbells. When he accepts it, he has accepted you. If he is empty-handed when it is time to proceed to the examination, and especially if a transition from another room has been made, reoffer a toy. When he accepts it, place a second introductory toy on the tabletop in plain view, and take your place at the left of the crib or examining table. If a clinical crib and chair are available, ask the mother, who is on the right of the crib, to place the infant in the chair and to "stand by" until all is well. The belt has been attached on the mother's side of the chair, left unfastened on the examiner's side. Secure the belt tightly around his chest; the infant is better able to tolerate what appears to be excessive compression than any degree of looseness which permits him to slump. Insufficient chest support interferes with adequate arm control. Move the tabletop into position, and if necessary, call the infant's attention to the toy on the table. As soon as he begins to play, the mother sits down at the right. If there is no crib, the infant examining chair and portable test table are utilized, on an available flat surface. If there is no special clinical examining equipment available, ask the mother to seat herself in a chair at a desk and hold the infant on her lap. The mother supports the infant firmly around the chest with both hands, leaving both of the child's arms free for exploitation. The appropriate Tabletop Situations follow.

40–56 Weeks Maturity. Offer the introductory toy as for the 24–36-week maturity levels; when the infant accepts it, ask the mother to place him seated on the crib platform or examining table before the tabletop. She stands by until all is well. The tabletop is moved into place by the examiner, who stands at the left (the mother again is at the right), and the infant's attention is called to the introductory toy on the tabletop. As soon as the infant begins to play, the mother sits down. The appropriate Tabletop Situations follow.

15 Months Maturity. At this age the size of the child is the chief factor in determining where the examination is done. If he is physically large, then placement in the kindergarten chair before the kindergarten table probably is best (18–36 Months, below). If he is small, then the examination is conducted best at the adjustable clinical table used for the interview, with the child on the mother's lap. The bag of varicolored building blocks which was on the table when mother and child entered the room, and with which the child was playing during the interview, is removed and is replaced by the Picture Book, which the examiner begins to demonstrate.

18–36 Months Maturity. The child is invited to play with some toys. He is shown the kindergarten table with a bag of varicolored blocks on it, and shown his chair. The mother seats herself at the right of the table, the examiner at the left. The mother may be asked to help the child into his chair. When the interview is over, the child is asked to help put the blocks back into the bag because there are more toys to play with. This task is completed, with or without the child's cooperation, and when the child is in position behind the table, seated or perhaps still standing, the examiner begins to demonstrate the Picture Book which follows.

Modifications for special circumstances. If the infant is emotionally fragile, cries and is unwilling to leave his mother, the examination is carried out at the adjustable clinical table with him on his mother's lap. Usually, by the time the postural situations are reached, the infant is sufficiently disarmed to accept placement in the crib; the mother keeps her hands on him and cuddles close when she first places him before the mirror. The examiner will have to decide in each instance whether or not to risk trying the examination in the crib first. He should not hesitate to return the infant to the mother's lap if necessary. A fragile older child also may need to start out on the mother's lap.

The best dictum when the child is suspicious is *"Examiner, withdraw!"* Sit back in your chair and increase the distance between yourself and the child. If the child is inhibited and won't participate, let the mother offer the test object at the beginning. If that fails, put one on the tabletop, pick up a book or papers, hand a book to mother, and *ignore him.* It may take 15–30 minutes and changes of the items offered, with occasional comments and demonstrations, before the child suddenly breaks through and participates. With an older child, the formboard often is successful as a last resort; with an infant, the bell.

If the child has a motor handicap for which he needs assistance with sitting, he is strapped into the supporting chair or held on his mother's lap, depending on his age and size. But the initial sequence may be the one appropriate to his chronologic rather than his motor age (Chapter 10).

§3. EXAMINATION SEQUENCES

So far as possible, the standard sequences should be followed in the administration of the examination situations. The standard sequence differs with the maturity and age of the child. There are three maturity zones: Supine; sitting, either with support or free; and locomotor. The recommended standard sequence for each of these maturity zones, presented in Table 4-1, is repeated here for readier reference. The table here also serves as a *finding list for all the examination situations,* each being assigned an identification number. This number refers to the procedural syllabus in Appendix A-4, where each situation is described separately.

Table A-1 (4-1).   EXAMINATION SEQUENCES

Supine (Crib)

4 Weeks Zone	16 Weeks Zone
0 - 4 - 8 weeks	12 - 16 - 20 weeks

Situation Number*	Situation Number
Supine-------------------------- 1	Supine-------------------------- 1
Dangling ring-------------------- 2	Dangling ring-------------------- 2
Rattle-------------------------- 3	Rattle-------------------------- 3
Social stimulation-------------- 4	Social stimulation-------------- 4
Bell-ringing-------------------- 5	Bell-ringing-------------------- 5
(Pull-to-sitting)--------------- 6	Pull-to-sitting---------------- 6
Sitting supported---------------50	Sitting supported---------------50
Standing supported--------------51	*Chair--Table top*-----------------
Prone--------------------------52	*Cube 1,(2)*----------------------7,8
	Massed cubes-------------------11
	(Cup)--------------------------16
	Pellet------------------------18
	(Bell)------------------------22
	Mirror------------------------24
	Standing supported--------------51
	Prone--------------------------52

Sitting (Chair) | *Sitting (Crib)*

28 Weeks Zone	40 Weeks Zone
24 - 28 - 32 weeks	36 - 40 - 44 weeks

Chair--Table top Situation Number	Table top Situation Number
Cube, 1,2,3--------------------7,8,9	Cubes 1,2,3--------------------7,8,9
Massed cubes--------------------11	Massed cubes--------------------11
(Cup and cubes)----------------17	Cup and cubes-------------------17
Pellet-------------------------18	Pellet-------------------------18
Bell---------------------------22	*Pellet beside bottle*------------19
Ring and String----------------23	*Pellet in bottle*---------------20
Mirror-------------------------24	Bell---------------------------22
Sitting supported---------------50	Ring and String----------------23
Standing supported--------------51	Mirror-------------------------24
Prone--------------------------52	*Mirror and ball*----------------25
(Supine)------------------------ 1	*Sitting free*--------------------53
(Dangling ring)----------------- 2	*Creeping*-----------------------54
(Rattle)------------------------ 3	*Rail*--------------------------55
Social stimulation-------------- 4	*Cruising*-----------------------56
Bell-ringing-------------------- 5	*Walking supported*--------------57
(Pull-to-sitting)--------------- 6	

( ) = Situation sometimes omitted for special reasons.
Italicized items appear for first time in this sequence.
*Situation number identifies the test situation described
in Appendix A, Examination Procedures.

§4. EXAMINATION PROCEDURES

The purpose of this section is to outline in detail the procedures used in administering the individual examination situations. The general character of these procedures already has been indicated in Chapters 3 and 4. The procedures described here are appropriate for children at the stated ages or maturity levels. For deviant children with motor or sensory handicaps, modifications may be necessary;

Table A-1 (4-1) *Continued*

Sitting (Crib)	*Locomotor (Child's Table and Chair)*
52 Weeks Zone	**18 Months Zone**
48 - 52 - 56 weeks	15 - 18 - 21 months

	Situation Number		Situation Number
Table top		*Picture book*---------------------40	
Cubes 1,2,3---------------------7,8,9		Cubes: Tower---------------------12	
Tower 2------------------------10		(*Train*)------------------13	
Massed cubes---------------------11		Cup and cubes---------------------17	
Cup and cubes---------------------17		Pellet beside bottle--------------19	
Pellet beside bottle--------------19		Drawing: *Spontaneous*-------------26	
Pellet in bottle------------------20		Scribble imitation------27	
Ring and String-------------------23		*Vertical strokes*-------28	
Drawing-Scribble imitation--------27		(*Circular scribble*)-----29	
Formboard-----------------------35		Formboard-----------------------35	
Ball play------------------------46		(*Picture card*)------------------41	
Mirror--------------------------24		(*Performance box*)----------------36	
Mirror and ball-------------------25		(*Test objects*)-------------------45	
Sitting free---------------------53		*Small ball: Throwing*-------------46	
Creeping------------------------54		*Directions*----------47	
Rail----------------------------55		(*In box*)------------48	
Cruising-------------------------56		*Kicking*-------------------------58	
Walking supported---------------57		*Sitting in chair*-----------------50	
		Walking, running-----------------59	
		Stairs-------------------------60	

Locomotor (Child's Table and Chair)	
24 Months Zone	**36 Months Zone**
21 - 24 - 30 months	30 - 36 - 42 months

	Situation Number		Situation Number
Picture book---------------------40		Picture book---------------------40	
Cubes: Tower---------------------12		Cubes: Tower---------------------12	
Train---------------------13		Train---------------------13	
(*Chimney*)----------------14		Chimney-------------------14	
Cup and cubes---------------------17		*Bridge*-------------------15	
Drawing: Spontaneous-------------26		Drawing: Spontaneous-------------26	
Vertical strokes--------28		Strokes-------------28,30	
Horizontal strokes------30		*Circle*-----------------31	
Circular scribble-------29		*Cross*------------------32	
(*Picture cards*)------------------41		*Incomplete man*----------33	
Formboard-----------------------35		*Trace diamond*-----------34	
Performance box-------------------36		(*Picture cards*)------------------41	
(*Name*)--------------------------42		Formboard-----------------------35	
(Test objects: Names)------------45		*Color forms*----------------------37	
Use)------------45		(Name, *sex*)----------------------42	
Small ball: Throwing-------------46		(*Comprehension*)------------------43	
Directions-----------47		(*Digits*)------------------------44	
(In box)------------48		*Geometric Forms*------------------38	
Kicking--------------------------58		*Weighted blocks*------------------39	
Sitting in chair-----------------50		*10 Pellets and bottle*------------21	
Walking, running-----------------59		(Test objects-use)---------------45	
Stairs--------------------------60		Small ball: Throwing-------------46	
		Prepositions--------49	
		Kicking--------------------------58	
		Running--------------------------59	
		Walking on tiptoe----------------61	
		Standing on one foot-------------62	
		Jumping-------------------------63	
		Stairs--------------------------60	

these in turn will need to be interpreted in light of the clinical nature of the abnormality.

Although the situations are discussed separately here, the examiner should not regard them as a series of rigidly separate tests. The examination should be conducted as an organic unit; the transition from one situation to the next should be accomplished in such a way that the child's working rapport is not only preserved but actually increased. The examiner should shift readily to a higher or lower maturity level when the child's performance indicates a change is necessary. On the other hand, the examination must not assume so much informality that the situations lose their integrity as diagnostic tools. They should be administered in the prescribed standardized manner. The examiner must strike a very careful balance between uniformity and variation.

For each situation, an opportunity for exhibiting the most advanced behavior should always be given, i.e., request and gesture before demonstration. Attention should be secured to all demonstrations. The examiner is not trying to trick the child. *Never* give the child a chance to refuse by asking "Do you want to . . .," "Would you like to . . ." *Always* phrase activities positively: "We are going to . . .," etc.

The examiner must maintain firm control of the situation at all times, and may have to ask the parent to desist from interfering. It goes without saying that he treats the child and the parents with courtesy, indicates his approval of the child's behavior and, of course, says "please" and "thank you."

In the following syllabus, each situation carries an identification number in the left margin; these assigned numbers are referred to in Chapter 3, in Table 4-1 and in Appendix A-3.

Supine Situations

1. Supine

4–20 WEEKS MATURITY. The examiner simply observes the child's posture and spontaneous activity. If necessary, he may be spoken to in a reassuring tone.

At *24 and 28 weeks* the infant may resent being placed down, and the supine situation follows all other situations. Offer the dangling ring or rattle immediately without preliminary observation. If infant is not appeased immediately, terminate the examination.

2. Dangling Ring

4–28 WEEKS MATURITY. The end of the string is held in the examiner's left hand, and the ring permitted to hang down. In this manner the ring is brought about 4–6 inches above the infant's feet and then moved headward. The ring is held 10–12 inches above the face. If the infant's head remains turned to the side, move the ring into the line of vision. Observe his reaction to the perception of the ring.

4–16 WEEKS MATURITY: RING FOLLOWING. Move the ring slowly through an arc of 180° from one side of the infant's head to the other, keeping the distance from the head about constant. If regard shifts to the examiner's hand, continue the arc until the hand rests on the crib platform. Repeated trials may be made, and every opportunity should be given the infant to demonstrate his optimal capacity to follow a moving object (ring or examiner's hand). The speed of the moving ring should be adapted to the infant's abilities in ocular pursuit.

12–28 WEEKS MATURITY: RING EXPLOITATION. If the infant reaches for the ring immediately, ring following is omitted. The ring is held suspended within reach above the upper chest, and the infant's prehensory efforts are observed. The ring may be steadied if he sets it swinging. If it is not grasped, it is then held about 1 inch from the *palm* to see if this distance can be completed. If necessary it is placed in his hand, selecting first the hand most favorable for ring regard. His perceptual and manipulatory exploitation of the ring is observed. Both hands are tried and any differences in control noted. If he drops the ring before observations are complete, it may be restored to his hand; otherwise it is gently recovered and the Rattle Situation (3) presented immediately. If regard for the examiner predominates, he steps out of range of the infant's vision. If tonic-neck-reflex positions persist after 16 weeks and interfere with exploitation, the examiner gently cradles the infant's head in his palm to assist in maintaining midpositions, at the same time allowing free head rotation. This technique permits distinguishing motor from adaptive components of behavior.

3. Rattle

4–28 WEEKS MATURITY. The rattle is held in the examiner's left hand, presented silently over the infant's feet and moved to within reaching distance over the upper chest of the supine infant. His perceptual response is observed; the rattle may be moved into the line of vision if the infant's head is averted, or it may be shaken gently to elicit attention. The infant is allowed to grasp the handle of the rattle if he can, or it is brought near his hand or finally placed in his hand. The hand most favorable for rattle regard is selected first, and the fingers may have to be opened. His exploitation of the rattle is observed and also his response to loss of the rattle. If he retains it, it is removed gently and placed at his side within his visual field to determine his ability to pursue the lost rattle and to roll to prone.

4. Social Stimulation

4–28 WEEKS MATURITY. The infant is shifted gently so that he lies across the table or crib; the examiner may make the shift himself, taking his position at the infant's feet. The examiner bends over the infant and smiles, talks and nods his head, endeavoring to elicit attention and social response. The situation is not prolonged; it is continuous with the Bell-Ringing Situation (5). After *24 weeks* social responses are elicited opportunistically.

5. Bell-Ringing

4–28 WEEKS MATURITY. While the infant is active and the examiner is talking to him, the rattle is shaken two or three times and then silenced. It is held 2–3 inches from first one ear and then the other, and the adaptive responses noted. The bell then is rung sharply in a similar manner. The examiner should take care that the infant does not spy the examiner's hand or the objects. If the infant is exploiting a toy and makes no response, the toy should be removed before repeating the procedure. If the infant objects to supine, the behavior should be elicited in the sitting position. After *28 weeks,* if there is any question of a hearing defect, this behavior should be elicited opportunistically.

6. Pull-to-Sitting

4–28 WEEKS MATURITY. Having secured the infant's attention, the examiner holds the infant's hands in his own and exerts gentle, steady forward traction on the arms. If the infant's head lags excessively, the traction is released and the infant raised to the sitting position with head supported. Otherwise, the pull-to-sitting is completed, and the infant's head control and participation in the pull are noted.

Tabletop Situations

Between *12 and 20 weeks,* the tabletop situations follow the Pull-To-Sitting Situation (6). At *24 weeks* of age and thereafter, the examination begins with the tabletop situations. At *24 and 28 weeks,* the postural and supine situations follow the tabletop situations. Thereafter, the supine situations are omitted.

Presentation. From *12 to 56 weeks,* a standard procedure is used to present all single test objects of this group. They are held in the examiner's left hand; the object is brought to the center of the far edge of the table; the infant's attention to the presentation is elicited, tapping the object against the table edge if necessary. In extreme cases it may be necessary to use other methods to elicit attention; their use should be noted. When attention is secured, the object is brought smoothly toward the infant and placed in easy reach on the table before him. In presentation, the object should be held so that it is more conspicuous than the examiner's hand. Placement should be central to favor a free choice of handedness in grasp. The examiner should withdraw his hand as inconspicuously as possible.

From *15 to 36 months,* the presentations are made by simply reaching in from the left and placing the test objects in easy reach on the table before the child. The presentation of multiple object situations will be described individually.

Transitions. In making the transition from one situation to another in the tabletop situations, the examiner should take advantage of the infant's dropping a toy to substitute the next. If it is necessary to remove a toy from the infant's hand, it should be grasped lightly, and then the examiner should wait until the infant releases the object. At times it is necessary to present the next object, permitting the infant to retain the one in hand until it can be withdrawn opportunistically. Transitions should be made smoothly; *the infant should never have to wait* for the next object.

No situation is prolonged. One or two minutes of exploitation is usually ample, but sometimes two or three demonstrations are necessary before the child performs.

7. First Cube

12–56 WEEKS MATURITY. The cube is presented and the infant's responses observed. Before *24 weeks* of age, the cube is offered to his hand or even placed in the hand.

8. Second Cube

20–56 WEEKS MATURITY. While the infant is holding the first cube, a second is presented in a similar manner and the response is observed. Before *28 weeks* of age, it may be placed in his hand.

9. Third Cube

20–56 WEEKS MATURITY. While the infant is holding two cubes, the third cube is presented and the response observed. Before *28 weeks* of age, the cubes may be placed in his hands or contact and grasp induced by placing the infant's hands on top of the cubes on the table.

10. Tower of Two

48–56 WEEKS MATURITY. The examiner secures the child's attention, then builds a tower of two cubes at the edge of the table, places a third cube within easy reach on the table and offers the child a fourth. He may point to the third cube, and he may dismantle and replace the demonstration tower once or twice to induce performance. Finally, the infant may be permitted to remove the tower cube, but initially the demonstration tower should be out of reach.

11. Massed Cubes

16–56 WEEKS MATURITY. The examiner arranges the ten cubes into a square of nine, the tenth cube surmounting the mass, and the cubes are advanced into position. Cubes that the infant pushes to the platform or floor are retrieved later; cubes that he pushes out of reach on the table may be moved nearer. If necessary, he may be helped to grasp a cube.

48 WEEKS–15 MONTHS MATURITY. If the tower building was not elicited during the Tower of Two Situation, another attempt may be made to elicit this behavior.

18–36 MONTHS MATURITY. The cubes are placed in position, and the child is asked to "make something." His spontaneous exploitation of the cubes is observed.

12. Tower

15–36 MONTHS MATURITY. While the child is holding a cube, the examiner points to a cube on the table, saying *"Put it here."* If the child does not comply, the examiner may start the tower, placing one or more cubes. Each time the child places a cube successfully, or at appropriate intervals, he is praised, *"Good!"* and encouraged to continue. If the child has difficulty with precise release but clearly understands the concept of building, the examiner may hold each succeeding cube the child himself puts into position.

13. Train

18–30 MONTHS MATURITY. The examiner says, *"I'll show you how to make a choo-choo train,"* and removes all the cubes. He then shows the child how to align four cubes, saying *"This is one car, another car and another car."* He pushes his train across the table, saying *"Choo-choo-choo,"* then dismantles the model and shoves the disarranged cubes toward the child, saying *"You make it."*

14. Train with Chimney

24–36 MONTHS MATURITY. The examiner says *"Now I'll show you a fancy choo-choo train,"* and removes all the cubes. As in the Train Situation, he shows the child how to align four cubes and then places a fifth on top of an end cube, saying *"These are the cars; this is the chimney for the smoke to come out."* He again pushes his train across the table, saying *"Choo-choo-choo,"* dismantles the model and shoves the disarranged cubes toward the child, saying *"You make it."* If the child fails to place the chimney, he may ask *"Where is the chimney?"*

15. Bridge

36–42 MONTHS MATURITY: COPYING. Behind a screen, or opportunistically while the child is still occupied with the train, the examiner builds a three-cube bridge (illustration, p. 103) and says *"See the house I've made. It has a downstairs, an upstairs and a door,"* pointing to each of the blocks and the separation in turn. Leaving the model in place, he gives the child three cubes, saying *"You make it down here."*

30–36 MONTHS MATURITY: IMITATION. The examiner says, *"Now I'll show you how to make a little house." "One like this, one like this and one like this,"* as he places each block in turn. *"See, it has a downstairs, an upstairs and a door,"* again pointing to each block in turn. He leaves the model in place and gives the child three cubes, saying *"You make it down here."*

16. Cup

12–20 WEEKS MATURITY. The cubes are removed and the cup is presented upright with the handle pointing directly toward the child. This situation is omitted if the infant already has contacted any of the cubes.

17. Cup and Cubes

28–56 WEEKS MATURITY. While the infant is holding at least one of the massed cubes, his attention is called to the upright cup tapped at the edge of the tabletop. The cup is then placed within reach to the left of the massed cubes, and the spontaneous play observed. After *36 weeks,* when the infant has a cube in his hand, the examiner points into the cup, saying *"Put it in there."* If he does not comply, the examiner takes a cube, and securing the infant's attention, drops the cube into the cup. His responses are then observed.

15–24 MONTHS MATURITY. The cup is added within reach to the left of the mass of cubes. If the child does not begin to insert the cubes, the examiner says *"Put the blocks in."* If the child hesitates, or starts removing the cubes after a few are inserted, he says *"More." "Put them all in,"* and pushes one cube after another toward the child by way of proffer. The examiner may pick up and hold cubes out to the child, or gently inhibit his removing them from the cup. When all the cubes have been put into the cup, he holds out his hands and says *"Give me the cup."*

18. Pellet

12–52 WEEKS MATURITY. The examiner presents the pellet, flat side up. If it is hit from position, it is restored. The examiner intervenes, if possible, before the infant carries the pellet to his mouth. If the infant is too quick, the mother is reassured that the pellet is harmless. Sooner or later, infants usually let the pellet slip out of the mouth, when it can be removed. The examiner may attempt to call the infant's attention to the pellet by tapping his finger near it. He must withdraw his hand slowly, since the younger infants tend to follow the moving hand. Usually it is best to wait until the infant spies the pellet when he looks down at the tabletop.

19. Pellet Beside Bottle

36–48 WEEKS MATURITY. The examiner places the pellet and the bottle on the tabletop, the pellet at the infant's right. He calls attention to the pellet, then to the bottle and to the pellet again, tapping back and forth. Pushing the pellet with thumb and index finger of his left hand and holding the bottle with his right hand, the examiner brings both simultaneously within reach and observes the spontaneous behavior. If the infant picks up only the bottle, attention may be directed towards the pellet again while the infant holds the bottle. As in the pellet situation, the examiner should forestall the infant from eating the pellet.

52 WEEKS–21 MONTHS MATURITY. The examiner presents the pellet and bottle simultaneously from the left, placing them side by side on the tabletop, the pellet at the child's right. The child is asked to put the pellet in the bottle; demonstration will be needed before *15 months*. After he has inserted the pellet, the examiner says *"Get it out." "Get the candy,"* demonstrating dumping if necessary. If the examiner is trying to induce placing the pellet into the bottle, the pellet is left *beside* the bottle following any demonstration; conversely, if he is trying to elicit dumping the pellet out, it is left *inside* the bottle.

20. Pellet in Bottle

36–56 WEEKS MATURITY. The examiner takes the top of the bottle in his left hand and holds it so the bottom is at about the level of the infant's eyes. The pellet, in the right hand, is held over the mouth of the bottle. Securing the infant's attention to the pellet in hand, he drops it into the bottle. The bottle is then placed on the table with the pellet visible to the infant, or he is allowed to take it from the examiner. If the pellet does not fall out of the bottle during exploitation, the examiner simulates this by tossing one on the tabletop, making sure that the infant does not see him do it.

21. 10 Pellets and Bottle

36+ MONTHS MATURITY. Ten pellets and the bottle are placed before the child, the pellets to the side of the preferred hand. *"Put them all in the bottle just as fast as you can, but one at a time."* Repeat instructions if the child dawdles or grasps several pellets at once. The time taken to complete the task is recorded, provided the pellets are put in singly. The pellets are then placed on the other side of the bottle, and use of the dominant hand is inhibited, unless this results in vigorous protest or refusal.

22. Bell

20–48 WEEKS MATURITY. The bell is presented without being rung and placed upright on the tabletop. At *20 weeks* the infant may be assisted to grasp it, and it always may be restored if dropped. Ringing is demonstrated if necessary; this requires a broad sweep of the examiner's whole arm.

23. Ring and String

28–56 WEEKS MATURITY. The examiner holds the ring in the left hand, the end of the string in the right, pulling the string taut. The ring is placed out of reach at the far edge of the table, the end of the string within reach obliquely toward the infant's right. The string is held in place on the table and attention called to the ring by tapping it up and down. If the string is flipped out of position it may be restored. If the string is ignored in the oblique position, it may be placed with the end of the string directly in front of the infant. If he is unable to secure the ring and threatens to cry, it is moved within reach. At *48–56 weeks,* dangling of the ring may be demonstrated, using an up and down movement and broad sweeps of the arm.

Mirror Situations

24. Mirror

16–56 WEEKS MATURITY. The roller shade is lifted, and the infant turned around to face the mirror. If the supporting chair was used, the infant should be removed and firm support around his chest maintained by the examiner. He should sit or be held very close to the mirror. If he stares at his feet or the image of his feet, the examiner may tap the glass to call the infant's attention to his face.

25. Mirror and Ball

40–56 WEEKS MATURITY. While the infant is looking in the mirror, the small ball is held behind him so that its image is visible in the mirror, and his reaction noted. If there is no response to the image of the ball, bring it slowly forward until he turns his head to look at it, as a gross test for visual fields. He is then given the ball to hold in his hand and exploit. If the infant has difficulty retaining the ball, substitute the ring.

Drawing Situations

In these situations, if the child objects to releasing the crayon, the examiner may use a second crayon. After each demonstration, he must conceal this crayon. Each demonstration should have the child's attention and be made so the child can see what is being done. Each demonstration should be done on a *fresh* side or piece of paper.

26. Spontaneous Drawing

15–36 MONTHS MATURITY. A piece of paper at least 5 by 8 inches is presented from the left and placed on the tabletop directly before the child. The examiner steadies the paper with his left hand, unless the child objects, and places the crayon in the center of the paper, pointing away from the child. He is asked to *"write on the paper"* or to *"make something."* At *24-36 months* he is asked what he has made. The crayon is handed to the child if he does not pick it up.

27. Scribble Imitation

52 WEEKS–18 MONTHS MATURITY. The examiner takes the crayon from the child with his right hand, and turns over the paper on which the child has been marking. Holding his arm elevated so that his arm and hand do not obstruct the child's view, and securing the child's attention, the examiner scribbles back and forth several times across the top of the paper with well-defined strokes. He then replaces the crayon in a central position, saying *"You make it."* He may put it in the child's hand in a position such that when the child pronates, the point of the crayon contacts the paper.

28. Vertical Stroke Imitation

15–36 MONTHS MATURITY. The examiner takes the child's crayon, draws one or two decisive strokes down the left margin of the paper, and releases the crayon centrally, saying *"You do it. Make one just like this."* The stroke movement may be slightly exaggerated. Rapid and slow movements may be tried to induce imitation.

29. Circular Scribble Imitation

18–24 MONTHS MATURITY. The examiner takes the child's crayon and makes a decisive circular scribble, going round and round at the top of the page. He releases the crayon centrally, saying *"You make it."* (Note: The words "circle" and "round" are never used unless the child says them first.)

30. Horizontal Stroke Imitation

24–36 MONTHS MATURITY. The examiner takes the child's crayon and draws one or two decisive strokes across the top margin of the paper, releases the crayon centrally, and says *"You make it. Make it just like this."* Rapid and slow strokes are tried, as for the vertical stroke. When it is included, the Horizontal Stroke Situation follows the Vertical Stroke Situation (28).

31. Copy Circle

30–42 MONTHS MATURITY. The examiner shows the child a card on which a circle (diameter 3 inches) has been drawn, saying *"Make one like this"* (pointing) *"on your paper"* (pointing). If the child's response is unsatisfactory, the circle is demonstrated, followed finally by the Circular Scribble Situation (29). (Note: The circle is never named to the child unless he says it first.)

32. Cross Imitation

30–42 MONTHS MATURITY. The examiner takes the child's crayon and makes a decisive cross at the top of the paper, vertical stroke first, saying with each stroke, *"One like this, and one like that."* He releases the crayon centrally, saying *"You make it."* (Note: The cross is never named unless the child says it first.)

33. Incomplete Man

36+ MONTHS MATURITY. The sheet with the outline of the Incomplete Man is placed before the child and he is asked, *"What is this?"* *"What do you call it?"* At this age he is unlikely to add any parts, even if they are indicated to him.

34. Tracing Diamond

42+ MONTHS MATURITY. Fold the paper so that only the diamond figure is showing and then say, *"Now take this pencil and draw a line right around here, but don't go outside of the lines."* *"Start right here, but be careful and don't go outside the lines."* The examiner may demonstrate by moving a pencil along the proper path without marking on the paper.

Form Perception Situations

35. Formboard

The examiner always introduces the formboard from the left and places it on the tabletop before the child, the round hole at the child's right, the apex of the triangular hole centered to the child's body and pointing away from him.

48–56 WEEKS MATURITY. The examiner holds the formboard securely on the table with his left hand and with his right offers the infant the round block, presenting it centrally. After the infant has looked over the board and manipulated the block, the examiner points to the round hole, saying *"Put it in."* The examiner then takes the round block and ostentatiously inserts it in its hole. If the infant cannot remove it, the examiner demonstrates how to lift one edge up with his thumb. Finally, the examiner takes the block out, restores it to the infant and again tries to induce insertion or removal.

15 MONTHS MATURITY. The examiner holds the formboard securely on the table with his left hand and with his right offers the child the round block, presenting it centrally. After the child has manipulated the block, the examiner points to the round hole, saying *"Put it in."* Either the child or finally the examiner inserts the block. The examiner then says *"Watch what I'm doing,"* lifts the board, leaving the block on the table, and turns the board slowly through an arc of 180°, keeping it flat. As he releases the board on the table, he shoves the block to the table edge at the right. The round block is now on the table directly in front of the square hole. If the child does not pick up the block, the examiner offers it centrally, saying *"Put it in."* The examiner may point to the correct hole if the child fails to respond, or place the block himself before repeating the rotation.

18–36 MONTHS MATURITY. The examiner places the formboard on the table and puts the three blocks in front of their respective holes between the board and the child. *"Put the blocks in."* Before the examiner makes any further moves, the child's spontaneous behavior with each of the three blocks in turn is observed. If the child has difficulty in adjusting corners in insertion, he may be assisted. If he piles all three blocks, then insertion is demonstrated, the examiner patting each block into place, and the situation is represented. When all three blocks are in (except at *18 months*), the examiner lifts the board, leaving the three blocks on the table, and turns the board slowly through an arc of 180°, saying *"Watch!"* In this maneuver he keeps the board flat. As he replaces the board on the table, he shoves the blocks back toward the edge of the table. The round block is now on the table directly in front of the square hole and vice versa. *"Put them in again—nicely."* If the child makes an error and persists in it, the examiner may say *"Where does it go?"* He may then run his fingers back and forth on the far side of the board and finally point to the correct hole. Repeated trials may be given.

36. Performance Box

18–24 MONTHS MATURITY. Holding the box in the left hand by the handle and keeping hold, the examiner presents the box from the left. The holes in the side of the box face the child. The examiner offers the square white block with his right hand. If the child does not bring it to the correct hole, it is indicated to him. *"Put it in."* *"All the way."* If necessary, the examiner completes or starts insertion. The open end of the box is then turned toward the child, and he is invited to get the block out. Tilt the box a little if necessary. Return the box to position and say *"Do it again."* In restoring the block to the child after demonstration, turn the block in handing it to him so that he must make a manual adjustment to insert it. If failure threatens to annoy the child, assist him to insert it. If the child holds the square block in his own right hand, the open end of the box is angled away from him; conversely, if he uses his left hand, insertion is facilitated by angling the open end of the box toward the child. It may be necessary to shift the box from one position to the other as the child transfers the block.

37. Color Forms

30–36 MONTHS MATURITY. The color card is placed on the tabletop, the circle in the upper right corner, and the child's attention is called to the forms on the card. He is given the cut-out *round* form and asked *"Where does it go?" "You put it on."* If he fails to place or misplaces it, the examiner demonstrates and allows the child to place it. He is then given, in order, the *square*, the *triangle*, the *semicircle*, and the *cross*. Vary the instructions. *"Look at all of them on the paper." "Put it where it fits," "Put it right on top of the one that looks just like it."* The round form is the only one demonstrated; all other placements or pointings are accepted by the examiner, who merely says *"Good,"* after each response, whether right or wrong.

38. Geometric Forms

36+ MONTHS MATURITY. The card with the ten geometric forms is placed before the child and the matching circle is laid on the X in the bottom row. *"Where is the other one?" "Show me the other one just like this." "Where does this one go?"* If the child fails to indicate or incorrectly indicates the circle, the examiner points to it. The child may be allowed to place the test form on its corresponding one on the card. The circle is the only one demonstrated; all other placements or pointings are accepted by the examiner, who merely says *"Good,"* after each response, whether right or wrong. Present in order the circle, square, triangle, oval, rectangle, hexagon, rhomboid, square with indented arc, trapezoid and irregular.

39. Weighted Blocks

42+ MONTHS MATURITY. Place the 3- and 15-gram weights before the child. *"See these blocks?" "They look just alike but they are not; one of them is heavy and one of them is light." "Try them and give me the heavy one."* If the child chooses a block without testing them, say *"No, like this,"* and demonstrate lifting the blocks pincerwise, one in each hand. *"Now you try them and give me the heavy one."* Juggle the blocks, reversing their position, for second and third trials.

Verbal Situations

If the child fails to talk, all the verbal situations except Picture Book (40), Picture Cards (41), and possibly use of Test Objects (45) are omitted.

40. Picture Book

15–36 MONTHS MATURITY. In this age range the examination begins at this point. The picture book *Goosey Gander,* is on the table, and the examiner starts by describing what is on the cover. He then may call attention to the salient features on each page, may ask for comments and responses on each page or may skip through the book rapidly. The situation is used to introduce the examination, to get the child talking, if he will, or to give the examiner a chance to disarm the child by responding for him. The examiner may ask the child to turn pages or to complete the turn he starts; he may need to do all the turning.

At *15–24 months* the child is asked first to name and then to point to eyes, shoes, hat, dog, spoon, baby, umbrella, etc. Failing both, the examiner himself points.

At *30–36 months* the child is asked to tell and then to indicate what the child is doing (crying, eating, sleeping). Again the examiner answers his own questions if need be.

At *36 months* he may be asked to recite a familiar nursery rhyme, with or without help.

41. Picture Cards

18–36 MONTHS MATURITY. Four pictures (cup, dog, shoe, house). The picture card is presented from the left, the examiner retaining hold of the card. The examiner points to the pictures, asking *"What is this?"* in the following order: (1) dog, (2) shoe, (3) cup, (4) house. For any the child does not name, ask in the same order, *"Where is the doggie (or bow-wow)?" "Show me where it is."* Failing both, the examiner may point before proceeding to the next situation.

24–36 MONTHS MATURITY. Six pictures (flag, clock, star, leaf, basket, book). The examiner says *"Here are some more pictures,"* presenting the card from the left and retaining hold of the card. The examiner points to the pictures, asking *"What is this?"* in the following order: (1) clock, (2) basket, (3) book, (4) flag, (5) leaf, (6) star. For any the child does not name, ask in the same order, *"Where is the clock (tick-tock)?" If he does not respond to the first two or three pictures, the remainder are omitted.*

42. Name and Sex

30–36 MONTHS MATURITY. The examiner says *"What is your name?"* If the child does not respond or gives only his first name (or nickname), the examiner says "(Johnny) What?" A response is never insisted upon. The examiner then says to a girl, *"Are you a (little) girl or a (little) boy?;"* to a boy, *"Are you a (little) boy or a (little) girl?"* He may also say *"Which are you?"* if the response is unsatisfactory. Do not say *"Are you a girl?"* If the question is to be repeated, give the full form.

43. Comprehension Questions A

36+ MONTHS MATURITY. The examiner asks, in order: *"What do you do when you are hungry?"* *"What do you do when you are sleepy?"* *"What do you do when you are cold?"*

44. Digit Repetition

30–36 MONTHS MATURITY. If the child is giving verbal responses fairly freely, say to him *"Listen, say 4–2."* *"Good."* *"Now say 6–4–1."* The numbers should be recited in a spaced manner. The following digit series are used: 641, 352, 837. Do not repeat a series. If necessary, ask the child to wait until you have finished, with *"I am going to say the numbers first and when I am through I want you to say them."* *"Listen carefully."*

45. Test Objects

18–30 MONTHS MATURITY. The examiner shows the child the following objects in order: pencil, shoe (the examiner's), key, penny and small ball, saying *"What is this?"* At *24–30 months,* if the child responds correctly, say *"What do you do with it?"* The child who does not talk may pantomime a correct response. The examiner retains possession of all the objects except the ball, which the child is allowed to take. If the 18–21-month child does not respond to the first two objects, skip to the small ball.

Ball Situations

46. Ball Play

48 WEEKS–15 MONTHS MATURITY. The test table is removed; the child remains seated on the examining table or crib. The examiner goes to the foot of the table or crib and casts the ball to the child, assisting him to grasp it if necessary. The examiner then holds out his hands and asks the child to throw the ball. He may take it and bounce it away from the child and back again once or twice to induce responsive release.

18–36 MONTHS MATURITY. The child has just been given an opportunity to name the ball. He is given the ball and the table is moved aside so that he is free to get up and walk around. The examiner holds out his hands and says *"Throw it."* It sometimes helps if the examiner squats down to the child's level.

47. Directions with Ball

18–30 MONTHS MATURITY. The examiner squats down, secures the child's attention and gives him the ball, saying *"Now we are going to play a game with the ball."* *"Don't throw it."* *"Put it on the TABLE."* The request may be repeated several times, but an incorrect response is accepted with *"Good."* Secure the ball again, and give it to the child, saying *"Put it on the CHAIR."* Then, warning the mother not to hold out her hands, *"Give it to MOTHER."* Then, *"Give it to ME."* *"Thank you."* If necessary, add *"I'll give it back to you."*

48. Ball in Box

18–21 MONTHS MATURITY. The examiner holds the performance box upright on the floor, tipping the open end toward the child, and invites him to throw the ball in. *"Can you get it?"* *"Get it out."* Safeguard the child when he leans into the box, when he lifts it and sets it down, when he pulls it over. He may be recalled to the task if he abandons it. If he is unsuccessful, the examiner says *"Turn the box over."* He may demonstrate and finally get the ball for the child. (Note: A very tall child can reach the ball, invalidating the situation.)

49. Prepositions with Ball

36+ MONTHS MATURITY. The child has just thrown the ball. The examiner takes the ball and gives it to the child, saying *"Put it ON the chair."* Then *"Put it UNDER the chair."* An incorrect response is accepted and the Directions with Ball Situation (47) given. Follow correct responses with additional prepositions: *"in back of, in front of, beside."*

Postural Situations

After *15 months,* the postural tests are so free as to be incidental rather than imposed formally. During the interview the child may have demonstrated most of his gross motor capacities. Items *61–63* are exceptions to this rule. If the infant of *36–56 weeks* is in the crib or on the floor during the interview, he also may demonstrate most of his locomotor abilities, and they need not be elicited formally.

From *4 to 56 weeks,* the infant's shoes and stockings are removed prior to the examination and the remainder of his clothes taken off prior to the postural situations. From *15 to 36 months,* he keeps his clothes throughout all situations. Depending on the indications, they then may be removed for further observation of locomotion and any necessary physical examination.

50. Sitting Supported

Note: This should *always* be carried out on a *hard* surface.

4–20 WEEKS MATURITY. After the Pull-To-Sitting Situation (6) is completed or the infant turned away from the Miror Situation (24), the examiner squats down to the infant's eye level and supports him by the sides of the thorax. Sitting posture and control are observed; the examiner may release his support slightly to determine the infant's participation in the sitting act. Of course, the infant should not be permitted to fall, nor to lean too far forward, nor should this test be at all prolonged.

24–36 WEEKS MATURITY. At the conclusion of the mirror situations, the examiner turns the infant on the platform, squats down to the infant's eye level, and removes his hands, though they remain protectively near. If necessary, the infant's legs should be arranged in flexion and abduction and his hands placed in a propping position alongside his feet. If he maintains his balance, a lure (tricolored rings or catbells) may be offered to test his ability to lift one hand and still maintain the position, and to induce, if possible, an erect sitting position. The examiner is on the alert to protect the infant from losing his balance.

51. Standing Supported

4–28 WEEKS MATURITY. The infant has been sitting, supported by a hand on either side of the chest. The examiner now lifts the infant to the standing position, holding him securely under the arms. He releases his support slightly to ascertain the infant's participation in the standing act. At *32 weeks,* the examiner shifts his hands, one at a time, and holds the infant's hands at shoulder height with elbows fully extended to provide only balance, not support.

52. Prone

4–20 WEEKS MATURITY. The examiner has been holding the infant facing him in standing. He now turns the infant away from him and adjusts his hands from behind so that his right hand is under the infant's right arm, the left under the left. Suspend the infant horizontally (face down) over the crib and lower him to the platform. As he is placed on the platform, adjust the infant's arms if necessary so they are not caught under his chest or extended footward. If the infant does not turn and lift his head, the examiner takes the head between his hands and gently turns it so that the infant's chin rests on the table. If the head lifts, dangle a lure (tricolored rings or catbells) before his eyes, raising it to induce optimal head lifting. Do not prolong this situation if there is any protest. At this age range, this situation concludes the examination.

24–32 WEEKS MATURITY. The infant has rolled to or is placed in the prone position on the crib platform by the maneuver described above. Dangle a lure (tricolored rings or catbells) before his eyes, raising it to induce optimal head lifting. Then put the lure on the platform just out of reach at the side; as the infant PIVOTS, keep the lure just out of reach. Try one side then the other. When the infant has exhibited his abilities in prone, reward him with the lure. At this age range, this situation concludes the examination.

53. Sitting Free

36–56 WEEKS MATURITY. The child sits on the crib platform or other *hard* surface. After his sitting posture has been observed, place the lure on the platform before him, just out of reach. Observe his ability to either lean forward and reerect himself or go over to the prone position.

15–36 MONTHS MATURITY. The child's ability to seat himself in an ordinary kindergarten chair and to get up again are noted, either at the beginning of the examination or opportunistically.

54. Creeping

36–56 WEEKS MATURITY. The infant either is placed in prone or has attained the prone position himself. Using a lure (tricolored rings or catbells) kept just out of reach, try to induce forward locomotion.

55. Rail

36–56 WEEKS MATURITY. If he does not creep over to the crib rail, the child is placed seated, facing it. The examiner dangles a lure at the top of the rail, just out of reach, to induce the standing position. If necessary, place the infant's hands on the rail; the mother may dangle the lure and call him. If he does not pull to his feet at the rail, place him standing, so that he may hold the rail, and release support. At *36 weeks,* this situation concludes the examination.

56. Cruising

40–56 WEEKS MATURITY. While the infant is standing holding the rail of the crib, dangle the lure just out of reach and to the side. If the infant steps sideward, keep the lure out of reach. Try one side, then the other. When his cruising ability has been observed, place the lure down on the platform of the crib and observe the infant's efforts to lower himself to sitting again.

57. Walking Supported

40–56 WEEKS MATURITY. The examiner takes the infant's hands and tries to induce him to walk. Many infants will perform better if allowed on the floor at this time; some will do better if the mother holds the hands. If he walks when both hands are supported at shoulder height, or overhead just for balance, try releasing one hand. At this age range, this situation concludes the examination.

58. Kicking

18–36 MONTHS MATURITY. The small ball is removed and the large ball handed to the child. After he has thrown it once or twice, it is placed on the floor before him and he is asked to *"Kick it." "Give it a good kick." "Kick it with your foot."* The examiner may take the hand of a younger child if he does not respond, and repeat the request. If he responds with the hand held, release his hand and repeat the request again. The examiner may also demonstrate kicking if the child does not respond; he must use a wide swing of the leg. (Note: The child should be in the center of the room so that he cannot hold wall or furniture to steady himself.)

59. Walking, Running

15–36 MONTHS MATURITY. Observed incidentally during the interview or ball situations.

60. Stairs

15–36+ MONTHS MATURITY. If stairs are available and the behavior has not been observed opportunistically prior to the examination, encourage the child to creep up or to walk up and down in the erect position, holding his hand when it is indicated. At *15–24 months,* this situation concludes the examination.

61. Walking on Tiptoes

30–36 MONTHS MATURITY. The examiner demonstrates walking on tiptoes, making sure to lift his heels clearly from the floor, saying *"You do what I'm doing."* He may hold the child's hand initially.

62. Standing on One Foot

30–36 MONTHS MATURITY. Lead the child to the center of the room so that he cannot hold wall or furniture for support. Stand facing the child and say *"Stand on one foot like this."* *"Pick up your foot."* The examiner demonstrates and encourages, *"That's the way!"* *"Keep it up."* Showing the child how to hold dress or trousers with both hands facilitates the performance. When the child lifts his foot, the examiner may time the performance in an approximate way by counting *"1–2–3"* at the rate of one per second.

63. Jumping

30–36 MONTHS MATURITY. The examiner jumps in place with both feet off the floor, saying *"You do what I'm doing."* If stairs are available, ask the child to jump off the bottom step. Occasionally an equivalent height is available for this purpose. At *30–36 months* this concludes the examination, except for Stairs (60).

§5. RECORD FORMS, RECORDING AND APPRAISAL

The sample record forms presented in this section are those which we have found most convenient for gathering complete information. The procedures are presented in the order in which they usually are carried out. The forms are designed for a minimum of writing and are almost completely precoded for IBM card punching. Data for a fictitious case have been entered on the specimen forms to illustrate their practical application. Reference should be made to Chapter 4 for a general discussion of the use of these forms in developmental diagnosis.

History

Historic information is acquired by two methods, and ideally should be obtained before proceeding to the examination. Items from the Developmental Screening Inventory (DSI) are mailed to the parents prior to their appointment in order to obtain information about the child's developmental progress. This inventory is found and discussed in Chapter 17, and in Appendix A-6. For older children the DSI questions generally cover all of past development. For children under 18 months of age, current behavior usually is sufficient, provided inquiry always is made about whether there has been any loss of behavior once acquired. When this information is available, it substitutes for page 8 of the Developmental History Form. The parents' answers to these questions are transferred to the corresponding items on the developmental schedules.

When the parents bring their child for his assessment, the Developmental History Form is completed. The information obtained should be recorded directly on the form as it is elicited from the parents. This form is self-explanatory and coding can be done after the entire examination is completed. Finally, additional items of behavior and any necessary clarification of the parents' responses to the DSI are recorded directly on the appropriate developmental schedules as they are being obtained.

CHILD DEVELOPMENT SERVICE
Department of Pediatrics
Medical College Hospital, U.S.A.

FORM 4B
2/73

DEVELOPMENTAL HISTORY

IDENTIFYING INFORMATION

Name: _John Doe_   Hospital #: _X-1234_   Case #: _0001_

Address: _3 James Street - Williamstown, N.Y._   Phone: _123-4567_
Father's name: _George_   Family physician: _Joseph Doctor, M.D._
Mother's name: _Mary_   Address: _Williamstown, N.Y._
Date of birth: _1-1-72_   Date of Interview: _7-28-72_

     CHIEF COMPLAINT:
       Told us he was mongoloid - but he's behaving so

      well we wonder.
     PARENTAL HISTORY:

COLS.
1-2. | 4 ¦ 1 | Father's age (in years)
3-4. | 3 ¦ 9 | Mother's age (in years)
5-6. | 1 ¦ 2 | Father's education (in years completed)
7. | | Father's occupation _Plumber_
       How long? _20 yrs._ Previous, if less than one year _____
8-9. | 1 ¦ 2 | Mother's education (in years completed)
10. | | Mother's occupation _Housewife_
       How long? _____ Prior to marriage _None_

HEALTH STATUS OF PARENTS:
(Code for each: 0-None; n-Decade of onset; 9-No data)   Record details briefly:

	Father	Mother		Father	Mother
11-12.	0	0	Epilepsy		
13-14.			Mental deficiency		
15-16.			Cerebral palsy		
17-18.			Mental disease		
19-20.			Diabetes		
21-22.			Heart deformities		
23-24.			Blindness		
25-26.			Deafness		
27-28.			Other; Specify:		

CONSANGUINITY:

29. | 0 | Are father and mother related except by marriage?
          0. No
          1. Yes: Specify:_____
          9. No data

CHILD DEVELOPMENT SERVICE
Developmental History--Page 2

FORM 4B
Case #: _0001_

OTHER PREGNANCIES: (Indicate ordinal position of patient)

	Name	Birth Date	Birth Wt. or L of G	Complications of Pregnancy, esp. bleeding and toxemia
1.	James	1957	6-10	-
2.	Anne	1960	7-0	-
3.	Miscarriage	1961	2 mos.	Bleeding first month
4.	Bruce	1962	7-3	-
5.	Pt.	1972		
6.				
7.				
8.				

	CP	MD	CONV	Congenital Anomalies	Death & Age	If applicable School & Grade
1.	-	-	-	Hare lip		10 Forrest
2.	-	-	-	-		7 Brooks
3.	-	-	-	-		-
4.	-	-	-	-		5 Brooks
5.						
6.						
7.						
8.						

(CP = CEREBRAL PALSY; MD = MENTAL DEFICIENCY; CONV = CONVULSIONS)

HEALTH STATUS OF IMMEDIATE RELATIVES:
Record existence of above conditions, those inquired about for parents and other possibly hereditary conditions in grandparents, aunts, uncles or cousins. Diagram family trees on other side if necessary.

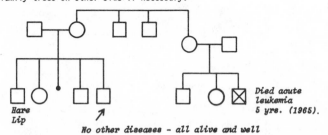

Hare Lip

Died acute leukemia 5 yrs. (1965).

No other diseases - all alive and well

CHILD DEVELOPMENT SERVICE   FORM 4B
Developmental History--Page 3   Case #: _0001_

OTHER PREGNANCIES: (Summarize from information on page 2)

COLS.
30-31. | 0,4 | Number of other pregnancies
32. | 1 | "   "   "   miscarriages
33. | 0 | "   "   "   stillbirths
34. | 0 | "   "   "   neonatal deaths
35. | 0 | "   "   "   later deaths
36. | 0 | "   "   "   living, "damaged"
37. | 0 | "   "   "   living and well
----
38. | 0 | "   "   "   prematures

PRESENT PREGNANCY:

                Birth Weight _5-8_   lbs. & oz.   Expected date of birth _1-15-72_
39-42. | 2 ¦ 4 ¦ 9 ¦ 5 | grams _2495_   Sure of expected date? _Yes_
                                                   Last periods normal? _Yes_
                Total weight gain _19_

                Gain of 5 pounds in one week? _0_

                Albuminuria _0_

                Edema (hands & face) _Feet only_

                Blood pressure _Normal_

                Convulsions or coma _0_

                Visual disturbances _0_

                Treatment for toxemia _0_

43. | 0 | Toxemia
               0. None
               1. Possible preeclampsia
               2. Preeclampsia
               3. Eclampsia
               9. No data

               (Code for following columns: 0-No; 1-Possible; 2-Yes; 9-No data)
               (1°, 2°, 3° = Trimester of Pregnancy)

44. | 0 | Chronic nephritis or hypertension

45-47. | 0 ¦ 0 ¦ 0 | Acute pyelonephritis
          1° 2° 3°
48-50. | 0 ¦ 0 ¦ 0 | Hyperemesis _____
          1° 2° 3°
51-53. | 0 ¦ 0 ¦ 0 | Medications--other than vitamins, Fe, Ca; Specify:_____
          1° 2° 3°
               _____

               Febrile illness_____

               Rash_____

               Diagnoses_____

CHILD DEVELOPMENT SERVICE
Developmental History--Page 4

FORM 4B
Case #: _0001_

COLS.

54-56.	$\lfloor 0 \mid 0 \mid 0 \rfloor$ $1°\ 2°\ 3°$	Rubella
57-59.	$\lfloor 0 \mid 0 \mid 0 \rfloor$ $1°\ 2°\ 3°$	Other febrile illness with rash
60-62.	$\lfloor 0 \mid 0 \mid 0 \rfloor$ $1°\ 2°\ 3°$	Other febrile illness without rash
63-65.	$\lfloor 0 \mid 0 \mid 0 \rfloor$ $1°\ 2°\ 3°$	Operation with general or spinal anesthetic
66-68.	$\lfloor 0 \mid 0 \mid 0 \rfloor$ $1°\ 2°\ 3°$	Any illness requiring oxygen
69.	$\lfloor 0 \rfloor$	Gestational diabetes (see Col. 20 for other diabetes)
70.	$\lfloor 0 \rfloor$	Maternal iso-immunization _0_ Blood type, if known _0+_

73. | $\lfloor 0 \rfloor$ | Status of patient: 0 ✓ Out-patient; 1 ___ In-patient. Check one.

75-78. $\lfloor 0 \mid 0 \mid 0 \mid 1 \rfloor$ Case Number
79-80. $\lfloor 4 \mid 1 \rfloor$ Card Identification

(Code for following columns: 0-No; 1-Possible; 2-Yes; 9-No data; IP-Intrapartum)

1-3.	$\lfloor 2 \mid 0 \mid 0 \rfloor$ $1°\ 2°\ 3°$	Spotting _At time first menstrual period_
4-7.	$\lfloor 0 \mid 0 \mid 0 \mid 2 \rfloor$ $1°\ 2°\ 3°\ IP$	Bleeding _Moderate - after membranes ruptured_
		Placenta previa _?_ or
8.	$\lfloor 9 \rfloor$	Abruptio placentae _?_
9.	$\lfloor 9 \rfloor$	Post-partum hemorrhage _?_
10.	$\lfloor 1 \rfloor$	Month prenatal care started _2nd_ (Code: 1,2,3-Appropriate trimester; 4-Labor; 5-None; 9-No data)
11.	$\lfloor 1 \rfloor$	Duration of labor _4 hours_ 0. None 1. Normal 2. Precipitate 3. Prolonged, disproportion 4. Prolonged, other reason
12.	$\lfloor 0 \rfloor$	Multiple birth 0. No 1. First twin 2. Second twin 3. Triplet
13.	$\lfloor 0 \rfloor$	Delivery 0. Normal vertex 1. Breech 2. Mid or high forceps 3. Cesarean section 4. Version and extraction
14.	$\lfloor 0 \rfloor$	Cord difficulty; Specify:

CHILD DEVELOPMENT SERVICE
Developmental History--Page 5

FORM 4B
Case #:___0001_____

NEONATAL PERIOD:
(Code: 0-No; 1-Possible; 2-Yes; 9-No data)

COLS.
15-16. | 0 ¦ 8 | Number of days infant stayed in hospital_____

17. | 0 | Delayed cry_____

18. | | Delayed respiration_____

19. | ↓ | Resuscitation used_____

20. | 1 | Cyanosis__*First day a little blue*_____

21. | 2 | Oxygen, not routine *For 2 days*_____

22. | 0 | Respiratory distress_____

23. | 2 | Apneic episodes *Stopped breathing once on first day*_____

24. | 0 | Abnormal cry_____

25. | | Twitching_____

26. | | Convulsions_____

27. | | Sucking difficulty_____

28. | | Gavage feeding_____

29. | | Dropper or Breck_____

30. | | Jaundice, not exchanged_____

31. | ↓ | Jaundice, exchanged_____

SUBSEQUENT COURSE: (If present essentially since discharge from hospital)
(Code: 00-No; nn-Duration in months; 99-No data)

COLS.
32-33. | 0 ¦ 0 | Sucking difficulty) Breast fed_____ Over 10 min. first oz._____

34-35. | ¦ | Swallowing difficulty) _____

36-37. | ¦ | Choking) In absence of obstructive_____

38-39. | ↓ ¦ ↓ | Vomiting) lesions_____

40-41. | 0 ¦ 1 | Crying, # of hours (Code actual hours; 00-not at all; 01-only if hungry or wet)

42-43. | 0 ¦ 0 | Crying, duration in months if 4 or more hours per day_____

44-45. | ¦ | Limpness_____

46-47. | ↓ ¦ ↓ | Stiffness (Distinguish strength from hypertonicity)_____

48-49. | 0 ¦ 0 | Other; Specify:_____

CHILD DEVELOPMENT SERVICE
Developmental History--Page 6

FORM 4B
Case #: _0001_

ILLNESSES:
Record information in spaces below and then code for each numbered item.
(Code, Col. 1: 0-No; 1-Possible; 2-Yes; 9-No data)
(Code, Cols. 2 & 3: 00-No; nn-Month of onset; 99-No data)

COLS.

Cols.	Code	Item	Description
50-52.	0|0|0	1.	Accident without CNS symptoms
53-55.	||||	2.	Accident with CNS symptoms
56-58.	||||	3.	General anesthetic
59-61.	↓|↓|↓	4.	Meningitis or encephalitis
62-64.	2|0|4	5.	Illness with encephalitic symptoms
65-67.	0|0|0	6.	Communicable disease without encephalitic symptoms
68-70.	0|0|0	7.	Communicable disease with encephalitic symptoms

---

Cols.	Code		Description
75-78.	0|0|0|1		Case Number
79-80.	4|2		Card Identification

Cols.	Code	Item	Description
1-3.	0|0|0	8.	Chronic or recurrent lower respiratory infection
4-6.	||||	9.	" " " gastro-intestinal disturbances
7-9.	||||	10.	" " " fever of unknown origin
10-12.	||||	11.	Visual problems (See page 8)
13-15.	||||	12.	Hearing problems (See page 8)
16-18.	||||	13.	Is diaper always wet (dribbles) or is there a poor urinary stream?
19-21.	||||	14.	Major chronic disease
22-24.	||||	15.	Congenital anomalies
25-27.	↓|↓|↓	16.	Other significant illness (include severe reactions to immunization)

ITEM #	AGE	HOSPITAL NAME, IF APPLICABLE	DURATION & DIAGNOSIS
62-64	4 mos.	Williamstown	Sick 3 days at home -
			hospital 3 days -
			Roseola and convulsion
___	___	_____	_____
___	___	_____	_____
___	___	_____	_____
___	___	_____	_____
___	___	_____	_____
___	___	_____	_____
___	___	_____	_____
___	___	_____	_____
___	___	_____	_____
___	___	_____	_____
___	___	_____	_____
___	___	_____	_____

CHILD DEVELOPMENT SERVICE
Developmental History--Page 7

FORM 4B
Case #: _0001_

SEIZURES:
(Code, Col. 1: 0-No; 1-Possible; 2-Yes; 9-No data)
(Code, Cols. 2 & 3: 00-No; nn-Month of onset; 99-No data)
Enter age of onset for each positive response for items in left hand
column, and record below for each the information specified in the
right hand column:

COLS.		TYPE OF EPISODE	DETAILS TO BE RECORDED
28-30.	2 0 4	1. Convulsions or fits	Number of item
31-33.	0 0 0	2. Spasms or jerking	Description of episodes
34-36.		3. Stiffening episodes	Age of onset
37-39.		4. Trembling episodes	Frequency of episodes
40-42.		5. Limp or falling episodes	Duration of longest episode
43-45.		6. Blue spells (No cardiac disease)	Presence of fever
46-48.		7. Loss of consciousness	Date of last attack
49-51.		8. Staring episodes	Medication and dosage
52-54.		9. Temper tantrums	Date treatment started
55-57.		10. Nightmares	Date treatment stopped
58-60.		11. Sleepwalking	Is patient in contact with
61-63.		12. Periods of unusual or variable behavior	environment during episodes?
64-66.		13. Recurrent abdominal pain (colic)	
67-69.		14. Recurrent vomiting	
70-72.		15. Recurrent headaches	

Item # _28-30_

At 4 mos. had high fever for 4 days. 3rd day generalized tonic

clonic seizure lasted 1/2 hour until we got him to hospital. -

gave him a shot. Rash next day.

Not on anticonvulsants

75-78. | 0 0 0 1 | Case number
79-80. | 4 3 | Card identification

CHILD DEVELOPMENT SERVICE
Developmental History--Page 8

FORM 4B
Case #: _0001_____

DEVELOPMENTAL PROGRESS: (Record age achieved in months, if no questionnaire available)

Motor behavior:

4	Holds head 90° in prone
4	Holds head steady mother's lap
5	Rolls to prone, arms out
7	Takes weight on feet when held
7	Sits, leaning on hands
9	Sits steady indefinitely
9	Creeps on hands and knees
	Rolls or arches to progress
9	Pulls to standing
11	Cruises around furniture
15	Gets up alone and walks
18	Walks upstairs, 1 hand held
24	Kicks ball well

Language behavior:

2	Smiles in response to person
4	Laughs aloud
8	Imitates sounds: cough, tongue-click
8	Knows name
9	Mama and Dada with meaning
9	1 other "word"
9	Nursery trick on request
13	Recognizes objects by name
15	Uses jargon
18	Recognizes pictures
21	Combines words
24	Uses pronouns
	Number of words used now

Adaptive behavior:

4	Holds & looks at objects placed in hand
6	Reaches and grasps object
7	Transfers hand to hand
9	Picks up crumbs and threads
9	Pokes with index finger
10	Takes things out of box
15	Piles objects
18	Scribbles spontaneously

See questionnaire

Personal-social behavior:

2	Follows moving person
5	Smiles at mirror image
7	Takes feet to mouth
8	Feeds self cracker
12	Cooperates in dressing
18	Hugs and loves doll
18	Feeds self with spoon
21	Pulls person to show something
24	Imitates household activity, play

HAS YOUR CHILD EVER FAILED TO MAKE PROGRESS, OR EVER LOST ANY BEHAVIOR ONCE ACHIEVED?

Describe: *Didn't use right arm as well after his convulsion but*

no real problem with it.

(Code, Col. 1: 0-No; 1-Possible; 2-Yes; 9-No data)
(Code, Cols. 2 & 3: 00-No; nn-Month of onset; 99-No data)

COLS.

1-3.	`1 0 4`	Failure to progress in motor development
4-6.	`0 0 0`	" " " " adaptive development
7-9.		" " " " language development
10-12.		" " " " personal-social development
13-15.		Regression in motor development
16-18.		" " adaptive development
19-21.		" " ability to hear
22-24.		" " ability to see
25-27.		" " ability to communicate
28-30.		Loss of recognition of familiar things or people

Change occurred following:
(Code: 0-No change; 1-Possible; 2-Yes; 9-No data)

31.	`0`	Illness
32.	`0`	Accident
33.	`1`	Convulsions
34.	`0`	No specific cause

How old was child when you began to worry about problems related to development?

35-36. `0 1` (Code: 00-No problems; nn-Month; 99-No data) *At birth, chromosomes abnormal*

CHILD DEVELOPMENT SERVICE   FORM 4B
Developmental History--Page 9   Case #: _0001_____

COLS.
37-38. |0¦0| Does your child relate to you and others as people with a social give and take?
              00. As persons
              11. Possibly "Autistic"
              nn. "Autistic," month of onset
              99. No data

39-40. |0¦0| Pica. (Code same as Columns 37-38)
              Does your child eat plaster, paint, dirt, etc? Specify:_____

              _____

       (Code for Cols. 41 & 42: 0-No; 1-Possible; 2-Yes; 9-No data)

41. | 0 | When child is well, do you consider he has any feeding problem? Specify:_____

              _____

42. | 0 | When child is well, do you consider he has any sleeping problem? Specify:_____

              _____

43. | 0 | When child is well, do you consider he is a happy baby?
              (Code: 0-Happy; 1-Variable; 2-Unhappy; 9-No data)

44. | 1 | What does child do when strangers come into the home?
              0. No strangers come
              1. Makes friends
              2. Makes friends unless picked up and handled
              3. Makes friends only if on mother's lap
              4. Cries in specific situations:_____
              5. Withdraws or cries even on mother's lap
              6. Ignores and disregards them
              7. Other; Specify:_____
              9. No data

45. | 1 | What does child do in strange places?
              (Code same as Col. 44)
              7. Other; Specify:_____

46. | 0 | Is there anything (else) about your child that worries you?
              (Code: 0-No; 1-Possible; 2-Yes; 9-No data. Code 1 & 2 only if not already
              coded)

              Specify:_____

              _____

47. | 0 | Do you and your husband have any disagreements about the child?
              0. No
              1. About what you think is wrong?   Describe:_____
              2. About management?
              3. Other; Specify   _____
              4. Code if more than one area
              9. No data   _____

              _____

CHILD DEVELOPMENT SERVICE   FORM 4B
Developmental History--Page 10   Case #: _0001_

List others besides parents and children living in household:

	NAME	AGE	RELATIONSHIP TO CHILD
	None		

Indicate if either parent or any of the children not living at home:

_____

_____

Number of rooms, excluding bathrooms _8_

COLS.
48-49. | 1 ¦ 3 | Code number of rooms per person (Code as 2.5, 1.0, 0.5, etc.)

50. | 0 | Is kitchen shared?

51. | 0 | Is bathroom shared? (Code for Cols. 50-52. 0-No; 1-Yes; 9-No data)

52. | 0 | Is home public housing?

53-55. | 1 ¦ 5 ¦ 0 | Rent per month in hundreds (or mortgage payments): e.g., 92.50=093

Total Income: per year _12,000_ or per month_____ or per week_____

56-57. | 2 ¦ 0 | Code per capita income in thousands and hundreds: e.g., 21=$2100, 09=$900

Person(s) interviewed _Mr. and Mrs. Doe_

58. | | Relationship(s) to child _Parents_

59. | 1 | Interviewer _HK_

60-63. | 0 ¦ 7 ¦ 7 ¦ 2 | Date of interview (Code month and year) _7/28/72_

75-78. | 0 ¦ 0 ¦ 0 ¦ 1 | Case number
79-80. | 4 ¦ 4 | Card identification

Developmental Schedules

Several possible methods of recording an examination are noted in Chapter 4 and Appendix C-3 and C-4. Videotape is the best. Even brief notes made by the examiner during the course of the examination are apt to disturb the flow of the infant's behavior. It is far better if he can train himself to retain a vivid memory picture of what the infant does and record it on the forms immediately after the examination, adding descriptive notes and comments.

No matter how the examination is recorded, the child's performance is always noted first on the developmental schedules. The examiner makes use of his clinical impression of the child in selecting the appropriate developmental schedule(s) for recording. He selects the schedules in terms of key ages and says to himself, "This child is best viewed in terms of 16 weeks—or 40 weeks—or 2 years," whatever the case may be.

On all developmental schedules, two columns are provided: H for history, and O for observation. The use of both history and observation columns allows the examiner to indicate that the information given by the parent has been confirmed. Some information is available only by report, particularly in language and personal—social behavior. In instances of disagreement, the parent's report is accepted and the observation column is left blank unless the examiner observes the pattern which was reported as lacking. A pattern is recorded as lacking in the face of a positive report only when there is overwhelming evidence that the parent's information is inaccurate. As already indicated in Chapter 4, rejection of parental information is a very risky venture.

In recording observed behavior on the chosen schedule(s), the examiner must remember that there are two types of behavior patterns: *permanent* patterns and *temporary* patterns. Temporary patterns are ones which transform or are replaced by different and more advanced patterns at later ages. Temporary patterns are indicated on the schedules by an asterisk; the age at which the pattern is replaced by a more advanced pattern also is given. Some temporary patterns form part of a sequence; an infant cannot sit indefinitely without first being able to sit for 10 minutes, or hold his head at a 90° but not a 45° angle in prone. Other temporary patterns are completely replaced by more mature patterns; the scissors grasp of 36 weeks is replaced by the inferior pincer grasp at 40 weeks. In a transitional phase, both may be seen. In addition to knowing whether the less mature pattern has been discarded completely, we wish to indicate if any particular item is an integral part of the child's behavior or merely incipient.

To record these complexities in observed behavior patterns adequately, the following code is provided:

A plus sign (+) is entered when any behavior pattern on the schedule is well established as an organic part of the child's working equipment.

A plus-minus (±) is entered for a pattern that is incidental or incipient, but not yet fully integrated. Circling this designation prevents confusion with adjacent entries.

Name: John Doe	CC Age: 28 Weeks	Date: 7/28/72	Case No: 0001

H = History
O = Observation

KEY AGE: 28 Weeks

24 Weeks (H O)

Adaptive (23–29) 27)
- ++ Dangling Ring, Rattle, Cube, Bell: approaches & grasps
- + Rattle: prehensile pursuit dropped rattle
- –|–(⊕) Cube: regards 3rd cube immediately (*18m)
- + Cube, Bell: to mouth (*18m)
- + Cube: resecures dropped cube
- ++ Massed Cubes: holds 1, approaches another (*28w)

Gross Motor (25)
- ++ Supine: lifts legs high in extension
- ++ Supine: rolls to prone
- –|– Pull-to-Sit: lifts head, assists (*40w)
- + Sit in chair: trunk erect (*36w)

Fine Motor (23)
- –(⊕) Cube: grasps palmarvise (*36w)
- + Rattle: retains   L >R

Language (26)
- ++ Bell-ringing: turns head to bell
- ++ Vocalization: grunts, growls (*36w)
- ++ Vocalization: spontaneous vocal-social (including toys)

Personal-Social (27)
- ++ Social: discriminates strangers
- ++ Play: grasps foot, supine (*36w)
- ++ Play: sits propped 30 minutes (*40w)
- ++ Mirror: smiles and vocalizes

KEY AGE: 28 Weeks (H O)

Adaptive (23–29) 27)
- + Rattle, Bell: 1-hand approach & grasp
- + Massed Cubes: holds 1, grasps another
- – M. Cubes: holds 2 more than momentarily
- + Bell: bangs (*40w)
- + Rattle: shakes definitely
- + Dangling Ring, Cube: transfers (awkward)
- – Bell: transfers adeptly (? disability)
- – Bell: retains

Gross Motor (25)
- –|– Supine: lifts head (*40w)
- –(⊕) Sit: briefly, leans forward on hands (*32w)
- – Sit: erect momentarily
- ++ Stand: large fraction of weight (*32w)
- –|– Stand: bounces actively (*36w)

Fine Motor (23)
- – Cube: radial palmar grasp (*36w)
- – Pellet: rakes with whole hand, contacts (*32w)

Language (26)
- + Vocalization: m-m-m (crying) (*40w)
- – Vocalization: controlled polysyllabic vowel sounds (*36w)

Personal-Social (27)
- – Feeding: takes solids well
- ++ Play: feet to mouth, supine
- ++ Mirror: reaches, pats image
- + Ring-string: fusses or abandons effort (*32w)

32 Weeks (H O)

Adaptive
- –|– Cube: grasps 2nd cube
- – Cube: retains 2 as 3rd presented (*36w)
- – Cube: holds 2 prolongedly
- + Cup-cube: holds cube, regards cup (*36w)
- – Ring-string: secures ring

Gross Motor
- – Sit: 1 minute, erect, unsteady (*36w)
- – Stand: maintains briefly, hands held (*36w)
- – Prone: pivots (*40w)

Fine Motor
- – Pellet: radial raking (*36w)
- –|– Pellet: unsuccessful inferior scissors (*36w)

Language
- Vocalization: single consonant, as da, ba, ka

Personal-Social
- –|– Play: bites, chews toys (*18m)
- – Play: reaches persistently for toys out of reach (*40w)
- – Ring-string: persistent

At times both a temporary pattern and its replacement are present, and both receive a plus (+) sign. However, when a behavior pattern on the schedule is not represented in the child's repertoire, the examiner must pause.

A *minus sign* (−) is entered when a permanent pattern (no asterisk) is not part of the child's behavior *or* when a lacking temporary pattern (asterisk) has not yet been superseded by its more mature pattern.

When a temporary pattern is lacking because the child is displaying more advanced superseding behavior instead, there are two possibilities:

A *double plus sign* (++) is used when the behavior is part of an obligatory sequence; e.g., sits 10 min⁺ *and* steadily at 36 and 40 weeks.

N (*no longer necessary*) is employed when the temporary pattern has been replaced entirely by the more mature pattern with which it is mutually exclusive; e.g., scissors grasp replaced by inferior pincer.

While the distinction between ++ and N may seem needlessly complicated, it does serve the examiner by emphasizing visually the developmental progressions and indicating clearly when the less mature pattern has been discarded completely. For computer analysis, when only individual items are examined and no total picture is in view, the nature of any given pattern is delineated more clearly by this device.

In summary, a + or ± sign entered for any pattern on the schedule means that the child displayed the pattern; a ++ or N sign means he displayed a more mature pattern instead; a − sign means that he is not yet mature enough with respect to that particular pattern to display it. By this device we preserve the fundamental connotation of the minus sign.

Other notations can be placed to the left of the history column to help add qualitative dimensions to the observed behavior.

A (*abnormal*) denotes that a pattern is present or incipient but abnormal in its expression.

D (*disability*) is entered if some item of behavior is not accomplished because of a motor or sensory handicap (e.g., no transfer in an infant with hemiplegia, or no words in a child with hearing impairment). D (disability) should not be entered for a motor behavior pattern; absence in itself constitutes disability. It is rarely possible to differentiate disability from immaturity when an item is just appearing at the child's chronologic age (e.g., the 32-week-old who does not grasp the second cube or the 15-month-old who does not build a tower of two cubes).

R (*refusal*) can be used when the child refuses a situation, usually at the very beginning of the examination before he has adjusted, or for gross motor activity. R (refusal) should not be substituted for a minus (−) sign when the child's behavior indicates that his typical reaction is to reject actively tasks he perceives as too difficult for him.

There is one further general principle to be followed. When recording performance in an area of behavior for any given age, enter some notation for every pattern in that specific area (other areas at that age may be completely blank). When you review the record at a later date, you will have no idea why there is a blank if you fail to take this simple precaution.

X indicates there is no information about a particular area because you deliberately or inadvertently omitted it, or no history was available.

? indicates you don't remember or can't interpret what the infant did.

For the novice's encouragement, it may be added that when there is familiarity with developmental sequences, and with a little practice, recording becomes faster and almost automatic.

To recapitulate:

1. On the basis of his modified first impression, the examiner selects the developmental schedule containing the most appropriate key age for recording.
2. He enters a + or ± sign whenever the child demonstrates the behavior pattern.
3. He enters a ++ or N sign whenever the child fails to display a temporary pattern *because he displayed a more mature pattern instead.*
4. He enters a − sign whenever the child fails to display a permanent pattern, or whenever he fails to display a temporary pattern *because he displayed less mature patterns instead.*
5. He enters qualifying notations or comments and indicates missing information.

The examiner now is ready to appraise the child's maturity level in each area of behavior. The developmental schedule is used to list the presence and absence of significant behavior. We prefer to say presence and absence rather than success or failure because fundamentally we are concerned with status and not with success. There are no right or wrong responses; any response is appropriate to some age level. When we list the presence and absence of behavior patterns, we do not censor the child's behavior, we judge it.

From the standpoint of developmental diagnosis, the significance of plus and minus signs is always relative rather than absolute. The final estimate of developmental maturity is based on the *distribution* of plus and minus signs. We do not sum and average the signs; it is the total clinical picture which is significant. Maturity is appraised by determining how well a child's behavior fits one age level constellation rather than another. *In any field of behavior the child's maturity level is that point where the aggregate of + signs changes to an aggregate of − signs.* The assignment of the specific developmental age between two adjacent levels on the developmental schedule depends on the nature of the positive and negative patterns present.

The plus and minus signs may be so irregularly distributed for a behavior area that this point of change becomes a band or zone of change, and no single age level can be determined. When this occurs, there are two possible ways of indicating it. A notation such as 35(26–38) denotes scatter and gaps but centering closer to the upper end of the range; 31(26–38) indicates the reverse. At times the behavior is so discrepant that the only adequate description is the range 26–38.

On occasion, only minimal information is available for any given area; the parents may not be available to provide a history of language or personal–social behavior, or the infant may be too ill or too inhibited to participate fully. For a 40-week infant, a notation such as 38-minimum would mean that the behavior is at least at the 38-week level, but the examiner feels that the optimum abilities have not been elicited. Such a notation is logical only when the behavior is in the normal range for the age of the child. For example, little information would be contributed to the assessment of the language behavior of a 40-week infant to record 26-minimum because you observed all of the 24-week behavior and heard polysyllabic vowel sounds. In such circumstances no maturity level should be assigned.

The maturity levels assigned for each of the five areas can be noted in the margins on the developmental schedules and later transferred to the first page of the developmental and neurologic evaluation form discussed below. A column is provided on this form to indicate, for later statistical analysis, whether the maturity level assigned is a single level, a minimum performance or a range of behavior. The final interpretation of these levels is not made until the qualitative aspects of the behavior and neuromotor patterns are recorded and appraised.

As discussed in Chapter 5, a general developmental level is assigned which represents the intellectual potential. It is not an average of all five areas of behavior and is never less than the adaptive level. The adaptive level may be raised one or two weeks on the basis of good quality, the presence of interfering motor handicaps not already taken into consideration or acceleration in language development. No general developmental level is assigned when language development is significantly more advanced than an adaptive level in the defective range. In such circumstances, there is obvious disorganization of behavior which requires further observation and investigation; language may be a better prognosticator of future potential than adaptive behavior.

Developmental and Neurologic Evaluation Form

This form is completed after the examination is finished and the observed behavior has been recorded on the developmental schedules. It is the basis for the formulation of a diagnosis and prognosis, and for the subsequent interview with the parents. It too is precoded. The form now includes virtually all the items which appeared originally in the diagnostic syllabus in Chapter 11 of the first two editions of this book. Selected items were incorporated in a simple form first used in 1952 in a study of prematures. In three or four subsequent revisions dictated by increasing clinical experience, the items were arranged by age groups, the material expanded, coding modernized and the diagnostic summary incorporated. The form has been employed in research investigations as well as in clinical teaching and diagnostic settings.

```
CHILD DEVELOPMENT SERVICE                                      FORM 5B
Department of Pediatrics                                       12/72
Medical School Hospital, U.S.A.
```

DEVELOPMENTAL AND NEUROLOGIC EVALUATION FORM

IDENTIFYING INFORMATION:

Name: _John Doe_   Case Number: _0001_

(Code month and year for birth and exam.)   Hospital Number: _X-1234_

COLS.
1-4. | 0 ¦ 1 ¦ 7 ¦ 2 | Date of Birth _1-1-72_   Expected Date of Birth: _1-15-72_

5-8. | 1 ¦ 0 ¦ 7 ¦ 2 | Examination Date _7-28-72_   Corrected Birth Date: _1-15-72_

9. | 1 | Race and Sex: ①-WM; 2-WF; 3-BM; 4-BF; 5-OM; 6-OF (Circle one.)

10-13. | 2 ¦ 4 ¦ 9 ¦ 5 | Birth Weight: grams (_5-8_   lbs. and ozs.)

14-15. | 1 ¦ 4 | Amount of Prematurity in Days

16-18. | 0 ¦ 2 ¦ 8 | Age in Weeks (Code 000 if months) Age is corrected for prematurity.

19-21. | 0 ¦ 0 ¦ 0 | Age in Months, to nearest half month (Code 000 if weeks) Corrected.

FIRST THREE PAGES ARE SUMMARY PAGES; TURN TO PAGE 4 TO BEGIN RECORDING.

DIAGNOSTIC SUMMARY: (after remainder of form completed)

   INTELLECTUAL: _Low Average_

   NEUROMOTOR: _Right spastic hemiplegia - mild_

   SEIZURES: _Grand Mal (by History)_

   SPECIAL SENSORY: _0̄_

   QUALITATIVE: _0̄_

   SPECIFIC DISEASES OR SYNDROMES: _Trisomy 21_

MATURITY LEVELS: (Note to Coder: For Range columns: 0-No range; 1-Minimum; 2-Range, age specified; 3-Range, extremes averaged; 9-No level assigned.)

COLS.	Range	Develop-mental Quotient	Weeks	Months	(Delete inapplicable word)
22-25.	0	0 ¦ 9 ¦ 6	27	...	...General Developmental Level
26-29.	1	0 ¦ 8 ¦ 9	25	...	...Adaptive Behavior
30-33.	↓	0 ¦ 8 ¦ 3	23	...	...Gross Motor Behavior
34-37.	2	0 ¦ 9 ¦ 6	27 (23-29)	...	...Fine Motor Behavior
38-41.	0	0 ¦ 9 ¦ 3	26	...	...Language Behavior
42-45.	0	0 ¦ 9 ¦ 6	27	...	...Personal-Social Behavior
46-49.	-	¦ - ¦	--	...	...Stanford-Binet Mental Age

50.   INTELLECTUAL POTENTIAL: (Circle one number in each column, 50 and 51.)

| 1 |
   0.   Felt to be adequately predictive
   ①   Indicative of present function but modifying factors present
   2.   Inadequate for precise evaluation   Specify: _Trisomy 21- expect deceleration_
   3.   Inadequate for evaluation

CHILD DEVELOPMENT SERVICE
Developmental and Neurologic Evaluation--Page 2

FORM 5B
Case Number: _0001_

COLS.

51. CLINICAL EVALUATION OF INTELLECTUAL POTENTIAL:

| 3 |

IN NORMAL RANGE
0. Superior
1. High Average
2. Average
③. Low Average
4. Dull Normal
5. Indeterminate, not Defective

MENTAL DEFICIENCY PRESENT OR LIKELY
6. Borderline Dull
7. Borderline Defective
8. Defective
9. Undecided

NEUROMOTOR STATUS: (Circle one number in each column, 52 and 53.)
Posture, locomotion, movement control, muscle tone, coordination and
manipulation, reflexes, etc.

----

52. TYPE OF NEUROMOTOR ABNORMALITY:

| 2 |

0. No abnormality
1. Due to disease outside of the central nervous system (e.g., renal or
        cardiac, marked malnutrition, acute disease, arthrogryposis, etc.)
        Specify:_____

② Indicative of Chronic Organic Brain Disease
3. Other central nervous system disease (e.g., anterior horn cell,
        degenerative disease, brain tumor, myelomeningocele, etc.)
        Specify:_____

4. Multiple conditions
        Specify:_____

9. Undecided

----

53. DEGREE OR NEUROMOTOR ABNORMALITY:

| 7 |

0. No abnormality

0. Motor behavior normal for chronologic age
1. Gross motor normal for chronologic age,
        minimal fine motor abnormalities
2. Gross motor normal for chronologic age,
        minor fine motor abnormalities
3. Motor retardation without abnormal signs
        for level of function

4. Abnormal neuromotor signs of
        no clinical significance
5. Abnormal neuromotor signs of
        minor degree
6. Abnormal neuromotor signs of
        marked degree

4. Motor retardation with abnormal signs
        of no clinical significance
5. Motor retardation with abnormal signs
        of minor degree
6. Motor retardation with abnormal signs
        of marked degree
⑦ Abnormal neuromotor signs of severe degree; qualitative change,
        e.g., "Cerebral Palsy," specific syndrome, etc.
        Specify type: _Mild right spastic hemiplegia_

9. Undecided

54. HISTORY obtained from parent(s): (Circle one number.)

| 1 |

0. No parents present
① Reliable
2. Reliable but not too many details recalled or available
3. Unreliable in details but generally satisfactory
4. Unreliable in most respects
9. Undecided

CHILD DEVELOPMENT SERVICE
Developmental and Neurologic Evaluation--Page 3   FORM 5B
                                                            Case Number: _0001_

COLS.
55-56.   EMOTIONAL STABILITY: Consider in terms of adaptive maturity if child mentally defective.
         (Check one item in applicable column at right, with or without "autism" or seizures.)
                                        0.   1.   2.   3.
                              No assoc. cond. with "autism" with seizures with both
  |0 ¦ 0| 0. Normal   ✓
           1. Minimal disturbance _____ _____ _____ _____
           2. Moderate disturbance _____ _____ _____ _____
           3. Apathetic and passive _____ _____ _____ _____
           4. Severe disturbance   _____ _____ _____ _____
           5. Other; specify: _____ _____ _____ _____

           9. Undecided _____
                              _____ _____ _____ _____

57-58.   QUALITY OF INTEGRATION: Consider in terms of adaptive maturity level if child defective.
         (Check one item in applicable column at right, as above.)
                                        0.   1.   2.   3.
                              No assoc. cond. with "autism" with seizures with both
  |1 ¦ 0| 0. Normal
           1. Mild disorganization   ✓
           2. Moderate disorganiz. _____ _____ _____ _____
           3. Severe disorganiz.   _____ _____ _____ _____
           9. Undecided   _____ _____ _____ _____

59.   TOTAL NEUROMOTOR POTENTIAL: by standard neurologic examination at school age.
         (Circle one number.)
  |2| 0. Normal
          1. No significant neuromotor sequelae
         (2.) Neuromotor sequelae of mild degree
          3. Neuromotor sequelae of moderate degree
          4. Neuromotor sequelae of severe degree
          9. Undecided

60.   TOTAL POTENTIAL OTHER THAN PHYSICAL: (Circle one number.)
         Intellectual, emotional, integrative.
  |4| 1. Above average
          2. Average
          3. Below average
         (4.) Markedly below average
          9. Undecided

         PARENTS' ESTIMATE OF CHILD'S FUNCTION:
         (Enter age in months, or qualitative statement, or circle applicable numbers.)

         Mother   Father   Mo.   Fa.
61-64. |0 ¦ 5| |7 ¦ 7| Motor   _5 mo._   00.--Wouldn't give level--00. _77_
65-68. |0 ¦ 6| |7 ¦ 7| Adaptive   _6 mo._   77.--Qualitative----------77. _77_
                                                       statement only
                                                  88.--Not present----------88.
                                                  99.--No data--------------99.
----
73. |0| Status of patient:(0-)Out patient; 1-In patient. (Circle one number.)

74. |1| Examiner: _M.D._

75-78. |0 ¦ 0 ¦ 0 ¦ 1| Case Number
79-80. |5 ¦ 1| Card Identification

CHILD DEVELOPMENT SERVICE   FORM 5B
Developmental and Neurologic Evaluation--Page 4   Case Number: _0001_

QUALITY OF INTEGRATION:
Consider in terms of adaptive maturity level if child mentally defective.
(Check one space for each numbered item in left hand column.)

COLS.		1. Above Average	2. Average	3. Below Average	4. Markedly Below Average	9. Undecided
2	1. Emotional Stability		✓			
3	2. Organization					
3	3. Attention			╱		
3	4. Interest			✓		
2	5. Maturity					
	6. Discrimination		╱			
	7. Judgment					
	8. Spontaneity					
	9. Exploitation					
	10. Rapport					
	11. General Adjustment		✓			

ABNORMAL BEHAVIOR PATTERNS:
Consider in terms of adaptive maturity level if child mentally defective.
(Check one space for each numbered item in left hand column.)

		0. Absent or Normal in Amount	1. Mild Degree	2. Moderate Degree	3. Severe Degree	9. Undecided
0	12. Perseveration	✓				
0	13. Irritability	✓				
1	14. Restlessness		✓			
1	15. Hyperactivity		✓			
0	16. Crying	✓				
0	17. Stereotyped Mannerisms	✓				
2	18. Scatter			✓		
0	19. Dependency on Mother	✓				

Specify Type of Mannerisms: _____

WRITE DESCRIPTIVE COMMENTS ABOUT EXAMINATION BELOW:

Clinically typical features Trisomy 21.

Rather impulsive and slightly disorganized. Attention and interest wander but easily recalled.

Mild right hemiparesis superimposed on mild generalized hypotonicity.

CHILD DEVELOPMENT SERVICE   FORM 5B
Developmental and Neurologic Evaluation--Page 5   Case Number: *0001*

20-51.   MUSCLE TONE AND MOVEMENT:
(Enter number for degree of abnormality in applicable spaces below.)
Degree of Abnormality

0. Normal
1. Questionably abnormal   HYPOTONICITY must be evaluated in terms of the
2. Mild involvement   adaptive maturity level of the infant; the others are
3. Moderate involvement   qualitative changes which are abnormal at any age.
4. Severe involvement   Example: 2 under RA and LA in line 4 if mild
9. No data   athetosis of both arms present.

COLS. | 3:2:0 0 | 3:2:0 0 | 1:2:0 0 | 1:2:0 0 | 1:3:0 0 | 1:2:0 0 | 0:0:0 0 | 0:0:0 0 |

	Abnormality	20-23 RA	24-27 RL	28-31 LA	32-35 LL	36-39 Back	40-43 Neck	44-47 Face	48-51 Other
	1. Hypotonicity	0	0	2	2	3	2	0	0
	2. Hypertonicity	0	0	0	0	0	0		
	3. Spasticity	2	2						
Dys-	4. Athetosis	0	0						
kinesia	5. Dystonia								
	6. Rigidity								
	7. Ataxia								
	8. Tremor								
	9. Flaccidity								

52-63.   SENSATION:
(Enter number for degree of abnormality in applicable spaces below.)
Degree of Abnormality

0. Normal
1. Questionably diminished   Example: 4 under RL, LL, Trunk in line 4 if
2. Hyperaesthesia   sensation absent up to thoracic level.
3. Diminished
4. Absent
9. No data

COLS. | 0:0 | 0:0 | 0:0 | 0:0 | 0:0 | 0:0 |

	Level	52-53 RL	54-55 LL	56-57 Trunk	58-59 RA	60-61 LA	62-63
	1. Caudal	0	0	0	0	0	
	2. Sacral						6. Other; Specify:
	3. Lumbar						
	4. Thoracic						
	5. Cervical						

75-78. | 0:0:0:1 | Case Number
79-80. | 5:2 | Card Identification

SPECIAL SENSORY:

1-8.   Strabismus
Enter number for degree of abnormality in applicable spaces below.
Degree of Abnormality

0. None
1. Mild degree   If questionably present, always enter 1 for mild degree.
2. Moderate degree
3. Severe degree
9. No data   COLS. | 2:2 | 2:2 | 0:0 | 0:0 |

		1-2 Right In	3-4 Left In	5-6 Right Out	7-8 Left Out
	Persistence	0	0	0	0
	0. None	0	0		
	1. Questionably present	0	0		
	2. Inconstant	2	2		
	3. Constant	0	0		
	9. No data	0	0		

CHILD DEVELOPMENT SERVICE   FORM 5B
Developmental and Neurologic Evaluation--Page 6   Case Number: _0001_

Other Eye Problems: (Check one space for each numbered item in left hand column.)

COLS.		0. Normal	1. Question. Present	2. Mild Degree	3. Moderate Degree	4. Severe Degree	9. No Data
0 | 9.	Nystagmus.....................R						
| 10.	L						
| 11.	Ptosis.......................R						
| 12.	L						
| 13.	Uses peripheral vision.......R						
| 14.	[ocular tilt present] L						
| 15.	Failure of fixation..........R						
| 16.	L						
| 17.	Spasmus nutans................						
| 18.	Visual field defect..........R						
| 19.	L						
| 20.	Other (e.g., random movements)R						
| 21.	L						
9 | 22.	Fundi........................R						
9 | 23.	L						
9 | 24.	Corneal reflexes..............						

Specify if items 9-10, 18-23: _____

_____

Visual Acuity:

0 | 25.	Below normal, but sees........R						
| 26.	L						
| 27.	Blind (always severe).........R						
| 28.	L						
| 29.	Abnormal, not blind...........						
	(e.g., visual cortical defect)						

Specify: _____

Hearing:

0 | 30.	Below normal, but hears.......R						
| 31.	L						
| 32.	Hearing defect...............R						
	L						
| 33.	Aphasia.......................						
| 34.	Abnormal, type undetermined....						

Specify: _____

35-36.   BABINSKI:
         Record presence or absence in spaces to right.
| 1; 1 | 0.   Not present   35.   36.
         1.   Equivocal   _1_ Right; _1_ Left
         2.   Present
         9.   No data

37-38.   FOOT GRASP:
         Record presence or absence in spaces to right.
| 9; 9 | 0.   Present   37.   38.
         1.   Equivocal   _9_ Right; _9_ Left
         2.   Not present
         9.   No data

CHILD DEVELOPMENT SERVICE   FORM 5B
Developmental and Neurologic Evaluation--Page 7   Case Number: _0001_

39-51. REFLEXES:
        (Record clinical evaluation of 0 to 4 at extreme right; code applicable
        number in left hand column if increased, in middle columns if decreased.
        Record 0 in both left and middle columns if reflexes clinically normal.)

        Increased   Decreased
        0. Not increased   0. Not decreased
        1. Questionably increased   1. Questionably decreased
        2. Increased   2. Decreased
        3. Unsustained clonus   3. Absent
        4. Increased stretch reflexes   9. No data
        5. Sustained clonus
        9. No data

                                                                    Clinical
                                                                    Evaluation
        COLS. | 1 : 1 : 2 : 1 | | 0 : 0 : 1 : 1 | | 0 : 0 : 0 : 0 | | 0 : 0 : 0 : 0 | 0 to 4
                  39-42   43-46   47-50   51-54
                 Right   Left   Right   Left   Right   Left
        Biceps....... 1 .... 0 .... 0 0   3+   2+
        Triceps...... 1 .... 0 .... | .... | 3+   2+
        Knee......... 2 .... 1 .... | .... | 4+   3+
        Ankle........ 1 .... 1 .... | .... | 3+   3+

        OTHER NEUROMOTOR ABNORMALITIES:

             The remainder of the abnormal neuromotor patterns must be considered in
             terms of the adaptive maturity age level of the child. An older child
             with a significant motor handicap may have abnormal patterns at some or
             all of the infant levels as well as in the patterns for children.
COLS.
 55.   AGE LEVEL selected for case: (Circle one number.)
| 3 | Asterisks below, and in margins, indicate age at which patterns become abnormal.
             4. 16 weeks (15-25)]....................... ***
            (3.) 28 weeks (26-35)]....................... **
             2. 40 weeks (36+)   ]....................... *
             1. Children (when independent locomotion
                          attained; usually 15 months)

        (CHECK ONE SPACE FOR EACH NUMBERED ITEM IN LEFT HAND COLUMN, at appropriate age levels.
        Cross out all the items above age level selected for the patient.)

        INFANT PATTERNS:

		Head	0. Normal	1. Question. Present	2. Mild Degree	3. Moderate Degree	4. Severe Degree	9. No Data
	0	56. Retraction......................	✓					
*	2	57. Backward sagging...............			✓			*
*	0	58. Forward sagging.................						*
*		59. Sideward sagging...............R						*
		60. L	✓					
		Supine						
	0	61. Persisting tonic-neck-reflex...R						
*		62. L						*
*		63. Extension of leg...............R						*
*		64. L						*
		65. Scissoring.....................	✓					

CHILD DEVELOPMENT SERVICE   FORM 5B
Developmental and Neurologic Evaluation--Page 8   Case Number: _0001_

(Check one space for each numbered item in left hand column.)

COLS.		Sitting	0. Normal	1. Question. Present	2. Mild Degree	3. Moderate Degree	4. Severe Degree	9. No Data
0	66.	Persisting tonic-neck-reflex....R	✓					
0	67.	L	✓					
3	68.	Extension of leg................R				✓		
2	69.	L				✓		
3	70.	Narrow base with leg adduction..R			✓	✓		
2	71.	L			✓			

76-78. |_0_:_0_:_0_:_1_| Case Number
79-80. |_5_:_3_| Card Identification

INFANT PATTERNS: (Continued)

COLS.		Sitting	0. Normal	1. Question. Present	2. Mild Degree	3. Moderate Degree	4. Severe Degree	9. No Data
3	1.	Flexion of knee and hip.........R				✓		
2	2.	L				✓		
0	3.	Hyperextension of back...........	✓		✓			
3	4.	Rounding of back................				✓		
		Standing						
2	5.	Extension of leg................R			✓			
0	6.	L						
	7.	Scissoring......................						
	8.	Plantar flexion of toes.........R						
	9.	L						
	10.	Abnormal postures of feet.......R						
	11.	L						

Specify abnormality for 10 and 11: _____

COLS.			0. Normal	1. Question. Present	2. Mild Degree	3. Moderate Degree	4. Severe Degree	9. No Data
2	12.	Standing on narrow base..........			✓			
	13.	Standing on wide base...........						
	14.	Standing on toes................R						
	15.	L						
	16.	Withdrawal of leg...............R						
	17.	L						
	18.	Flexion at knee and hip.........R						
	19.	L						
	20.	Knee hyperextended, hip flexed..R						
	21.	L						
	22.	Knee hyperextended and hip						
	23.	extended................R L						

CHILD DEVELOPMENT SERVICE   FORM 5B
Developmental and Neurologic Evaluation--Page 9   Case Number: _0001_

           (Check one space for each numbered item in left hand column.)

		0. Normal	1. Question. Present	2. Mild Degree	3. Moderate Degree	4. Severe Degree	9. No Data
Arms and Hands:							
COLS.							
2	24.	Adduction of arm...............R			✓			
0	25.	L	✓					
2	26.	Flexion of elbow...............R			✓			
0	27.	L						
*	28.	Flexion of wrist...............R						*
*	29.	L						*
*	30.	Pronation of arm...............R						*
	31.	L						
	32.	Extension of elbow............R						
	33.	L						
	34.	Abnormal posturing............R						
↓	35.	L						
		Specify abnormality for 34 and 35:						

3	36.	Fisted hand....................R				✓		
* 2	37.	L			✓			*
* 3	38.	Thumb adducted in palm.........R			✓	✓		*
* 2	39.	L			✓			*
0	40.	Withdrawal from grasp..........R						
	41.	L						
	42.	Excessive strength of grasp.....R						
↓	43.	L						

0	44.	Abduction of arm...............R	✓					
3	45.	L				✓		
* 0	46.	Failure to use arms independent..	✓					*
* 3	47.	Maldirected reaching...........R				✓		*
2	48.	L			✓			
0	49.	Requires support to move.......R						
0	50.	L						
3	51.	Difficulty retaining...........R				✓		
2	52.	L			✓			

	53.	Excessive extension in or.......R						
	54.	abruptness of release L						
	55.	Incoordinated transfer.........R						
	56.	L						
	57.	Exaggerated casting............R						
*	58.	L						*
	59.	Cascading......................R						
	60.	L						
	61.	Difficulty in release..........R						
	62.	L						
	63.	Poking, tipping................R						
	64.	L						
	65.	Whole hand grasp...............R						
	66.	L						
	67.	Curling fingers into palm.......R						
	68.	for pellet L						

75-78. |0 | 0 | 0 | 1 | Case Number
79-80. |5 | 4 | Card Identification

CHILD DEVELOPMENT SERVICE
Developmental and Neurologic Evaluation--Page 10

FORM 5B
Case Number: *0001*

PATTERNS IN CHILDREN: (Check one space for each numbered item in left hand column.)

		0. Normal	1. Question. Present	2. Mild Degree	3. Moderate Degree	4. Severe Degree	9. No Data
COLS.	**Lower extremities**						
1.	Walking on wide base.............						
2.	Hyperextension of knee..........R						
3.	L						
4.	Standing or walking on toes.....R						
5.	L						
6.	Incoordination gross movement...R						
7.	L						
8.	Circumduction...................R						
9.	L						
10.	Mincing gait....................						
11.	Scissoring......................						
12.	Lack of assoctd. arm movement...R						
13.	L						
	Arms and Hands						
14.	Abduction......................R						
15.	L						
16.	Adduction......................R						
17.	L						
18.	Persistence scissors grasp......R						
19.	L						
20.	Persist. inferior pincer grasp..R						
21.	L						
22.	Persistence palmar grasp.......R						
23.	L						
24.	Difficulty retaining...........R						
25.	L						
26.	Difficulty in precise release...R						
27.	L						
28.	Awkward manipulation, small.....R						
29.	obj. (e.g., cubes, pages) L						
30.	Awkward manipulation, large.....R						
31.	obj. (e.g., formboard blocks) L						
32.	Incoordinated movements..........						
	(e.g., drawing lines)						
33.	Perceptual-motor difficulties....						
	(e.g., form reproduction)						
	Speech (For maturity age)						
34.	Immature........................						
35.	Stuttering......................						
36.	Retarded........................						
37.	Dysarthric......................						
38.	Absent (always severe)..........						

(CHECK REMAINING COLUMNS FOR ALL CASES.)

39. DROOLING:
(Abnormal in children; at 40 weeks if constant. Cross out at 16 and 28 weeks.)

0 40. MISCELLANEOUS ABNORMALITY: ✓

Specify:_____

CHILD DEVELOPMENT SERVICE   FORM 5B
Developmental and Neurologic Evaluation--Page 11   Case Number: _0001_

	(Check one for each item.)	0. Normal	1. Question Present	2. Mild Degree	3. Moderate Degree	4. Severe Degree	9 No Data
COLS.	SUBSTITUTIVE PATTERNS:						
2 41.	Reaches with mouth.............			✓			
0 42.	Progresses by rolling...........						
43.	Arches in supine using feet......						
44.	Hitches in sitting..............						
45.	Crawls, dragging legs...........						
46.	Casting or cascading............						
47.	Poking or tipping...............						
✓ 48.	Other;..........................	✓					
	Specify:_____						

SEIZURES: (Observed)

		0.	1.	2.	3.	4.	9
0 49.	Abortive grand mal..............						
50.	Psychomotor.....................						
51.	Myoclonic.......................						
52.	Grand mal.......................						
✓ 53.	Other;..........................	✓					
	Describe seizures:						

54. LOCOMOTION: (Circle one number.) (Not applicable at 16 and 28 weeks; cross out.)
   0. Normal
   1. Questionably abnormal; specify:_____
   2. Retarded
   3. Abnormal; specify:_____
   9. No data

_4_ 55. HANDEDNESS: (Circle one number.)
   0. Ambidextrous
   1. Right
   2. Left
   3. Right, due to disability on left
   ④. Left, due to disability on right

PHYSICAL DEFECTS:

	(Other than neurologic)	0. None	1. Question.	2. Present	9. No Data	
0 56.	Temporary or acute condition....	✓				Check one for
0 57.	Minor defect....................	✓				each item at
2 58.	Major defect....................			✓		left

Specify: _Congenital Heart Disease - V.S.D., small_

PHYSICIAN'S ESTIMATE OF MOTHER:

	(In handling child)	0. No	1. Yes	9. Not Present	
1 59.	Relaxed.........................		✓		Check one space
1 60.	Self-assured....................		✓		for each numbered
0 61.	Tense...........................				item in left
62.	Uncertain.......................				hand column
63.	Unperceptive....................				
✓ 64.	Other;..........................	✓			
	Specify:_____				

75-78. | 0 ┊ 0 ┊ 0 ┊ 1 | Case Number
79-80. | 5 ┊ 5 | Card Identification

Several aspects of the developmental and neurologic form require elaboration; other sections are self-explanatory. In spite of its formidable appearance, the form requires a minimum of writing, and a little practice results in facility in its use. The clinician need be concerned only with checking the appropriate blanks or items in the body of the form. A secretary can transform this information into the correct codes and enter them in the appropriate boxes. The identifying information is entered at the top of page 1. Recording then begins on page 4, since the remainder of the first three pages are summary. Recording of abnormalities does not by itself explain them.

QUALITY OF BEHAVIOR (page 4). If only the chronologic age of the child were taken into consideration in evaluating the quality of behavior, all children with mental deficiency would be markedly below average. No distinction could be made between those infants who showed behavior that was reasonably well integrated for the age level at which they were functioning and those with varying degrees of disorganization associated with their mental defect. Consequently, a 40-week-old with adaptive behavior of 24 weeks must be viewed in terms of responses appropriate to 24 weeks. He is abnormal, but how he responds to situations has an important bearing on his utilization of his potentialities, just as it does for a child with normal intelligence.

MUSCLE TONE AND MOVEMENT (page 5). The same 40-week infant might have gross motor behavior which is also at the 24-week level. In terms of 40 weeks, one might be tempted to say he is hypotonic because of failure to sit and bear weight. He is abnormal, but his muscle tone is appropriate for 24 weeks. In contrast, if gross motor behavior were 12 weeks, associated with decreased resistance to passive motion and decreased spontaneous activity, he would be hypotonic, in addition to having mental deficiency. In the illustration recorded for muscle tone and movement, the infant has mild hypotonicity of the left side and the neck, and moderate hypotonicity of the trunk, associated with mild spasticity of the right side of the body.

STRABISMUS (page 5). The coding illustrated for strabismus indicates a moderate degree of alternating esotropia. A code of 3 under right eye out, constant, would indicate severe exotropia of one eye only.

INFANT NEUROMOTOR ABNORMALITIES (pages 7–9). Whether a neuromotor pattern is abnormal depends on the age of the infant. It is not possible to make a list and apply all items at all ages. It is not abnormal for a 16-week-old to have a rounded back in sitting or a 28-week-old to have a whole-hand grasp; these are immature patterns which are appropriate for the respective chronologic ages. Further, there may be mental deficiency with retarded motor development but no other distortion of motor integration. The 40-week-old discussed above is abnormal because of his mental deficiency, but his 24-week-old motor behavior may show that there are no abnormal neuromotor patterns for his 24-week level of function. A 2-year-old with adaptive behavior at 11 months is not ataxic if he does not walk alone; he requires time, not referral to a cerebral palsy treatment center, to achieve independent locomotion.

The first step, then, in evaluation of neuromotor patterns is the selection of the appropriate *adaptive* age level. Those items bracketed with three asterisks in the margins are abnormal if they are present when the infant is in the 16-week zone (15–25 weeks). In this youngest maturity group, the remainder of the patterns are crossed out and disregarded. The items with two asterisks are not abnormal until the 28-week zone (26–35 weeks) is reached; the three- and two-asterisk items both are considered in evaluating an infant of this maturity. When the 40-week zone (36+ weeks) is attained, the items with one asterisk are added; then, all the infant patterns are applicable in the evaluation of abnormal behavior.

Caution must be used in the interpretation of the infant neuromotor patterns prior to 16 weeks of age. Obviously, the very young infant normally has imperfect head control, persistence of the tonic-neck-reflex and fisted hands. This part of the form is not entirely applicable at the youngest ages. However, certain neuromotor patterns are abnormal at any age: retraction of the head, scissoring, persistent flexion or extension of extremities (except for legs in sitting) and adduction of the thumb into the palm. For the most part, these are items 5–11 on page 8 and items 24–35 on page 9; most of these abnormal patterns are present whenever there is a qualitative change in movement control, such as spasticity or dyskinesia.

PATTERNS IN CHILDREN (page 10). Once independent locomotion has been attained, the infant patterns should be crossed out and any abnormalities recorded under the patterns for children. However, an older child with adaptive behavior above 15 months but with a significant motor handicap, may have abnormal patterns at some or all of the infant levels, as well as in the patterns for children. Items 12, 13, 32 and 33 on page 10 are not abnormal until 2 years of age.

After completing the remainder of the form for patients of all ages, the examiner is ready to summarize and appraise the child's total behavior and formulate diagnosis and prognosis. In appraising maturity, the examiner also must undertake to explain, or at least give weight to, discrepancies—behavior patterns seriously out of line with the child's total picture. He must take into account factors that might influence the behavioral responses: illness, fatigue, apprehension, insecurity, unhappiness, visual and hearing defects, motor handicaps, seizures, language difficulties, etc. The child always is interpreted in terms of his age, his experiences, his fitness and his environment. A penetrating appraisal of this kind tells much more than the child's maturity status; it sums up his characteristics, the integrity of his organization and his latent and realized potentialities.

MATURITY LEVELS (page 1). The examiner returns to the bottom of page 1 of the form and transfers the maturity levels for each area of behavior noted on the developmental schedules, assigning a general maturity level if he has not already done so.

INTELLECTUAL POTENTIAL: ADEQUACY OF PREDICTION (page 1). A statement that the examination is adequately predictive assumes that the environment and subsequent educational opportunities will be optimum, or at least satisfactory. For a normal infant, the precise IQ attained at school age will depend on the sociocultural status of the parents. Later experience will affect the function of a child with mental deficiency also, but an enriched environment will not make him normal. A statement that the examination is indicative of present function but modifying factors are present implies that the behavior elicited is fairly typical and that the infant has exhibited this to the best of his ability, but that a diagnosis or a firm prognosis for the future cannot be given. A child who has spent his life in an institution can improve after placement in a good foster home. An infant with frequent seizures may appear grossly defective but show a few fragments of age-appropriate behavior; he may well function entirely normally when his seizures are controlled. Conversely, an infant with trisomy 21 may have normal adaptive behavior at 6 months of age, but deceleration and subsequent mental deficiency of some degree are the rule. A statement of inadequate examination means that the infant is not participating fully. Enough behavior may be elicited to indicate that mental deficiency is not present, but a precise maturity level representing optimum performance cannot be determined. In rare instances (less than 1%) the child simply refuses to cooperate, the examination is entirely inadequate and few or no details of any kind can be recorded.

INTELLECTUAL POTENTIAL: CLINICAL EVALUATION (page 2). The clinical evaluation of intellectual potential is a qualitative description of the performance which obviously is related to the developmental quotient, but is not rigidly defined by the numerical value calculated. Marked acceleration in itself does not indicate superiority; conversely, moderate acceleration combined with unusual maturity and novel exploitation might be so designated. A decision between dull normal and borderline dull is made on the basis of the quality and integration of the behavior. The category indeterminate, not defective, usually is employed when the examination is inadequate for precise evaluation but behavior is in the normal range. Undecided generally indicates that behavior is qualitatively abnormal but the extent of the mental deficiency is in doubt.

NEUROMOTOR STATUS (page 2). The examiner makes his diagnosis of neuromotor status on the basis of both the maturity level of the child and the abnormal patterns recorded. If he determines that some neuromotor disorganization is present, he must decide on its nature and degree. The definitions of the various degrees of abnormality are delineated in Chapter 10. When the intellectual potential has been recorded at the top of the page as Normal, recording is done in the left column under Item 53. When intellectual potential is recorded as Mental Deficiency, the appropriate item is recorded in the right column under Item 53. A diagnosis of abnormal signs of severe degree, with qualitative changes in movement control, is made independently of the intellectual potential.

With the recording form in front of him, the clinician automatically relates intellectual potential and neuromotor status to each other. For computer analysis, columns 50–53 must be analyzed as a single four-digit unit.

QUALITATIVE ASPECTS (page 3). A summary of the emotional stability and quality of integration permits the examiner to indicate at least two of the most important possible explanations for abnormalities in behavior recorded on page 4. Seizures may affect the behavior continuously or intermittently. An "autistic" child may have well-organized exploitation of the test objects in the absence of an awareness of people.

NEUROMOTOR POTENTIAL (page 3). The neuromotor potential is summarized in terms of what is to be expected when a standard neurologic examination is done at school age. Normal includes those children with no neuromotor abnormality and those with abnormal signs of no clinical significance. Those children with abnormal signs of minor or marked degree, with the hypotonic type of "cerebral palsy," or with other clinical conditions in which recovery or gross compensation is expected, would be expected to have no significant neuromotor sequelae. If some degree of abnormality would be detected by the classical neurologic examination, one of the last three categories is applicable.

TOTAL POTENTIAL OTHER THAN PHYSICAL (page 3). The major factor influencing the potential other than physical is the child's intelligence, which presupposes no subsequent noxious events. The infant with "autism" usually compensates; seizures are treatable. Below average is used for the clinical designation of dull normal or borderline dull, and markedly below average when a definite diagnosis of mental deficiency has been made.

DIAGNOSTIC SUMMARY (page 1). As a final step, a brief notation is made in each of the six major areas in the Diagnostic Summary. Although it is completed last, it occupies the position of prominence on the first page to provide a quick overview when the chart is perused later.

If the infant is entirely normal, the experienced clinician might elect to make a few descriptive notes on the back of the developmental schedule before writing a final report and omit the detailed form. Less skilled examiners always should complete the entire form. In this way they will incorporate observation and interpretation of any possible abnormalities as an integral and routine part of their examination procedure.

Final Report of the Evaluation

The appended format was evolved as a guide for students, house staff and fellows. The purposes of a report are to clarify what has been heard and observed, to give the data on which diagnosis, prognosis and recommendations for treatment are based and to transmit this information in a clear and understandable way to others. Certain basic information is included for all patients, but the report is geared toward a specific description of the distinctive abilities and disabilities of the infant under consideration.

Under Parts V.A and VI, instructions to number items on the Developmental and Neurologic Evaluation Form and the Developmental Schedules are present for use by a secretary who has been trained to follow a prepared list of neuromotor abnormalities and behavior patterns and incorporate them into the report. When the behavior is markedly atypical, this numbering procedure should be avoided and the examiner's own words used. It is also possible to devise a form that provides a number of choices in each of the paragraphs from which a skilled clinician can select appropriately for a secretary's guidance in typing the report. Again, this procedure is useful only in relatively uncomplicated cases. It should not be used by a beginner; it prevents him from really thinking about what he has heard and seen.

I. Identifying information: Record patient's name, case number, birthdate, age (or corrected chronologic age), person to whom original copy of report goes and persons to receive carbon copies.

II. Reason for examination.

III. History (use past tense):

A. Birth weight and duration of gestation. Note if amount of prematurity was assigned arbitrarily because of discrepancies between history of gestation and birth weight, and reason for making adjustment.

B. Pregnancy, labor and delivery and neonatal period. Mention abnormalities specifically associated with high risk.

C. Significant illnesses.

D. Convulsions: type of episodes, age of onset, frequency, duration, association with fever and treatment.

E. Developmental history: indicate if normal or in what areas significant deviation occurred, and age at which deviation first was noted. Note specifically if deterioration has occurred.

IV. Qualitative description of behavior (use present tense for remainder): Mention specific patterns which characterize the behavior of this infant, as well as physical anomalies that will call him to mind, if any are present. Include both unusual distortions in sequences (e.g., exploits on touch rather than on visual perception) or outstandingly mature patterns. Comments on general description, adjustment to the examination, interest and attention and quality of exploitation are included as a rule.

V. Neuromotor abnormalities:

A. Abnormal patterns to be included in the report may be numbered on the Developmental and Neurologic Evaluation Form for the secretary's guidance. Some will warrant description in the examiner's own words, being specific rather than general; e.g., "shows incoordination in the use of a pencil in drawing."

B. Describe any seizures observed during the examination.

C. Where speech development is a problem, comment on the comprehension of language as well.

D. Mention visual or auditory deficits.

E. If there are no significant neuromotor abnormalities, a sentence to this effect at end of paragraph IV is sufficient.

VI. Behavior characteristics (do not use "he is able to ..."): Mark the developmental schedules for the items to be typed in the report. Each area is taken separately, in order: adaptive behavior, gross motor behavior, fine motor behavior, language behavior and personal–social behavior. Within each area, number observed items first, then reported behavior. Group together related behavior: e.g., cube, pellet, supine, prone, etc. Not all items necessarily are included, and negatives are mentioned only if they are particularly pertinent to the problem. Do not include the less mature item of a sequence if a more advanced one is positive; e.g., omit "stands and supports large fraction of his weight" (28 weeks) if infant also stands with hands held (32 weeks). The assigned maturity level for each area is placed in parentheses after each field subheading.

VII. Diagnosis:

A. The following three items are detailed first: the general maturity level, the quality of the behavior and the level of development indicated. If development is average, include only a qualitative statement, such as high average, average, etc. If it is not average, give the percentage of normal development, followed by a qualitative phrase; e.g., "Maturity is 55–60% of normal and a mild degree of mental deficiency is indicated."

B. Do not list maturity levels in all areas of behavior in the diagnostic paragraph. Unless there is an indication, such as is specified below, other areas are not mentioned.

C. Gross motor behavior is mentioned specifically if it has diagnostic importance; e.g., "Gross motor behavior is approximately X weeks, and John has 'cerebral palsy,' which is an athetoid quadriplegia." Give the neuromotor diagnosis when it is abnormal. For normal infants, proceed as in V.E.

D. Language development is mentioned in three circumstances: if the child is referred specifically for a language problem, regardless of the findings; if language behavior is significantly accelerated and may be a better prognostic indicator than the current adaptive behavior; if an unsuspected abnormality is detected.

E. If seizures are present, whether by history and/or observation, state the type and give the specific dosage schedule of phenobarbital recommended. Depending on the situation, this may better be deferred to paragraph VIII.

F. Etiology: Rarely can this be specified precisely. If antecedent factors are present, indicate that etiology may be related to them; e.g., toxemia, bleeding, prematurity, illness during pregnancy. If not, indicate if the damage appears to have arisen prenatally (the usual), postnatally or at birth.

VIII. Prognosis and Recommendations:

Indicate if average, normal or slower than normal development is to be expected. If prognosis is guarded, state reasons. Separate intellectual from motor development when appropriate.

B. Make specific recommendations for immediate treatment (e.g., cerebral palsy clinic, seizure control, auditory training) and for the type of educational placement that might be anticipated (e.g., school at regular age, regular school with younger children, slow-learners classes in the public schools, community classes for the retarded or rarely, institutionalization).

IX. Reexamination:

A. Thank you sentence: "We appreciate the opportunity of seeing John and would like to be kept informed of his progress."

B. State the specific time for reexamination, and whether by you or by other agencies at school age to determine educational placement. Alternatively, state no further examination is indicated unless special problems arise.

X. Indicate for secretary what diagnoses should be entered on the patient's file card.

Illustrative Case Report (based on data entered in specimen forms)

Joseph Doctor, M.D.	Re: John Doe
High Street	Birth Date: 1/1/72
Williamstown, New York 12201	CCAge: 28 weeks
	Case #: 0001

7/28/72   Developmental Consultation

John Doe is examined because the parents are puzzled about his progress in the face of a chromosomally confirmed diagnosis of trisomy 21.

John is the fifth pregnancy of this 39-year-old mother. The 15-year-old brother had a hare lip repaired with good cosmetic results. There was a miscarriage at two months of gestation between the births of the 12- and 10-year-olds, who are entirely normal. There is no other relevant family history. John was born 2 weeks before the expected date with a weight of 5 lb 8 oz. There was spotting at the time of the first missed menstrual period and moderate bleeding after the onset of labor. Immediate neonatal condition was good, but there was one apneic episode on the first day of life with perhaps some subsequent cyanosis. Oxygen was given for 2 days, and he was discharged on day 6. A report from the genetics laboratory indicated the presence of trisomy 21.

John did well until 4 months of age when he had a tonic-clonic generalized seizure lasting about 30 minutes on the 3rd day of what proved to be roseola. He was discharged from the hospital after 3 days on no medication. The mother feels that after this he did not use his right arm and leg as well as before, but is not really handicapped significantly, and his progress has been about the same as that of her other children. There is no history of any other seizure activity, and he has had no difficulty as a result of his heart disease (a small ventricular septal defect).

John has the typical clinical appearance of trisomy 21. He makes a stable adjustment to the examination and establishes a friendly social rapport with the examiner after first sizing her up. Behavior is slightly disorganized, and exploitation is impulsive. Attention and interest tend to wander but are easily recalled to the examination situations. No seizure activity is observed.

Abnormal neuromotor patterns are present. There is mild hypotonicity of the left arm and leg and the neck, with moderate hypotonicity of the back. The right extremities show mild spasticity with increased resistance to rapid movement but no limitation of the full range of motion. There is a moderate alternating internal strabismus. In sitting, there is mild extension and adduction of the legs or flexion of the knees and hips, greater on the right, and moderate rounding of the back. In standing, the right leg is mildly extended and the base slightly narrow. The right arm is held slightly adducted with the elbow flexed, while the left arm has moderate abduction. There is fisting, thumb adduction, maldirected reaching and difficulty retaining, all of which are mild on the left and of moderate degree on the right.

John shows the following behavior characteristics: *Adaptive behavior* [27 (23–29) weeks]: He resecures a dropped cube, occasionally takes the cube to his mouth, has a one-hand approach and grasp, holds one and grasps another of the multiple cubes and regards the cup while holding a cube. He bangs the bell, shakes the rattle and transfers the dangling ring, but awkwardly. *Gross motor behavior* (25 weeks): He lifts his legs high in extension, rolls to prone, holds his trunk erect in the supporting chair, is beginning to sit leaning forward on his hands and supports a large fraction of his weight when held in standing. *Fine motor behavior* (23 weeks): He grasps the cube palmarwise, more effectively on the left, and retains the rattle. *Language behavior* (26 weeks): He turns his head to the bell-ringing, grunts and growls, has spontaneous vocal socialization, and is reported to say "m-m-m." *Personal–social behavior* (27 weeks): He discriminates strangers, vocalizes and pats at his mirror image and abandons his effort with the ring and string. He is reported to sit propped for 30 minutes, and to take his foot to his mouth in supine.

On the Gesell Developmental and Neurologic Examination, John's general maturity level is approximately 27 weeks with some scatter; behavior is fairly well integrated, and a low average development is indicated at the present time. He has a mild right spastic hemiplegia, superimposed on mild generalized hypotonicity, probably secondary to the grand mal convulsion at 4 months of age.

Many children with trisomy 21 show average development in early infancy and do not begin to evidence the deceleration that invariably occurs until 9–12 months of age. The functional level John will attain at maturity cannot be predicted precisely, but it is anticipated that he will have a mild degree of mental deficiency, provided no adverse circumstances supervene. He should be able to participate in special classes in the public school system. His hemiplegia should not interfere with the acquisition or exercise of motor control, but he must be observed carefully and a program of physical therapy instituted immediately if there is the slightest hint of limitation of motion. His strabismus should be evaluated by an ophthalmologist. The most important measure for maximizing his developmental potential is the prevention of subsequent convulsions, especially since his first seizure left neuromotor residua. John should be placed on daily doses of phenobarbital at 10 mg/kg and maintained on medication for at least 2 seizure-free years. A copy of the seizure control regimen we have found effective is enclosed.

The diagnosis and prognosis were discussed with the parents, who appear to have a realistic acceptance of the situation. They might benefit from contact with other parents through the local chapter of the National Association for Retarded Children, and were given the address.

We appreciate the opportunity of seeing John and would like to be kept informed of his progress. Unless special problems arise, reevaluation by us is not indicated. He should have psychologic examinations at later ages in order to make plans for the best educational placement, initially in a nursery school, should the parents wish it, and later in a formal academic program.

Jane Roe, M.D.
Director, Child Development Services
Professor of Pediatrics

cc: Division of Medical Genetics

§6. QUESTIONS FOR THE DEVELOPMENTAL SCREENING INVENTORY (DSI)

Because of space limitations, items on the Developmental Screening Inventory (DSI) and its supplementary page, presented in Chapter 17, are necessarily very abbreviated. The words used have been chosen as carefully as possible to indicate the exact meaning. The items are expanded more precisely in the form at the end of this section. The questions correspond to those items on the DSI for which the history column has not been blocked out. Within each of the five areas of behavior they are arranged sequentially by age, which is indicated in the left margin. The clinician should become familiar with this expanded version to avoid incorrect

QUESTIONS FOR THE DEVELOPMENTAL SCREENING INVENTORY (DSI)

		Group I--(Adaptive)	AGE FIRST ATTAINED

DOES YOUR CHILD.....

			AGE FIRST ATTAINED
(4w)	A.	Follow a toy you dangle in front of his eyes to the midline but not past it?---	_____
		Drop a toy you put into his hand at once?--------------------	_____
(8w)	B.	Follow a toy you dangle in front of his eyes past the midline?---	_____
		Hold on to a toy you put in his hand for a few moments?------	_____
(12w)	C.	When he is on his back, follow a toy you dangle over his face from one side all the way over to the other side?-----	_____
		Glance at a toy briefly when it is put in his hand?----------	_____
(16w)	D.	Wave his arms and move his body at the sight of a toy dangled in front of him when he is lying on his back or when you support him in a sitting position?-------------------------	_____
		Look directly at a toy which you have put in his hand so you are sure that he is looking at it?-------------------------	_____
		When he is lying on his back, take a toy which you have put in his hand to his mouth?-----------------------------------	_____
(20w)	E.	Bring both his hands directly up toward a toy dangled or held in front of him when he is lying on his back or when you support him in a sitting position?-------------------------	_____
		Get hold of a toy if you hold it near his hand (approximately one inch away)?---	_____
		When he is on his back, turn his head to look for a toy that he drops?---	_____
(24w)	F.	Usually reach for and pick up a toy in front of him with both hands at once?---	_____
		Reach for a toy he has dropped if it is within his sight?----	_____
		When you support him in a sitting position, put a toy into his mouth?---	_____
(28w)	G.	Usually reach for and pick up a toy in front of him with only one hand?--	_____
		Put a toy back and forth directly from one hand to the other?	_____
		When you support him in a sitting position, bang a toy up and down on a table or his lap?--------------------------	_____
(32w)	H.	Pick up one small toy (about one inch in size) in one hand and then pick up a second one with his other hand without dropping the first?--	_____
		Hold these two toys he has picked up himself, one in each hand, for more than a minute?-------------------------------	_____
(36w)	I.	Hit a toy he holds in his hand against one on the table?-----	_____
		Hold a toy that has a string attached in one hand and play with the string with the other hand?---------------------	_____
(40w)	J.	Touch and play with a toy that he has watched you put inside a cup or a box?---	_____
		Hold a small toy (about one inch in size) in one hand and at the same time try to or pick up a smaller object such as a crumb, small button or thread with the other?-----------	_____
		Poke at things or into holes with a single finger?----------	_____
(44w)	K.	Take a small toy out of a cup or box after he has watched you put it in?---	_____
		If you drop a small toy (about one inch in size) inside a cup or box first, put it back in but not let go of it?-----	_____

Group I--(Adaptive Behavior)

		AGE FIRST
DOES YOUR CHILD.....		ATTAINED

(48w) L.	Play with one toy after another in a similar way so that you are sure he is repeating the same action each time? For example: Drop one toy on the floor, then drop a second, and a third; or move them one after another from one area of the table or floor to another.-------------------------- _____
(52w) M.	If you show him first, try to pile one small toy such as a small block or small box on top of another one, but without success? (May do this by holding both toys in his hands while trying.)-- _____
	Put a small toy into a cup or a box after he watches you put one in first? (You have to start each time you play this game with him.)-- _____
	Hold a toy up by a string attached to it and watch the toy move as he intentionally pulls the toy up and down?-------- _____
(56w) N.	Put a small toy into a cup or a box just if you point and ask him to do it?-------------------------------------- _____
	Scribble back and forth with a crayon or pencil (after you have done it first to show him how)?------------------- _____
(15m) O.	Succeed in piling one small toy such as a small block or small box on top of a second one?-------------------------- _____
	Put 5 or 6 of a pile of small toys into a cup or box but start to take them out again before the whole pile is in?-- _____
(18m) P.	Watch a pea-sized crumb fall out of a bottle when he turns it upside down to get it out? (It doesn't just fall out by accident when he shakes the bottle.)----------------------- _____
	Scribble back and forth when you hand him a crayon or pencil and just ask him to write?----------------------------------- _____
(21m) Q.	If you line up four blocks to make a train, saying "here's one car, another and another," then push it while saying "choo-choo," imitate the motion by pushing at least one block, with or without saying "choo-choo" also?------------ _____
(24m) R.	If you line up four blocks to make a train, saying "here's one car, another and another," clearly imitate your train by aligning at least two blocks?-------------------------- _____
	If you make a vertical stroke on a piece of paper for him, make a definite vertical stroke in imitation?-------------- _____
	If you make a circular scribble on a piece of paper for him, make a definite circular scribble in imitation?------- _____
(30m) S.	If you make a horizontal stroke on a piece of paper for him, make a definite horizontal stroke in imitation?------------ _____
	If you make a cross on a piece of paper for him, make two or more separate strokes in an attempt to imitate you?-------- _____
	If you line up four blocks to make a train and then put a fifth block on top of one of the end blocks saying "and here's the chimney for the smoke," align the blocks in imitation and then add the chimney. (You may say "Now put the chimney on," without pointing, if he only aligns the blocks)?--- _____
(36m) T.	Give a name to something he draws?-------------------------- _____
	Make a cross if you draw one first and ask him to imitate it? _____
	Make a circle if you draw one out of his sight and ask him to copy it?-- _____

		Group 2--(Gross Motor)	AGE FIRST ATTAINED
	DOES YOUR CHILD.....		
(4w)	A.	When he is lying on his abdomen, lift his head enough to clear his nose from the bed?-------------------------------	_____
(8w)	B.	When he is lying on his abdomen, lift his head up so his chin is 3-4 inches from the bed?--------------------------	_____
(12w)	C.	When he is lying on his abdomen, hold his head up for more than one minute so his chin is 3-4 inches from the bed?----	_____
(16w)	D.	Hold his head steady when you support him in a sitting position?---	_____
		When he is lying on his abdomen, hold his head straight up for more than one minute and look directly ahead?----------	_____
(20w)	E.	When he is lying on his abdomen, straighten both elbows out and push his whole chest off the bed?----------------------	_____
(24w)	F.	When he is lying on his back, get hold of his foot?---------	_____
		Roll from his back to his abdomen and get both arms out from under himself?--	_____
(28w)	G.	When he is lying on his back, lift his head off the bed as though trying to sit up?-------------------------------	_____
		Sit briefly leaning forward on his hands when you place him in this position on a hard surface such as the floor or a table?---	_____
		Support most of his weight while standing if you balance him by holding him around the chest under his arms?------------	_____
(32w)	H.	Sit up straight for about one minute without leaning on his hands for support when you place him on a hard surface such as the floor or a table?---------------------------	_____
		Stand and support his full weight if you hold his hands at shoulder height out in front of him only to balance him?---	_____
		While he remains on his abdomen, move about in a circle by means of crossing and uncrossing his arms?-----------------	_____
(36w)	I.	Sit up straight for more than 10 minutes without leaning on his hands for support when you place him on a hard surface such as the floor?-------------------------------	_____
		If you put him there, stand holding on to furniture or his crib rail without leaning his chest against it for support?	_____
(40w)	J.	Sit up straight and steady indefinitely without leaning on his hands so you can put him on the floor and go away and leave him?--	_____
		Go straight forward from sitting over to his abdomen or his hands and knees without going to the side first or falling over?--	_____
		Move forward while up on his hands and knees?----------------	_____
		Pull himself up to a standing position on the furniture or his crib rail?---	_____
(44w)	K.	Stand at furniture or his crib rail without leaning against it and lift a foot up and down?----------------------------	_____
(48w)	L.	Hold on to furniture or his crib rail and walk around it?----	_____
		Walk well if you hold both of his hands to balance him but without helping him to support his weight?----------------	_____
(52w)	M.	Walk well when you hold only one hand to balance him?--------	_____
		Forget to hold on and stand alone for a moment?-------------	_____
(56w)	N.	Take a few steps alone if you put him in standing or he pulls himself up on some furniture?-------------------------	_____
		Fall "flat on his face" if he loses his balance while walking alone without holding on to anything?--------------	_____

Group 2--(Gross Motor)

DOES YOUR CHILD.....	AGE FIRST ATTAINED

(15m) O.
Get up in the middle of the floor and walk alone, without having to pull himself up on something first?-------------- _____

No longer go about on his hands and knees but walk <u>alone</u>, without holding on to things?------------------------------ _____

Catch himself and sit down while walking <u>alone</u>, without holding on, rather than lose his balance and "fall flat on his face?"--- _____

(18m) P.
Try to run, but with a stiff quality like a fast walk?------- _____

Fall very little when walking?-------------------------------⸺ _____

Climb into a couch or an adult chair?------------------------ _____

<u>Walk</u> upstairs when you hold only one hand?-------------------- _____

(21m) Q.
<u>Walk</u> upstairs by himself if he holds on to the railing or wall?--- _____

<u>Walk</u> downstairs if you hold one hand?------------------------ _____

Squat down and rest on his heels, and play in this position without having to sit down on the floor?-------------------- _____

(24m) R.
<u>Walk</u> downstairs by himself if he holds on to the railing or the wall?--- _____

Run well and stop himself without having to run into a wall or piece of furniture?------------------------------------- _____

Kick a ball with a good leg motion and without holding on just if you ask him to, without demonstrating first?------- _____

(30m) S.
Walk on tiptoe in imitation of your doing it?---------------- _____

Jump and get both feet off the floor at the same time?------- _____

Try to stand on one foot without holding on for support?----- _____

(36m) T.
Ride a tricycle using the pedals?--------------------------- _____

Jump off the bottom step with both feet, without falling?---- _____

Stand balanced on one foot for a moment without holding on?-- _____

Group 3--(Fine Motor)

DOES YOUR CHILD.....	AGE FIRST ATTAINED

(4w) A. Hold both hands tightly fisted when he is awake?------------- _____

(12w) B.
Hold his hands open or loosely closed instead of tightly fisted?-- _____

(16w) C.
Scratch and clutch at his clothes?-------------------------- _____

Bring his hands together over his chest and play with his own fingers?-- _____

(24w) D.
Pick up a small toy (about one inch in size) and hold it in the center of his palm with all of his fingers?----------- _____

(28w) E.
Succeed in touching a pea-sized crumb with his whole hand (usually his whole arm moves while he tries to do this)?--- _____

(32w) F.
Try to pick up a pea-sized crumb by curling his fingers and bringing his thumb against them?----------------------- _____

(36w) G.
Pick up a small toy (about one inch in size) with the ends of his fingers?--- _____

Pick up a pea-sized crumb by bringing his thumb and one finger (usually the first finger) together?---------------- _____

(40w) H.
Put a small toy down and take his hand off of it, not just drop it?-- _____

(48w) I.
Pick up a pea-sized crumb easily with his thumb and a single finger (usually his first finger), without resting his arm or hand on the table top as he is doing it?--------------- _____

Group 3--(Fine Motor)

DOES YOUR CHILD.....		AGE FIRST ATTAINED
(56w) J.	Pick up two small toys (about one inch in size) in the same hand at one time, meaning to and not just by accident?-----	_____
(15m) K.	Drop a small pea-sized crumb into a bottle just if you point and ask him to?-------------------------------------	_____
	Help you turn the pages of a book or magazine?----------------	_____
(18m) L.	Pile 3 or 4 small toys such as small blocks or boxes on top of each other?---	_____
	Turn pages of a book or magazine two or three at a time?-----	_____
(24m) M.	Turn pages in a child's book one at a time?------------------	_____
(30m) N.	Hold a pencil or crayon with his fingers the way an adult does?---	_____

Group 4--(Language)

DOES YOUR CHILD.....		AGE FIRST ATTAINED
(4w) A.	Make small indefinite sounds in his throat?--------------------	_____
(8w) B.	Make single vowel sounds, such as "ah, eh, uh?"---------------	_____
(12w) C.	Make cooing sounds like "gooooo, aaaaah, oooooh," or have the beginning of a laugh that doesn't quite come out?-------	_____
	Make sounds back to you as if he were trying to talk if you just nod your head and talk to him?---------------------	_____
(16w) D.	Laugh out loud?--	_____
(20w) E.	Squeal by making his voice go up high like a little pig?------	_____
(24w) F.	Grunt, growl or make other deep-toned sounds?-----------------	_____
	Make babbling sounds to you or his toys as if he were starting a "conversation?" (If to you, without your nodding or making sounds to him first.)-------------------------------	_____
(28w) G.	Make "mum-mum-mum" sounds, especially when crying (sounding somewhat like a mama doll)?--------------------------------	_____
	Make the same vowel sounds in a series with control of his voice? For example: "ah-ah-ah," "oh-oh-oh," "uh-uh-uh."----	_____
(32w) H.	Make a sound like "da, ba, ka, or ga?"------------------------	_____
(36w) I.	Definitely combine two similar sounds like "ba-ba, ga-ga, da-da," even though he doesn't mean anything by them?-------	_____
	Imitate sounds you make by repeating them after you? For example: A cough, tongue click, razz, etc.-------------	_____
	Know his own name (or nickname) when you call him?------------	_____
(40w) J.	Combine two "ma" sounds into "ma-ma" and mean his mother when he does it?--	_____
	Combine two "da" sounds into "da-da" and mean his father when he does it?--	_____
	Play any games like "pat-a-cake," "peek-a-boo," "so big," or "bye-bye" if you just ask him to, so you are sure he knows what the words mean?---------------------------------------	_____
	Say a "word" besides "ma-ma" and "da-da" to mean something? What word or words?_____	_____
(52w) K.	Put a toy down in your hand if you ask him for it and hold out your hand (not just let you take it out of his hand)?---	_____

Group 4--(Language)

DOES YOUR CHILD.....	AGE FIRST ATTAINED

(56w) L. Know any objects by name (light, shoe, ball, T-V, etc.); that is, look at them when you ask him to without your pointing to them or looking at them yourself?----------------------- _____

(15m) M. How many words does he say?_____
What are they?_____

Jabber in a way that is different from baby babbling so that it sounds like sentences in a foreign language, raising and lowering his voice and pausing as though ending a "sentence?"--- _____

Pat at, or try to pick up, large colored pictures in the pages of a book or magazine?------------------------------- _____

(18m) N. Watch your hand and look at different things in a picture, as you point back and forth from one thing to another in a book or magazine?-- _____

Point to a picture when you just ask him to (for example: "show me the dog") without your pointing or looking at it first?--- _____

(21m) O. Combine 2 to 3 words which have different ideas, such as "daddy bye," "go car" (Not "all right" "what's this")?----- _____

(24m) P. If you give him directions one at a time, without pointing or using gestures, carry them out?
"Put the ball (or some other toy you hand him)"
    On the table--- _____
    On the chair--- _____
"Give it to mommy (or daddy)"------------------------------ _____
"Give it to me"--- _____
Make 3-word sentences?------------------------------------ _____
Give example:_____
Use pronouns such as I, you, me, mine?-------------------- _____
Name the following objects if you show them to him?----------
    Pencil_____ _____
    Key_____ _____
    Penny_____ _____
    Ball_____ _____

(30m) Q. Tell you what you do with any of the above objects?---------- _____
Show you in pantomime what you do with any of the above objects?-- _____
Tell you his first and last name if you ask him?------------- _____

(36m) R. Tell you what is happening in a picture book; (for example: eating, sleeping, etc.)?------------------------------------ _____
Use plurals correctly; (for example: babies, shoes, etc.)?--- _____
Tell you if he is a boy or a girl?-------------------------- _____
Carry out the following directions if you ask him to, without pointing or using gestures? "Put the ball (or other object you give him)"
    On the chair--- _____
    Under the chair-------------------------------------- _____
    In back of the chair--------------------------------- _____
    In front of the chair-------------------------------- _____

<u>Group 5--(Personal-Social)</u>

AGE FIRST
ATTAINED

DOES YOUR CHILD.....

(4w) A. Stare vaguely at his surroundings?--------------------------- _____

(8w) B. Smile back at you if you just nod your head and talk to him?- _____
          Follow a person moving around the room with his eyes?-------- _____

(12w) C. Hold his hand up and look at it?----------------------------- _____
          Get hold of his clothes or blankets?------------------------- _____

(16w) D. Start to smile at people just when they come up and stand
          beside him even if they don't talk or nod to him first?----   _____
          Recognize his bottle when he sees it, before you put it in
          his mouth?--- _____

(20w) E. Smile at himself when you put him close to a large mirror
          (Dresser or bathroom cabinet size)?------------------------- _____
          Put both hands on his bottle when you are feeding him?------ _____

(24w) F. Know the difference between strangers and people who belong
          in the house?--   _____
          Talk to himself when you put him close to a large mirror
          (Dresser or bathroom cabinet size)?------------------------   _____

(28w) G. When he is lying on his back, put his foot in his mouth?----- _____
          Reach out and pat himself in the mirror when you put him
          close to a large mirror (Dresser or bathroom cabinet
          size)?---   _____

(32w) H. Bite and chew on his toys, not just lick at them?------------ _____
          Keep on reaching for toys that are out of reach?------------- _____

(36w) I. Hold his own bottle and pick it up again if it drops before
          he is finished?--   _____
          Feed himself a cracker, taking definite bites until it is
          pretty well finished?--------------------------------------   _____

(40w) J. Play any games like "pat-a-cake," "peek-a-boo," "so big,"
          or "bye-bye" in imitation of you after you do them first?--   _____

(44w) K. Hold a toy out to you but not let go of it into your hand
          (unless you take it from him) even if you ask him for it?--   _____
          Reach into the mirror for the image of a toy he is holding
          when you put him close to a large mirror (Dresser or
          bathroom cabinet size)?------------------------------------   _____

(48w) L. Intentionally take toys off a table to another surface
          (for example: his chair or the floor) and then play with
          them there after he has done this, not just go after them
          if they drop down and bring them back up?-----------------   _____

(52w) M. Help when you dress him by pushing his arm through his
          sleeve or holding his feet up for a shoe or his diaper?----   _____
          Try to give a toy that he is holding to his mirror image
          when you put him close to a large mirror (Dresser or
          bathroom cabinet size)?------------------------------------   _____

(56w) N. Play ball with you, using a small throwing movement to
          throw the ball toward you?---------------------------------   _____

(15m) O. Indicate which thing he wants by pointing to it, or looking
          at it and making some sound to call your attention to it,
          so you don't have to guess what he wants?------------------   _____
          Leave his dish on his tray when you are feeding him, not
          throw it off?--   _____

	Group 5--(Personal-Social) DOES YOUR CHILD.....	AGE FIRST ATTAINED
(18m) P.	Pull a toy on a string after him while he walks or crawls around the house?--	_____
	Hug and kiss a doll or stuffed animal or carry it about with him as he walks around?------------------------------	_____
	Feed himself part of his food with a spoon, although it may spill when he does it?-------------------------------	_____
(21m) Q.	Handle a cup well and put it down when he is finished?-------	_____
	Pull you by the hand or clothes to show you some specific object or activity?--------------------------------------	_____
(24m) R.	Dress himself a little; for example, put on a hat or pull up his pants?---	_____
	Imitate the things you do around the house, such as sweeping, dusting, hammering nails?-----------------------	_____
	Get the spoon to his mouth right side up when he is feeding himself?---	_____
	Usually tell you when he has to go to the bathroom to urinate?--	_____
(30m) S.	Usually refer to himself by pronoun, saying "I want," or "me want," rather than using his name?---------------------	_____
	Help put his things away, if you ask him to or do it with him?--	_____
	Push a doll carriage or wagon with good steering and be able to back out if he gets stuck?------------------------------	_____
(36m) T.	Feed himself with a spoon with very little spilling?---------	_____
	Put on his shoes, not necessarily on the correct feet?-------	_____
	Understand taking turns?-------------------------------------	_____
	Unbutton, not merely pull apart, buttons he can reach?-------	_____

Table A-2. Range of Maturity Levels (columns) and Corresponding Expected Developmental Quotients (body of table) Determining the Selection of Questions from the Developmental Screening Inventory to be Sent to Parents at Specified Chronologic Ages (rows).

CHRONOLOGIC AGE	MATURITY LEVEL															
	Weeks														Months	
	4	8	12	16	20	24	28	32	36	40	44	48	52	56	15	18
4w	100	(200)														
8w	50	100	150													
12w		67	100	133												
16w			75	100	125	150										
20w			60	80	100	120	140									
24w				67	83	100	117	133								
28w				57	71	86	100	114	128							
32w					63	75	88	100	113	125						
36w						67	78	89	100	111	122	133				
40w						60	70	80	90	100	110	120				
44w							64	73	82	91	100	109	118	127		
48w								67	75	83	91	100	108	117		
52w								62	69	77	84	92	100	107	125	
56w									64	71	78	86	93	100	116	139
15m											68	74	80	86	100	120
18m											56	62	67	72	83	100

1. SAMPLE COVER LETTER FOR SURVEY OF PAST DEVELOPMENT.

   In order to decide whether it will be necessary to see your child we would like to have in advance some information in regard to his (her) development.
   If on the basis of your answers we decide a formal examination is needed this will save time when your child is examined.
   Please complete these questions by entering the age at which your child first achieved the behavior mentioned. If there are any about which you are really uncertain, please state so. If there is anything not covered by the questionnaire on which you would like to comment, please write your remarks on the back of the pages.

PLEASE MAIL QUESTIONNAIRE BACK AS SOON AS COMPLETED.

   After you have answered all of the questions please reply also to the questions below (use back of page if necessary):

Does (s)he turn to look at you when you talk in a normal voice?_____
Do you think (s)he hears?_____
Has (s)he ever had any convulsions or fits?_____
Does (s)he ever stare off into space and keep right on staring if you put your hand in front of his eyes and hold it there?_____
Does (s)he ever start to cry for no apparent reason and keep right on crying no matter what you do to try to comfort him?_____
Is there anything about your child that worries you?_____

Has (s)he ever lost any behavior once achieved?_____

What age child do you think your child is acting like in:
   Controlling his (her) body and hands------------------_____

   How his (her) mind works-----------------------------_____

   Making sounds or talking-----------------------------_____

   Understanding what you say---------------------------_____

Child's Name:_____ Date:_____

Birth Date:_____ Birth Weight:_____

Day YOU expected baby to be born:_____

Baby's Physician:_____

Your Telephone Number:_____

2. SAMPLE COVER LETTER FOR SURVEY OF CURRENT BEHAVIOR.

We are enclosing some questions about various things that babies do. Some
we would not expect your child to do yet and some will have been accomplished
long ago. Please check one of the two spaces after the questions. If you
cannot check either "Yes" or "No" you may write what you feel is the best
answer on the back of the sheet.

We have grouped together the questions about generally similar behavior;
for example, one group is about the use of the large muscles of the body and
another is about sounds and the understanding of words. Each of the five groups
we have made is divided into several sections, but sometimes there is more
than one group on a page. Start answering questions in Section A of Group 1
on the first page and continue until <u>all</u> the answers in <u>one</u> Section of Group 1
are "No." Go on to Section A of Group 2 and do the same; then answer
Groups 3, 4 and 5.

After you have checked the spaces for all of the questions that you need
to answer, please write your answer to the questions below also (use back of
page if necessary).

PLEASE MAIL QUESTIONNAIRE BACK AS SOON AS COMPLETED.

PLEASE COMPLETE A DAY OR TWO BEFORE YOUR APPOINTMENT
AND BRING THE SHEETS WITH YOU.

Does (s)he turn to look at you when you talk in a normal voice?_____
Do you think (s)he hears?_____
Has (s)he ever had any convulsions or fits?_____
Does (s)he ever stare off into space and keep right on staring if you <u>put</u> your
    hand in front of his eyes and <u>hold</u> it there?_____
Does (s)he ever start to cry for no apparent reason and keep right on crying no
    matter what you do to try to comfort him?_____
Is there anything about your child that worries you?_____

Has (s)he ever lost any behavior once achieved?_____

What age child do you think your child is acting like in:
    Controlling his (her) body and hands------------------_____

    How his (her) mind works------------------------------_____

    Making sounds or talking------------------------------_____

    Understanding what you say----------------------------_____

Child's Name:_____ Date:_____

Birth Date:_____ Birth Weight:_____

Day <u>YOU</u> expected baby to be born: _____

Baby's Physician:_____

Your Telephone Number:_____

paraphrasing in obtaining information from the parents. The glossary accompanying each developmental schedule in Chapter 3 explains the items on the DSI which are not included in the form in this appendix.

The expanded questions can be used with parents in a variety of ways. In the form illustrated, they provide a longitudinal survey of developmental progress from birth, as well as an indication of the current level of function. The parents are asked to indicate the age at which the child first acquired each behavior pattern. This version is most appropriate for sending as the first contact to parents of children over 18 months; it can also be used for 4- or 5-year-olds when there is good indication significant retardation is present. The ages which correspond to each item should not be included for parents.

For the evaluation of behavior in the first 1½ years of life, or for following the subsequent course of previously examined infants, YES and NO columns can replace the Age First Achieved column. The table following the DSI questions illustrates how a series of questionnaires can be prepared to permit estimation of developmental quotients varying from approximately 60 to 140, by selecting a range of questions at each chronologic age. A screening survey of a large population at any given ages also can be done by selecting appropriate questions.

Two sample cover sheets are presented after the DSI questions and the table. Each contains a brief explanation of the questions which follow, requests information about a few specific aspects of behavior and asks the parents' opinion about the age at which they think the child is functioning in several areas of behavior. One form is appropriate when all past development is surveyed, and the second is geared to evaluation of current behavior.

§7. TABLE OF TEMPORARY BEHAVIOR PATTERNS

In estimating the developmental significance of any given behavior, it is necessary to know whether the behavior is a permanent part of the child's equipment, whether it is undergoing augmentation or whether it is altering its form and will be replaced. This requires us to recognize two types of patterns, conveniently known as *permanent* and *temporary*. A temporary pattern, designated by an asterisk on the developmental schedules, is replaced by a more mature pattern of the same nature at a later age, also indicated on the schedules. For example, radial raking of the pellet at 32 weeks is superseded by scissors grasp of the pellet at 36 weeks. A permanent pattern, once in the behavior picture, stays in or augments. For example, a child builds a tower of two at 15 months, a tower of three or four at 18 months.

For convenience of reference and for comparative study, it is desirable to have the complete syllabus of the temporary patterns and the patterns which replace them at successive ages. The counterpart items are listed in parallel columns side by side, and classified both by key age and by behavior field. The age of replacement also is indicated. A temporary pattern, of course, may be replaced by another temporary pattern and finally by a permanent pattern. A few of the replacement patterns listed do not appear as items on the developmental schedules. They usually are qualitative rather than quantitative changes in behavior.

For a further visualization of these items and their developmental transformations at various ages, the student may examine the comprehensive Growth Trend Chart in Appendix B with profit.

TEMPORARY PATTERN	REPLACEMENT PATTERN

4 WEEKS

Adaptive
D. Ring, Ra: Regards in line vision only . . . . . . Delayed midline regard, 8 wk
Ra: Drops immediately . . . . Retains briefly, 8 wk
Bell-r: Attends, activity diminishes . . . . Turns head to bell, 24 wk

Gross Motor
Su: Side position head predominates . . . . Midposition head predominates, 16 wk
Su: t-n-r postures predominate . . . . Symmetric postures predominate, 16 wk
Su: Rolls partway to side . . . . Back flat, no rolling, 8 wk
P. Sit: Complete or marked head lag . . . . Moderate lag, 8 wk
Sit: Head predominantly sags . . . . Head predom. bobbingly erect, 8 wk
Pr: Head droops, ventral suspension . . . . Head compensates, ventral susp., 8 wk
Pr: (placement) Head rotates . . . . Head in midposition, 8 wk
Pr: Crawling movements . . . . Head up, legs flexed, externally rotated, no crawling, 8 wk

Fine Motor
Su: Both hands fisted . . . . Hands open or loosely closed, 12 wk
Ra: Hand clenches on contact . . . . Rattle placed with ease, 8 wk

Language
Express: Impassive face . . . . Alert expression, 8 wk
Express: Vague, indirect regard . . . . Direct, definite regard, 8 wk
Vo: Small, throaty noises . . . . Single vowel sounds, ah–eh–uh, 8 wk

Personal–Social
So: Regards ex. face, activity diminishes . . . . . Facial social response, 8 wk
Su: Stares indefinitely at surroundings . . . . . . Regards examiner, 8 wk
Feeding: 2 night feedings . . . . 1 night feeding, 8 wk

8 WEEKS

Adaptive
D. Ring: Delayed midline regard . . . . Prompt midline regard, 12 wk
Bell-r: Facial response . . . . Turns head to bell, 24 wk

Gross Motor
Sit: Head bobbingly erect . . . . Head steady, set forward, 16 wk
Pr: Lifts head Zone II, recurrently . . . . Head Zone II, sustained, 12 wk

Language
Vo: Single vowel sounds, ah,eh,uh . . . . da-da, 36 wk

Personal–Social
Feeding: Only 1 night feeding . . . . No night feeding, 28 wk

TEMPORARY PATTERN	REPLACEMENT PATTERN

12 WEEKS

Adaptive
D. Ring: Prompt midline regard . . . . Regards immediately, 16 wk

Gross Motor
Su: Head predominantly half-side . . . . Midposition head predominates, 16 wk
Sit: Head set forward, bobs . . . . Head steady, set forward, 16 wk
St: Lifts foot . . . . Feet on platform, sustained, 28 wk
Pr: On forearms . . . . Arms extend, on hands, 20 wk
Pr: Hips low, legs flexed . . . . Creeps, pelvis elevated, 40 wk

Language
Vo: Coos . . . . da-da, 36 wk

Personal—Social
Play: Hand regard . . . . Hand play, mutual fingering, 16 wk
Play: Pulls at dress . . . . Prefers toys, 24 wk

16 WEEKS

Adaptive
D. Ring. Ra, Cube, Cup: Arms activate . . . . . . Approaches and grasps, 24 wk
D. Ring: Free hand to midline . . . . Transfers, 28 wk
Cube, Cup: Looks from hand to object . . . . . . Hand on object, 20 wk

Gross Motor
Su: Hands engage . . . . Foot play, 24 wk
Sit: Head steady, set forward . . . . Head erect, steady, 20 wk
Pr: Legs extended or semiextended . . . . Creeps, legs flexed, 40 wk
Pr: Verge of rolling . . . . Stable position, arms extended, 20 wk

Fine Motor
Su: Fingers, scratches, clutches . . . . Grasps on visual cue, 24 wk

Language
Express: Excites, breathes heavily, strains on
  sight . . . . Competence and facility in grasp, 32 wk

Personal—Social
So: Vocalizes or smiles pulled-to-sit . . . . Effort to attain sitting, 24 wk
Play: Sits propped 10—15 min . . . . Sits alone indefinitely, 40 wk
Play: Hand play, mutual fingering . . . . Grasps foot, 24 wk
Play: Dress over face . . . . Prefers toys, 24 wk

20 WEEKS

Adaptive
Ra, Bell: Two-hand approach . . . . One-hand approach, 28 wk
Ra, D. Ring: Grasp only if near hand . . . . Approaches and grasps, 24 wk
M. Cubes: Grasps one on contact . . . . Grasps on visual cue, 24 wk

Fine Motor
Pr or TT: Scratches TT or platform . . . . Demands toys, 28 wk
Cube: Precarious grasp . . . . Palmar grasp, 24 wk

Language
Vo: Squeals . . . . da-da, 36 wk

Personal—Social
Feeding: Pats bottle . . . . Holds bottle, 36 wk

| TEMPORARY PATTERN | REPLACEMENT PATTERN |

24 WEEKS

Adaptive
Cube, Bell: To mouth .... Habitual inhibition, 18 mo
M. Cubes: Holds one, approaches another .... Grasps second cube, 28 wk

Gross Motor
P. Sit: Lifts head, assists .... Attains sitting independently, 40 wk
Sit chair: Trunk erect .... Sits independently, 36 wk

Fine Motor
Cube: Grasps, palmarwise .... Radial digital grasp, 36 wk

Language
Vo: Growls, grunts .... da-da, 36 wk

Personal-Social
Play: Grasps foot (supine) .... Sits, prefers toys, 36 wk
Play: Sits propped 30 min .... Sits indefinitely unsupported, 40 wk

28 WEEKS

Adaptive
Bell: Bangs .... Waves, shakes, 40 wk

Gross Motor
Su: Lifts head .... Attains sitting, 40 wk
Sit: Briefly, leans forward (on hands) .... 1 minute, erect unsteady, 32 wk
St: Large fraction weight (trunk supported) .. Briefly, hands held, 32 wk
St: Bounces actively .... Briefly, hands held, 32 wk

Fine Motor
Cube: Radial palmar grasp .... Radial digital grasp, 36 wk
Pellet: Rakes, whole hand contacts .... Radial raking, 32 wk
    Unsuccessful inferior scissors grasp, 32 wk

Language
Vo: m-m-m (crying) .... ma-ma, 40 wk
Vo: Polysyllabic vowel sounds .... da-da, 36 wk

Personal–Social
Play: With feet, to mouth (supine) .... Sits and prefers toys, 36 wk
Ring-str: Fusses or abandons effort .... Persistent, 32 wk

32 WEEKS

Adaptive
Cube: Retains 2 as 3rd presented .... Grasps 3rd cube, 36 wk
Cup-cu: Holds cube, regards cup .... Hits cube against cup, 36 wk

Gross Motor
Sit: 1 min, erect, unsteady .... Steady, 10 min, 36 wk
St: Maintains briefly, hands held .... Stands holding rail, 36 wk
Pr: Pivots .... Creeps, 40 wk

Fine Motor
Pellet: Radial raking .... Prehends, scissors grasp, 36 wk
Pellet: Unsuccessful inferior scissors grasp .... Prehends, scissors grasp, 36 wk

Personal–Social
Play: Bites, chews toys .... Habitual inhibition mouthing, 18 mo
Play: Reaches persistently toys out of reach ... Insight, creeps to toy, 40 wk

TEMPORARY PATTERN	REPLACEMENT PATTERN

36 WEEKS

Adaptive
Cube: Grasps third cube . . . . Retains two, exploits 3rd with cubes in hand, 40 wk
Cube: Hits, pushes cube with cube . . . . Builds tower or casts, 15 mo
Cup & cube: Cube against cup . . . . Cube into cup without release, 44 wk
Pellet and bo: Approaches bottle first . . . . Approaches pellet first, 40 wk

Gross Motor
St: Holds rail, full weight . . . . Cruises at rail, 48 wk

Fine Motor
Pellet: Prehends, scissors grasp . . . . Inferior pincer grasp, 40 wk

Language
Vo: da-da (or equivalent) . . . . Ma-ma and da-da with meaning, 40 wk

Personal–Social
Feeding: Holds bottle . . . . Bottle discarded, 15 mo

40 WEEKS

Adaptive
Cube: Matches two cubes . . . . Tower of 2 cubes, 15 mo
Cup & cube: Fingers cube in cup . . . . Removes cube from cup, 44 wk

Gross Motor
St: Pulls to feet at rail . . . . Attains standing independently, 15 mo
Pr: Creeps . . . . Walks alone, creeping discarded, 15 mo

Fine Motor
Cube: Crude release . . . . Controlled release (tower, casting), 15 mo
Pellet: Inferior pincer grasp . . . . Neat pincer grasp, 48 wk

Personal–Social
So: Waves bye and patacakes . . . . Too sophisticated

44 WEEKS

Adaptive
Cup & cube: (dem.) Cube into cup
 without release . . . . Releases cube into cup, 52 week
Pellet in bo: Points at pellet thru glass . . . . Dumps pellet out, 18 mo

Gross Motor
St: (at rail) Lifts, replaces foot . . . . Cruises at rail, 48 wk
 Walks, two hands held, 48 wk

Personal–Social
So: Extends toy to person without release . . . . Gives toy, 52 wk
Feeding: Milk from cup (in part) . . . . Bottle discarded, 15 mo
Mirror: Reaches image ball . . . . Offers ball to image, 52 wk

48 WEEKS

Adaptive
Cube: Sequential play . . . . Builds buildings, 48 mo
Pellet & bo: Takes pellet only . . . . Tries to insert in bottle, 52 wk

Gross Motor
St: Cruises at rail . . . . Walks alone, 15 mo
Walks: Needs both hands held . . . . Needs only one hand held, 52 wk

Personal–Social
Play: Toys to side rail . . . . Casts to floor, 15 mo
Play: Platform play . . . . Casts to floor, 15 mo

TEMPORARY PATTERN   REPLACEMENT PATTERN

52 WEEKS

Adaptive
Cube: (dem.) Tries tower, fails . . . . Tower of 2, 15 mo
Cup & cube: (dem.) Releases one cube in cup . (no dem.) Releases cube in cup, 56 wk
Pellet & bo: Tries inserting, releases, fails . . . . . Inserts pellet in bottle, 15 mo
Formboard: Looks selectively round hole . . . . Inserts round block (dem.), 56 wk

   Gross Motor
Walks: Needs only one hand held . . . . Walks alone, 15 mo

   Personal–Social
Dressing: Cooperates in dressing . . . . Dresses, undresses, supervision, 48 mo

56 WEEKS

Adaptive
Formboard: (dem.) Inserts round block . . . . . . (no dem.) Inserts round block, 15 mo
Drawing: Vigorous imitative scribble . . . . Drawing, scribbles spontaneously, 18 mo

   Gross Motor
St: Momentarily alone . . . . Walks alone, 15 mo

   Language
Vo: Incipient jargon . . . . Uses jargon, 15 mo

   Personal–Social
Ball: Releases with slight cast toward ex. . . . . . Hurls ball, 18 mo

15 MONTHS

Adaptive
Cup & cube: 6 cubes into cup . . . . 10 into cup, out inhibited, 18 mo
Drawing: Incipient imitation stroke . . . . Definitive stroke imitation, 18 mo

   Gross Motor
Walks: Falls by collapse . . . . Seldom falls, 18 mo
Stairs: Creeps up . . . . Walks up, one hand held, 18 mo

   Fine Motor
Book: Helps turn pages . . . . Turns 2–3 at once, 18 mo

   Language
Vo: Uses jargon . . . . Jargon discarded, sentences, 24 mo
Book: Pats pictures . . . . Looks selectively, names or points, 18 mo

   Personal–Social
Toilet: Partial regulation . . . . Verbalizes needs fairly consistently, 24 mo
Toilet: Indicates wet pants . . . . Regulated daytime, 18 mo
Communication: Indicates wants (points or
   vocalizes) . . . . Asks for food, toilet, drink, 21 mo
Play: Shows or offers toy . . . . Pulls person to show, 21 mo
Play: Casts object in play or refusal . . . . Inhibits, plays on table, 18 mo

18 MONTHS

Adaptive
Drawing: Scribbles spontaneously . . . . Names own drawing, 36 mo
Drawing: Makes stroke imitatively . . . . Imitates vertical stroke, 24 mo
Formboard: Piles 3 blocks . . . . Places single blocks on, 24 mo

   Gross Motor
Walks: Fast, runs stiffly . . . . Runs well, 24 mo
Stairs: Walks up, one hand held . . . . Walks up, holds rail, 21 mo
Adult chair: Climbs into . . . . Sits down

TEMPORARY PATTERN   REPLACEMENT PATTERN
18 MONTHS (Cont'd)

Ball: Hurls .... Throws overhand, 48 mo
Large ball: Walks into .... (dem.) Kicks, 21 mo

Fine Motor
Book: Turns pages, 2–3 at once .... Turns pages singly, 24 mo

Personal–Social
Feeding: Hands empty dish .... Inhibits
Feeding: Feeds self in part, spills .... Feeds self, spills little, 36 mo
Toilet: Regulated daytime .... Verbalizes needs, 24 mo
Play: Pulls a toy .... Pushes toy with good steering, 30 mo
Play: Carries or hugs doll .... Domestic mimicry, 24 mo

21 MONTHS

Adaptive
Cube: Imitates pushing train .... Aligns 2 or more cubes, 24 mo
Formboard: Places 2–3 blocks .... Inserts 3 on presentation, 30 mo
Performance box: Inserts corner of square .... Inserts square, 24 mo

Gross Motor
Walks: Squats in play .... Sits or leans over
Stairs: Walks down, one hand held .... Down alone, 24 mo
Large ball: (dem.) Kicks .... (no dem.) Kicks, 24 mo

Language
Speech: Combines 2–3 words spontaneously.. 3-word sentences, 24 mo

Personal–Social
Communication: Echoes 2 or more last words . Verbalizes immediate experiences, 24 mo
Communication: Pulls person to show .... Asks (for another, etc.), 24 mo

24 MONTHS

Adaptive
Cube: Aligns 2 or more, train .... Adds chimney, 30 mo
Drawing: Imitates circular stroke .... Copies circle, 36 mo
Formboard: Places single blocks on .... Inserts 3 blocks on presentation, 30 mo
Formboard: Adapts after 4 trials .... Adapts repeatedly, error, 30 mo

Personal–Social
Toilet: Dry at night, taken up .... Dry all night, 36 mo
Toilet: Verbalizes toilet needs .... Takes toilet responsibility, 42 mo
Communication: Verbalizes immed. exper .... Inhibits
Communication: Refers to self by name ..... By pronoun, 30 mo
Play: Parallel play predominates .... Associative play, 42 mo

30 MONTHS

Adaptive
Drawing: 2 or more strokes for cross .... Imitates cross, 36 mo
Formboard: Adapts repeatedly, error .... Adapts, no error, 36 mo

36 MONTHS
Adaptive
Cube: Imitates bridge................... (no dem.) Bridge from model, 42 mo
Drawing: Imitates cross .... Copies cross, 48 mo

42 MONTHS
Personal-Social
Play: Associative replaces parallel play .... Cooperates with children, 48 mo

Appendix B

Growth Trend Chart

The growth trend chart provides a comprehensive overview of the entire area of development from 4 weeks through 36 months. It is a single integrated chart which exhibits the continuity of the growth trends for this period. For convenience, however, the chart is separated into five subdivisions as follows:

> First Quarter: 4, 8, 12, 16 weeks
> Second Quarter: 16, 20, 24, 28 weeks
> Third Quarter: 28, 32, 36, 40 weeks
> Fourth Quarter: 40, 44, 48, 52 weeks
> Later Infancy: 15, 18, 21, 24, 30, 36 months

All diagnostically significant behavior, including that explored by the interview as well as by the examination, is represented in the chart. Characteristic behavior (that is, present in 50% or more of all cases) is shown for each of the age levels, both key ages and intermediate ages. The growth trends for any given behavior are readily ascertained by reading horizontally across the chart from age to age. The lines of continuity are represented by serial dots (. . . .). In the first column of each page, the continuity of an earlier item of behavior is indicated by reprinting the item in *italics*. The italics, by convention, therefore are equivalent to serial dots. When any given behavior no longer is significantly present in the examination and is not replaced, the termination is designated by a bracket sign].

To illustrate, consider the Cup and Cubes situation. The first significant behavior appears at 32 weeks. The infant holds the cube and regards the cup. At 36 weeks he brings the cube against the cup. At 40 weeks he reaches into the cup and fingers the cube. At 44 weeks he not only fingers but removes the cube from the cup; he can also put the cube into the cup but without release. At 52 weeks he releases the cube into the cup. This developmental progression is summed up succinctly on the chart as follows:

32 Weeks	*36 Weeks*	*40 Weeks*	*44 Weeks*	*48 Weeks*	*52 Weeks*
holds cube, regards cup. . . .	brings cube against cup. . . .	fingers cube in cup.	fingers cube and removes.		releases cube into cup

470

If the reader is curious to follow the genetic trends still further, the chart will show continuations of this patterning of cup-cube behavior at 15, 18, 21 and 24 months.

The chart also serves to visualize and to codify the numerous temporary patterns of behavior which were tabulated in the previous Appendix (A). The beginning, the developmental transformation, and the fate of each temporary pattern is shown in horizontal progression.

The chart lists not only the behavior patterns which appear on the developmental schedules but all other patterns of characteristic behavior elicited by the examination situations. Although the standard developmental schedules are ample for routine purposes, the systematic organization of the growth trend chart will make it serviceable for detailed analysis of cases which require special study. Finally, the chart serves as a compendium for the student who wishes to become more familiar with developmental relationships of the behavior characteristics which have diagnostic significance.

A Growth Trend Chart for the period of **EARLY INFANCY** is presented in four sections as follows:

§1. First Quarter: 4, 8, 12, 16 weeks
§2. Second Quarter: 16, 20, 24, 28 weeks
§3. Third Quarter: 28, 32, 36, 40 weeks
§4. Fourth Quarter: 40, 44, 48, 52 weeks

§ 1. GROWTH TREND CHART. *FIRST QUARTER: 4-16 WEEKS*

	4 WEEKS	8 WEEKS	12 WEEKS	16 WEEKS
Supine	Head side predom. T-n-r pos. predom. Windmill mvts.] Hand to mouth.] Both hands fisted. Legs fl. heels on platf.] Legs fl. & ext., sl. lifted. Rolls partway to side.] Impassive face. Indirect regard. Stares indef. at surr.	Alert face. Direct regard. Looks at Ex.	Head ½ side predom. H. midl. & sym. postures seen. Hands open or loosely cl. Predominant regard Ex.	Head midl. predom. T-n-r posit. seen. Sym. postures predom. Hands engage. Fingers, scratches, clutches. Smiles at Ex.
D. Ring	Regards line vis. only. Follows to midl., not beyond.	Delay reg. midl. Follows past midl. Regards Ex. hand.	Prompt midl. regard. Follows 180°. Regards Ex. face.	Arms activate. Regards ring in hand. Mouths ring. Free hand approaches. Retains.
Rattle	Regards line vision only. Hand clenches contact.] Placed with difficulty. Drops immediately. Drops rattle.	Placed with ease. Retains briefly.	Delay midl. regard. Holds actively. Glances at Ra in hand.	Prompt midl. regard. Arms activate. Regards Ra in hand.

Bell ring			
Attends, reduced activity	Facial response.		
Social stim			
Regards Ex., reduct. activ	Facial soc. resp.	Vocal social response.	Spontaneous soc. smile.
	Follows moving person		
Pull-sit			
Complete or marked lag.	Moderate lag.		Slight lag.
			Voc. or smiles on att. sit'g.
Sit			
Head sags.		Head set forward.	
Erects head.	Head predom. bob. erect.	Set fwd., bobbing.	Set forward, steady.
Head predom. sagging.			Lumbar curv. only.
Back rounded.			
Standing			
No weight support.		Small fraction wt. briefly.	
Sl. resist. platform.	]		
Legs extend briefly.		Legs ext. recurrently.	
Curls toes.		Lifts foot.	Rises to toes.
Prone			
No head compensation.	Head compensation.		
Head rotated (placement).	Head midl. (placement).		
Lifts to Zone I moment.	Zone II recurrently.	Zone II sustained.	Zone III, sustained.
Head returns to side.			
Lowers to platform.			
Hips high.	]	Hips low.	
(see next page)			

GROWTH TREND CHART. FIRST QUARTER: 4–16 WEEKS (Continued)

	4 Weeks	8 Weeks	12 Weeks	16 Weeks
Prone (Continued)	Kneeling position........ Crawling movements.......]	Legs fl., ext., rot........	Rests on forearms, fl........	Legs ext. or semi-ext........ 1 arm fl., 1 ext........ Verge of rolling........
Language	Sm. throaty noises........	Ah-uh-eh........ Smiles........	Coos........ Chuckles........	Laughs........ Breathes heavily, excites........
Interview	2 night feedings........ Startle, sneeze, jaw clonus.......]	1 night feeding........	Pull at dress........ Hand regard........	Dress over face........ & play, with mut. fingering........ Sits propped 10–15 min........ Antic. on sight food........
Chair			Slumps........ Erects head, nodding........ Regards Ex........ Fingers TT........	Regards TT or hands........
Cube			Follows Ex. withdr. hand........ Reg. own hand........ Reg. cube prol........	Shifts reg. hand to cube........ Reg. cube recurrently........ Arms activate........ Contacts cube........

	16 Weeks	20 Weeks	24 Weeks	28 Weeks
Pellet			Follow Ex. withdr. hand No regard pellet Hand regard	Delayed rec. regard
Cup			Immed. prolong. regard Hand regard Contacts cup	Shifts reg. hand to cup Arms activate
Bell				Prompt prol. regard Arms activate

§ 2. GROWTH TREND CHART.   *SECOND QUARTER: 16–28 WEEKS*

	16 Weeks	20 Weeks	24 Weeks	28 Weeks
Chair Slumps *Erects head, nodding* Regards TT, hands *Fingers TT* *Regards Ex.*		Head steady Regards toy on table Scratch TT	Trunk erect Grasps toy on TT	Dangles or bangs toy on TT
Cubes: First *Follows Ex. withdraw'g hand* Regards cube recurrently Arms activate Contacts cube Reg. shifts cube to hand⎤		⎤	Delayed 1 hand appr. & grasp Palmar grasp Cube to mouth Drops cube	Immed. 1 hand appr. & grasp Radial palmar grasp Retains cube
Second	Retains 1st as 2nd presented Regards 2nd			

(see next page)

GROWTH TREND CHART. SECOND QUARTER: 16-28 WEEKS (Continued)

16 WEEKS	20 WEEKS	24 WEEKS	28 WEEKS
Second Cube (Continued)	Drops 1st. Approach, contact 2nd.		
Third	Drops 1 immed. Regards dropt cube. Drops other cube. Delayed regard 3rd.	Rescures dropt cube. Immediate regard 3rd. Delayed appr., contact 3rd.	Holds 2 cubes more than mom. Immed. appr. contact 3rd. Transfers cube.
Massed Cubes	Visual pursuit screen. Approach. Grasps 1, tactile cue. Precarious grasp..] Drops immed. In all, grasps 1 cube.	Reaches for screen. Scatters cubes. Delayed grasp 1, visual cue Holding 1, appr. another. Drops. In all, 2 cubes.	Immed. grasp 1, visual cue. Mouths cube. Holding 1, grasps another. In all, 3 cubes.
Pellet Follow Ex. withdraw'g hand Delayed, recurrent regard. Hand regard.		Delayed intent regard. Whole hand approach.	Contacts. Rakes.
Cup Immed. regard. Arms activate.	Immed. approach.		

Contacts

Regard shifts cup to hand...... | | Hands on sides...... | Lifts & uprights cup......
| | Grasps handle......
| | Lifts cup......
| | Cup to mouth......
| | Drops......

Bell

Prompt regard...... | 2 hand appr., contact...... | Immed. 2 hand appr., grasp... | Immed. 1 hand appr. & grasp.
Arms activate...... | | Bell to mouth...... |
| | Free hand engages...... | Adept transfer......
| | Two-stage transfer...... | Bangs......
| | | Retains......
| | Drops......

Supine

Head midline predom...... | | | Lifts head from platf......
T-n-r positions seen...... |
Sym. positions predom...... |
Hands engage...... | Hands open...... |
Hands open or loosely cl....... |
Finger, scratch, clutch...... |
Legs flex & ext. sl. lifted....... | | Legs lifted high in ext...... | (Situation curtailed)
Smiles at Ex. spontan...... | Regards Ex...... |
| Rolls to side...... | Rolls to prone......

D. Ring

Prompts midl. regard...... | Approach, contact...... | Immed. appr. & grasp...... | Immed. appr. & grasp......
Arms activate...... | Grasps near hand only...... |
Placed in hand...... |
Regards ring in hand...... |
Mouths ring...... | | | Transfers......
Free hand approaches...... | | Holds with 2 hands...... |
Retains...... |

GROWTH TREND CHART. SECOND QUARTER: 16–28 WEEKS (Continued)

	16 Weeks	20 Weeks	24 Weeks	28 Weeks
Rattle	Prompt midl. regard.	2 hand appr., contact.	Immed. appr. & grasp.	Immed. 1 hand appr., grasp.
	Arms activate.	Grasp near hand only.		
	Placed with ease.			
	Regards Ra in hand.	Mouths Ra.	Free hand fingers.	Shakes activ. & vigor'sly.
		Free hand approaches.	Retains.	
	Drops	Visual purs. lost Ra.	Prehensory purs. lost Ra.	
Bell Ring	*Attends, activity reduced.*		Turns head to bell.	
	Facial response.			
Pull Sit	*Slight head lag.*	No head lag.	Lifts head, assists pull.	
	Vocalizes or smiles, attains sitting.			
Sit	*Head set forward, steady.*	Head erect, steady.	Sits v. mom., leaning forward.	Sits mom. +, lean forw. prop. on hands.
	Lumbar curvature.		Brief passive balance.	Sits erect v. moment.
				V. brief active balance.
				Active in sitting.
Stand	*Small frac. wt. briefly.*			Large frac. wt.
	Legs extend recurrently.			Bounces.
	Curls toes.			

Rises to toes ....

Lifts foot ....

Prone

Head compensates .... Head compensates ....

Holds head in Zone III, sust ....

Arms flexed on forearms ....

1 arm flexed, 1 extended .... Arms extended, on hands ....

Verge of rolling .... Scratch platform ....   Lifts arm to lure ....

Legs extended or semi-ext .... Legs extended ....

Attempts pivot, unsuccess ....

Mirror

Regards own image .... Regards own image ....

Smiles .... Smiles ....

Vocalizes ....   Pats mirror ....

Language (include report)

Ah-uh-eh ....

Smiles ....

Coos ....   Polysyllabic vowel sounds ....

Laughs ....

Breathes heavily, strains, excites ....

Squeals .... Squeals ....

Grunts, growls ....   M-m-m sound (crying) ....

Personal-Social Interview

Dress over face .... Discriminates stranger ....

Hand play, mutual fingering .... Grasps feet ....   Feet to mouth ....

Sits propped 10-15 min .... Sits propped 30+ min ....

Anticipates on sight food ....

Pats bottle .... Pats bottle ....   Takes solids well ....

Spontan. vocal-social ....

§ 3. GROWTH TREND CHART.   THIRD QUARTER: 28–40 WEEKS

Chair

28 WEEKS	32 WEEKS	36 WEEKS	40 WEEKS
Head steady	}	Sits on platform, good control	
Trunk erect	]	Holding 1, grasps 2nd	
Grasps toy on TT			
Dangles or bangs toy	Transfers toy		

Cubes: First

28 WEEKS	32 WEEKS	36 WEEKS	40 WEEKS
Immed. appr. & grasp			
Radial palmar grasp		Radial digital grasp	
Cube to mouth		]	
Retains cube		Transfers cube	

Second

28 WEEKS	32 WEEKS	36 WEEKS	40 WEEKS
Retains 1st during presenta.	Retains 1st throughout		
Regards 2nd	Appr., grasps 2nd		
Appr., contact 2nd	Mouths cube		
	Holds 2 cubes briefly		Holds 2 cubes prolongedly
Drops cube		Drops and resecures	Retains both cubes

Third

28 WEEKS	32 WEEKS	36 WEEKS	40 WEEKS
Drops 1 immed.	Retains both on presenta.		
Immed. regard 3rd		Grasps cube 3rd	
Immed. appr., contact 3rd	Appr. 3rd with cube in hand	Hits or pushes with cube in hand	Matches 2 cubes
Drops cube			
Resecures dropt cube			
Transfers cube			
Holds 2 cu. more than moment	Holds 2 cubes prolongedly		

Massed Cubes			
Reaches screen.................	....	....	....
Follows screen.................	....	....	1 hand appr.................
2 hand appr.................	....	Immed. grasp 2 cubes.........	Immed. grasp 1 cube.........
Immed. grasp 1 cube.........	....	....	Selects top or corner cube....
Scatters cubes.................	....	....	Controlled play..............
Holding 1, grasps another......	....	....	....
Mouths cube..............	....	....	....
Grasps 3 or more in all........	....	Drops and rescues............	Crude release............
Drops cube.............	....	....	....
Cup & Cubes			
Approaches cubes first........	Approaches cup first..........	....	....
Takes cup by rim............	....	....	....
Drops cup.............	....	....	....
Takes cube.............	....	Brings cube against cup......	....
Holds cube, regards cup......	....	Drops 1 for other...........	....
Drops cube............	....	No alt. behav., command, gest.	....
		No alt. behav. demonstra.....	Reaches into cup, fingers cube
Pellet			
Follows Ex. withdr. hand.........	....	....	....
Delayed intent regard............	Immed. regard and approach.	....	Index finger approach........
Appr. & contact.................	....	....	....
Whole hand raking............	....	....	Prehends promptly, inf. pincer.
Radial raking...............	....	....	....
Unsuccess. scissors attempt....	Prehends, scissors grasp.......	....	....
Pellet in bottle			
	Eyes drop..................	....	....
	Takes bottle................	....	....
	To mouth..................	....	....
	Quest. regard pellet in bo......	....	....
	(P. falls out) disregards P......	....	Regards pellet (fallen).........

GROWTH TREND CHART.   THIRD QUARTER: 28-40 WEEKS (Continued)

28 Weeks	32 Weeks	36 Weeks	40 Weeks
Pellet beside bottle			
		Reaches bottle first.	Reaches pellet first.
		Disregards pellet.	Takes pellet, drops.
		Takes botle.	
Bell			
Immed. 1 hand app. & grasp.			
Grasps bowl or junction.			By handle.
To mouth.			
Transfers adeptly.			
Bangs.			Shakes or waves.
Retains.]			
Ring-string			
Regard ring first.			
Reach toward ring.			
Slap, scratch TT...]			
Regard string.	Rakes at string.	Prehends string, pulls in.	Plucks string easily.
Contact string.	Pulls or drags in.		
	Secures ring.		
	Transfers ring.	Manipulates string.]	
Fuss or abandon effort.	Persistent, difficulty.		
Sitting			
Sits very momentarily.	1 min. or more.	10 min.+ (thru exam.)	Indefinitely.
Sits leaning fwd. onto hands.]			
Erect momentarily.	Erect.		
Almost active balance.	Active balance.		
Unsteady.		Steady.	
Active in sitting.		Leans fwd. and re-erects.	
Falls.			Sitting to prone.

Standing			
Support by trunk	Support by hands	Full weight, sustained	Pulls to feet at rail
Large fraction weight	Full weight briefly	Stands holding rail	
Legs ext. recurrently	Legs ext., hips sl. flexed	Legs extended	Lowers self from rail
Bounces			
Prone			
On abd. & ext. arms			On hands & knees
Lifts arm			
Unsuccess. attempt pivot	Pivots	Creeping position (boys)	Creeps
		Collapses to prone (boys)	
Mirror			
Reg. own image			
Smiles			
Vocalizes			Leans forward
Pats mirror			
Language			
Smiles			
Laughs			
Squeals			
Grunt			
M-m-m crying		Dada	Mama
Polysyll. vowel sounds	Da, ka, ba, ga, etc.	Imitates sounds	
		Understands name, no-no	And bye & patacake
Breathes heavily, strains, excites			One "word"
Personal-Social			
Discrim. strangers			
Feet to mouth			
(see next page)			

GROWTH TREND CHART.   THIRD QUARTER: 28-40 WEEKS (*Continued*)

28 Weeks	32 Weeks	36 Weeks	40 Weeks
Personal-Social (Continued)			
Sits propped 30 min.+			
Pats bottle			
Takes solids well			
	Bites, chews toys		
	Reach persist. toy out of reach		
		Holds bottle	
		Feeds self cracker	
			Sits indef. unsupported
			Pat-a-cakes
			Waves bye

§ 4. GROWTH TREND CHART.   FOURTH QUARTER: 40-52 WEEKS

40 Weeks	44 Weeks	48 Weeks	52 Weeks
Sits on platform, good control			
Holding 1 toy, grasps 2nd			
Transfers toy			
	Dangles or bangs toy		
Cubes: First			
Immed. appr. & grasp			
Radial digital grasp			
Transfers cube			
Retains cube			
Second			
Retains 1st throughout			
Appr. & grasp 2nd			
Mouths cube			
Retains both cubes			

Third			
Retains 2 on presentation....	Retains 2 throughout....	Retains 2 on presentation....	
Hits, pushes cube with cube....			
Match 2 cubes			
Drops cube		Drops cube....	
Tower			
		Cube to model....	Takes cube from model....
			Cube on cube without release....
			Attempts tower, it falls....
Massed Cubes			
Reaches for screen....			
1 hand approach....		2 hand approach....	
Takes 1 cube first appr....		Takes 2 cubes....	
Selects top or corner cube....			
Holding 1, grasps another....			
Controlled play....		Sequential play, 1 by 1	
Releases cube....			
Grasps 3 or more in all....			4 or more in all....
Cup & Cubes			
Grasp cup first, by rim....			
Takes cube....			
Fingers cube in cup....	Removes cube from cup....		
Cube against cup....	Cube into cup without release		Release 1 cube into cup....
Pellet			
Index finger approach....		Thumb and index approach....	
Prehends promptly....			
Inferior pincer grasp....		Neat pincer grasp....	
Pellet in bottle			
Eyes drop....			

GROWTH TREND CHART. *FOURTH QUARTER: 40-52 WEEKS (Continued)*

40 WEEKS	44 WEEKS	48 WEEKS	52 WEEKS
Pellet in bottle (Continued)			
Questionable regard P in Bo	Definite regard P in Bo		
	Points at P through glass		
Takes bottle....]			
Bottle to mouth....]			
Regards P if drops out	Grasps P if drops out		
Pellet beside bottle			
Reaches pellet first			
Takes pellet	Retains pellet	Takes pellet only	
Drops pellet		To mouth	Pellet over bottle
Takes bottle....]			Tries insert, unsuccessful
Bell			
Grasps by handle	Grasp by top of handle		
To mouth			
Transfers			
Shakes or waves	Regards & pokes clapper		
Ring and String			
Approach ring first	Approach string first		
Plucks string easily			
Secures ring			
Transfers ring			Dangles ring by string
Manipulates string			
Formboard			
Pulls at formboard			
Accepts round block			

Transfers round block...Looks selectively round hole...

Releases round block...

(Examiner inserts)

Removes with difficulty.....................................Removes easily.....................................Looks selectively round hole...

Transfers round block...Bang or release near round hole

Releases round block...

Ball

Accepts...

Mouths ball...Extends to Ex., no release.......

Releases ball...Casts ball.......

Mirror & Ball

Regards own image...

Leans forward...

Pats mirror...

Smiles, vocalizes...

Accepts ball...

Reach mirror for image ball.....................................Ball to mirror.......

Retains ball.....................................Release ball.....................................Retains ball.......

Posture & locomotion

Sits indefinitely.....................................Pivots in sitting.....................................

Goes from sitting to prone...

Creeps...

Pulls to feet at rail.....................................Cruises at rail.....................................Lifts foot, full wt., at rail.......

Lowers self from rail.....................................Walks 2 hands held.......

Full wt., hands held.....................................Lifts foot, hands held.....................................Walks 1 hand held.......

Language

Dada...

Mama...

GROWTH TREND CHART. *FOURTH QUARTER: 40–52 WEEKS (Continued)*

40 WEEKS	44 WEEKS	48 WEEKS	52 WEEKS
Language (Continued)			
1 word....................			2 words....................
Imitate sounds..................			
Comp. no, name, bye & patacake....			And also "give"...........
Personal–Social			
Holds own bottle..............	Drinks some milk from cup.....		
Feeds self cracker.............			
Patacakes & waves bye..........		Toy to side rail.............	
		Platform play............]	
	Extends toy to Ex. or mother,		Co-operates dressing........
	no release...........		Gives to Ex. or mother......

The Growth Trend Chart for the period of LATER INFANCY is continued in less detail on the next two pages, and includes the following age levels:

15 months
18 months
21 months
24 months
30 months
36 months

5. GROWTH TREND CHART.

	15 Months	18 Months	21 Months
Book	Helps turn pages.......... .... Pats pictures.........................	Turns 2-3 pages...................... Looks selectively.................	....
Cubes	Tower of 2.......................	Tower of 3-4........................	Tower of 5-6.......... Train—pushes cube....
Cup & cubes	6 cubes, in and out.................	10 cubes in..........................	....
Pellet & bottle	Inserts, no demonstration.............	Dumps pellet.......................	
Drawing	Holds crayon in fist.................... *Imitates scribble*...................... Incipient imitation stroke..............	Spontaneous scribble................ Imitates stroke.....................	....
Color forms			
Formboard	(Round block only given at 15 mos.) Places round block................... Adapts round block.................. Casts round block...................	(3 blocks given) Piles 3 in tower formation........... Inserts one........................ No adaptation.....................	Inserts two..........
Picture card		Names or points 1 picture...........	....
Digits			
Name, Sex			
Performance box		Square block flat against box.........	Inserts corner of block.
Test objects		Names ball........................	....
Comprehen. Question			
Ball	Casts........................	Hurls. Walks into.........................	Kicks (demonstration).
Directions		2 directions with ball...............	3 directions..........
Ball in box		Reaches........................... Abandons..........................	Gets ball............
Stand—1 foot			
Walking, Running, etc.	Alone several steps................. Falls by collapse...................	Well, seldom falls.... Walks fast, runs stiffly.............	Squats in play........
Stairs	Creeps up flight...................	Walks up, 1 hand held..............	Up, holding rail....... Down, 1 hand held....
Chair		Seats self in small chair............ Into adult chair....................	....
Vocabulary & Speech	Jargon........................... 4-6 words.........................	10 words..........................	20 words or more...... Joins 2 words.........
Feeding	No bottle........................ Inhibits grasp dish.................	Feeds self in part, spilling........... Hands empty dish to mother.........	Handles cup well...... ....
Toilet	Bowel control.................... Partial toilet regulation............. Indicates wet pants...............	Daytime regulation................	....
Dress	*Co-operates in dressing*.............		....
Communication	Indicates wants, points & vocalizes.... Shows or offers toy.................	....	Pulls person to show... Echoes 2-3 last words.. Asks for food, toilet, dri
Play	Casts toy........................	Pulls toy........... Carries, hugs doll...................	....

24 Months	30 Months	36 Months
Turns pages singly................. Names pictures....................	....	Gives action...................
Tower of 6-7...................... Aligns 2 cubes....................	Tower of 8.................... Adds chimney...............	Tower of 9-10................ Imitates bridge...............
Hands full cup to Ex....		
....	Holds crayon in fingers............	Names own drawing...........
Imitates vertical stroke............ Imitates circular stroke...........	And horizontal stroke............ Strokes twice for cross...........	Copies circle............... Imitates cross...............
	Places one....................	Places 3...................
Places separately on board.......... Inserts all..................... Adapts after 4 trials...............	Inserts all on presentation.......... Adapts repeatedly, persist, error.......	Adapts, no error or immed. correct...
Names 3, points 5..................	Names 5, points 7................	Names 8...................
	Repeats 2 digits..................	Repeats 3 digits...............
	Full name....................	And sex...................
Inserts square block.............. Names two......................	Gives use....................	
		Answers one..................
Kicks (command)................	....	....
4 directions....................	....	2 prepositions, ball & chair..........
	Tries to stand on 1 foot............ On tiptoe....................	Stands on 1 foot, mom. balance......
Runs fairly well..................	Jumps on both feet................	Rides tricycle................
Up alone.................... Down alone...................	....	Up, alternates feet............... Jumps from last step...............
3 word sentence or better........ Pronouns....................	....	Plurals....................
Inhibits turning spoon............	....	Pours from pitcher............ Feeds self well, no spilling..........
Dry nights, taken up........... Verbalizes needs consistently........	....	Assuming responsibility...........
Pulls on simple garment...........		Shoes on, unbuttons acces. buttons...
Asks for "another"............. Soliloquizes on experiences..........	Speech repetitious...............	Knows a few rhymes............
Refers to self by name............	Self by pronoun...............	Understands taking turns..........
Plays with domestic mimicry...... Parallel play with other children.....	Pushes, good steering............ Helps put things away............ Carry breakable object.............	....

Appendix C

Examination Equipment

§1. ARRANGEMENTS FOR HOSPITALS AND INSTITUTIONS

The basic procedures of developmental diagnosis are so simple that arrangements for examination can be set up with very little equipment. In Chapter 2 we showed how the ordinary furniture of a physician's office and a portable test table can be made to serve the needs of a formal behavioral examination. Once the examiner is well versed in the principles and methods of diagnosis, simple expedients can be used successfully in the home and on a children's hospital ward.

In hospitals and child care institutions, there is no need to depend on improvised and makeshift arrangements. If developmental examinations are made routinely and systematically, it is advisable to set aside a separate room or suite of rooms especially equipped for the purpose. The necessary apparatus is comparatively inexpensive. Much is gained by conducting the examination under standardized conditions in simplified surroundings which insure a minimum of distraction for the child. The furnishings of the room should be limited to essentials. Murals, pictures and special toys are not advised. The examination affords ample stimulation.

The room arrangements depend primarily on the recording facilities available. At the present time, videotape recording (Section C-3) is the ideal method, and one room roughly 14 feet square can contain all of the necessary equipment. The examination room should be as soundproof as possible. Observers should be seated in a conference room a short distance away in which simultaneous teaching can be carried out via the TV monitor. It is advisable to have an office interposed between the conference and examining rooms so that a postevaluation conference can be held without the parents hearing the discussion.

Fig. C-1 shows the arrangement of the furniture at the beginning of an infant evaluation. It is easily rearranged for different aged children or for shifts which may be necessary within a single examination. The child's table and chairs used for older children are an advantage for those occasions when a mother must bring other preschool children who will not leave her but will play quietly in the same room.

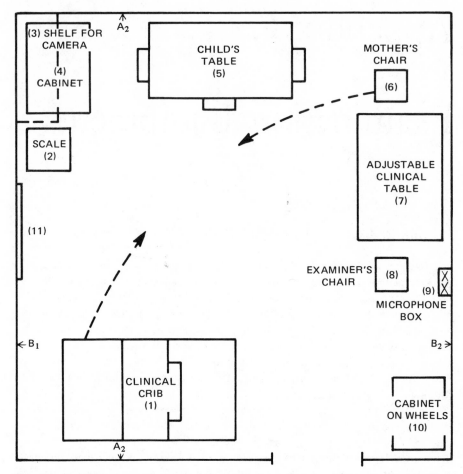

Fig. C-1. Examining room: Arrangement for start of an infant examination. Numbered objects are described in text.

The interview is conducted in the examining room, to minimize the number of adjustments the infant must make. The mother, with the infant on her lap, takes her place in chair (6), the examiner in chair (8); all three are within camera range at the adjustable clinical table (7). The camera (3) is mounted on a high shelf in the far left corner of the room, and the microphone outlet box (9) on the wall near the clinical table. If indicated, the crib (1) can be brought forward slightly and the infant placed in it during the interview. When it is time for the examination to start, the clinical crib (1) is moved into the center of the room facing the camera. The examiner takes his place to the left of the crib somewhat behind the infant's range of vision. The mother, after placing the infant satisfactorily in the crib, moves her chair (6) to the right side of the crib, also slightly behind the infant's position. If the infant must be placed back on the mother's lap, the crib easily can be pushed back toward its original position, leaving the shoe bag filled with examining materials angled toward the examiner for easy access. The mother is seated behind the adjustable table (7) facing the camera, and the examiner places his chair (8) to the left of the table, between it and the crib.

Other furniture includes an adult-type clinical scale (2) on which the infant can be weighed in the mother's arms, a storage cabinet (4) on which a small TV monitor is placed during the examination, the child's table and three chairs (5), one 14 inches high and two 12 inches high. The six-drawer file cabinet (10) on wheels (with lock), containing the examining materials for older children, is kept in the corner behind the door. Outer clothing should be left outside the room and the necessary baby bags and purses put on the child's table (5) or on an optional shelf or additional cabinet in the far right corner, if the room is large enough to accommodate one.

The room should be lighted with ranks of fluorescent tubes with the egg-crate shields removed, no closer to the camera than the level marked A1–A2. Adequate lighting for videotaping, without excessive heat, is provided by this arrangement; there is greater flexibility if each row of tubes has its own switch. Windows should be curtained with blackout material, since fluctuations in natural light adversely affect the videorecording. If adequate ventilation and cooling is provided by other means, a window is not needed. The walls should be painted a very light pastel with a nonglare finish; the ceiling should be sound-absorbent. A curtain may be hung across the right wall for a better photographic effect.

If desired, a movable nylon mesh curtain can be hooked back at point B1 and pulled across to point B2 to accommodate observers, should the recording equipment break down. If such observers are absolutely quiet, they do not interfere with the examination, even if not hidden from view; the curtain is a psychologic barrier for them rather than for the child.

For older children, the room should be rearranged in advance of the examination as shown in Fig. C-2. For both interview and examination the child sits in the larger 14-inch-high chair, mother and examiner in the 12-inch chairs, the examiner on the left. For active children who want to leave the room, a simple hook-and-eye on the door at a sufficient height serves the purpose of confining them; the lock on the examining cabinet needs to be used occasionally.

If videotape recording is not available, then two rooms separated by a one-way-vision screen (described in Section C-4) is most satisfactory. One room is set up for the examination of infants, and the other for older children, as in Fig. C-3. Minimum width for the infant's room should be $8\frac{1}{2}$ feet, and for the child's room, 7 feet. The room not in use serves as the observation area by adjusting the lighting appropriately, The chairs and stools used to seat the observers must be moved accordingly. Strict silence is an extremely important rule. The injunction to the observer who enters the observation room should be, "Be absolutely quiet. The child can hear you even though he cannot see you."

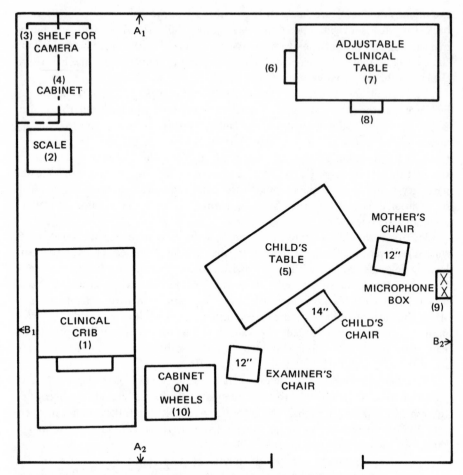

Fig. C-2. Examining room: Arrangement for start of an older child's examination.

§2. SPECIAL CLINICAL EQUIPMENT

CLINICAL CRIB. A hospital crib (Simmons Model #HC 240-2-6209-2, 30" X 54") with side panels adjustable by means of a hand-operated catch at the base of the panel is modified slightly, as shown in Fig. C-4. Additional panel heights are provided by drilling extra holes in the upright rods on which the side panels ride. A sturdy wooden platform is used instead of a mattress; it may replace the springs entirely if desired. The foot end panel is sawed off to provide a clearer view of the infant in the crib. The short spikes which are the remnants of the foot railings are capped with a wooden cover made to measure. An ingenious machine shop can remove the foot corner uprights while still permitting the side panels to be raised and lowered. If this is done, the view of the infant is entirely unobstructed.

A mirror, large enough to cover completely the head end panel of the crib, is

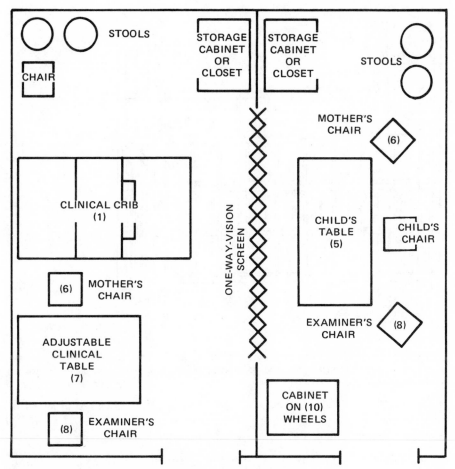

Fig. C-3. Two-room examining suite with one-way-vision screen.

fastened securely in place and a roller shade attached. The test objects are kept most conveniently in a shoe bag hung on the back of the crib head. A four-tier one may be purchased and one row of pockets modified to hold the formboard and picture book.

The tabletop is sturdy plywood 18 inches deep, the width fitted to the crib size. Strips of quarter-round on the short edges hold it in place on top of the crib side rails while permitting it to slide back and forth freely.

INFANT EXAMINING CHAIR.   The construction of the chair is indicated in Fig. C-5. The chair is provided with a removable washable cover of canvas weight; it slips over the top of the chair back, slings forward loosely and hooks over the pairs of screws at the front of the side panels. The infant is secured in place with a broad canvas band around his chest. Several buttonholes are made in each side of the band to fit over one of the screws on the side uprights and allow adjustment. For the

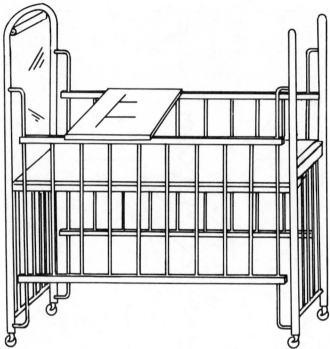

Fig. C-4. Clinical crib showing platform, tabletop 18 inches deep on adjustable side panels, roller shade covering mirror and end panel removed, with wooden box made to measure covering residual spikes.

infant unable to sit alone, the chest band must be tight enough to provide firm support and prevent any slumping, so that the arms can be used freely. Usually this is at least one buttonhole tighter than you think would be comfortable.

PORTABLE TEST TABLE. This table's construction is shown in Fig. C-6. In the event that a hospital crib with more than two panel heights is not available, the portable test table replaces the sliding tabletop, the other procedures remaining unchanged. The indicated height has been found adaptable for children of all sizes on a hospital ward. For very small infants, the entire chair is elevated on a suitable number of folded sheets or blankets. For the older infant who sits independently but is still too short to reach the table top properly, the chest band is fastened loosely merely to prevent him from getting out of the chair accidentally.

ADJUSTABLE CLINICAL TABLE. This table is shown in Fig. C-7. It has a plywood top 2 by 3 feet. The stem consists of two telescoping metal pipes attached to metal plates. The height is regulated by a plumber's joint on the outer pipe. The base is cross bars of two-by-fours to allow room for comfortable foot placement. This table is used (1) for conducting the interview with the parents; (2) for the situations when the mother must hold the child, e.g., the infant who will not leave her, the toddler too old for the crib but too small for the kindergarten

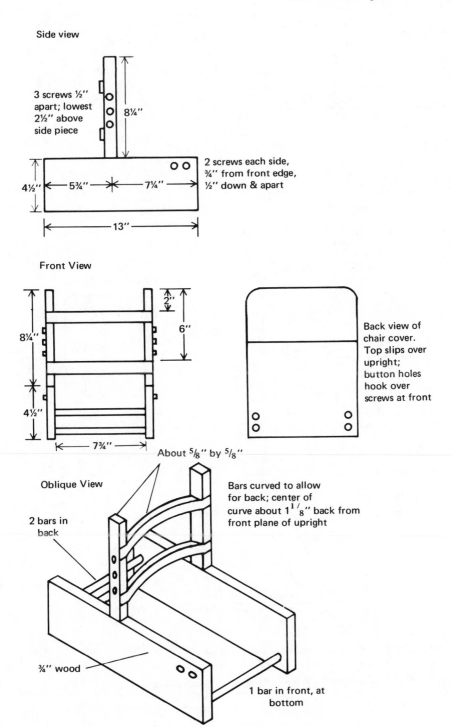

Side view

3 screws ½"
apart; lowest
2½" above
side piece

8¼"

2 screws each side,
¾" from front edge,
½" down & apart

4½"   5¾"   7¼"

13"

Front View

2"

6"

8¼"

4½"

7¾"

About ⅝" by ⅝"

Back view of
chair cover.
Top slips over
upright;
button holes
hook over
screws at front

Oblique View

2 bars in
back

Bars curved to allow
for back; center of
curve about $1^{1}/_{8}$" back from
front plane of upright

¾" wood

1 bar in front, at
bottom

Fig. C-5. Plans for infant examining chair.

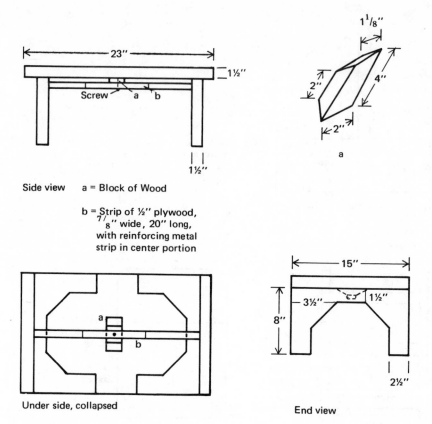

Side view   a = Block of Wood

b = Strip of ½" plywood,
    $^7/_8$" wide, 20" long,
    with reinforcing metal
    strip in center portion

Under side, collapsed

End view

One end of under side, open

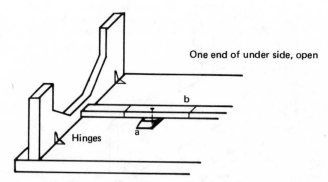

Hinges

Fig. C-6. Plans for portable examining table, made of ¾-inch plywood.

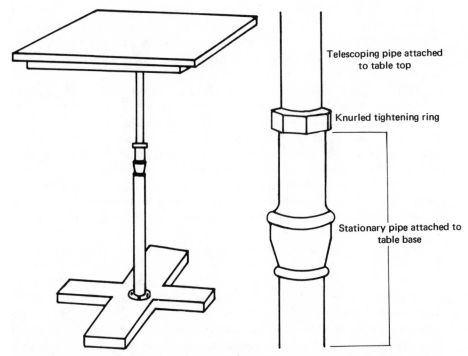

Fig. C-7. Adjustable clinical examining table, showing details of plumber's pipe joint used to regulate height.

chair, the handicapped child too big or too impaired for the infant examining chair; and (3) in conjunction with an adult chair, as a substitute for kindergarten furniture for the older child.

§3. VIDEOTAPE RECORDING

At the present time, videotape recording is the ideal method for chronicling an examination. It has the disadvantages of a relatively expensive initial investment and a varying amount of difficulty in maintaining the equipment in good working order and repairing it promptly However, its advantages are legion.

Videotape permits immediate playback of the material recorded, without an intervening week or more for processing of film. Specific behavior which you wish to preserve usually can be reelicited and retaped if technical imperfections occur. This immediate playback is also an invaluable teaching tool. Even an experienced examiner misses some facets of behavior because he is concentrating on other aspects. The camera records it all; furthermore, it provides a frontal view which is not obtained in the examining room. Points missed by a trainee can be demonstrated "live"; disagreements about what did or did not occur are settled quickly. A student can do an examination by himself for later review with the supervisor. The behavior can be seen later by others involved in the care of the child if they cannot be present at the actual examination. A conference room with a closed-circuit monitor can permit a teacher to discuss events with students as they occur.

Permanent and serial records can be made by editing the original material, and a variety of teaching tapes of both normal and abnormal behavior prepared. The tapes, which are reusable, can be converted into 16-mm sound film for outside distribution. Action pictures are unquestionably superior to the printed word; 1000 words cannot describe a staring episode as effectively as 20–30 seconds of tape. The closeup views provided by the camera reveal greater detail than can be afforded by the distance of an observation alcove; but by the same token they eliminate some of the interplay with mother and examiner that a wider angle gives. Videorecording can be made with ordinary fluorescent lighting, without uncomfortable heat and glare.

No attempt will be made to give precise specifications for all the components of the recording system, but a few points are worthy of comment. It has been our experience that many people tend to economize by getting a less expensive camera and lens, since there is greater latitude in the prices of these items. This is false economy; probably one of the most important factors in high-quality pictures is a high-quality camera and zoom lens. A second important feature is the incorporation of a remote control unit with a pan-and-tilt mechanism. This permits complete remote operation of the camera from the conference room; no one but mother, child and examiner need be in the examining room. The choice of videorecording system should depend on a variety of factors, including local availability of service; there is considerable difference of opinion about which is best. Tapes made on one system cannot be played directly on machines of another, although they can be transcribed electronically Even within brands there is not always intermachine compatibility. It is a worthwhile investment to have two recorders, although both need not be of similar degrees of sophistication. Two are needed to edit the tapes, and are insurance against complete machine failure when a particularly crucial examination is scheduled. Two monitors are desirable; a large one for the conference room is a necessity, while a second smaller (but not necessarily less expensive) one is put on the cabinet in the examining room. The examiner then can see what his confreres are recording and suggest technical corrections if necessary.

A traveling, wall-mounted microphone is the examiner's means of communicating with observers, dictating the behavior seen during the examination and recording the interview with the parents. Reverse communication from the conference room to the examining room also is necessary, and is easily installed with the television cables between the rooms. The teacher in the conference room has an amplifier and microphone, and the examiner an ear plug. The mother knows there is communication but cannot hear what is said. Comments and questions on technique as well as on the behavior can be made to a student examiner without interfering with the examination. This same system can be employed if a one-way-vision screen is used, since the microphone can be fitted with a padded mouthpiece to dampen the sound of the instructor's voice.

If a videotape system is installed, budgetary provision should be made for an assistant whose chief responsibility will be caring for and operating the machines. The assistant soon will gain enough experience with the examination procedures to know which parts should be included in the recording. With this combination of technical and behavioral knowledge, she then will be able to edit the tapes of examinations.

§4. ONE-WAY-VISION FACILITIES

The one-way-vision screen is so named because, with proper adjustment of lighting, it is transparent in one direction only. When videotape is not available, such a screen can be placed between the observation and examining areas. An arrangement of this sort can permit a whole group of persons to watch an examination without being seen and without disturbing the rapport between examiner and child.

A screen is preferable to a one-way mirror, even if its use prohibits talking in the observation area. Infants and young children tend to be preoccupied by their own mirror images. Further, the sounds most likely to be picked up from the examining room by the recording equipment are the banging of the test objects rather than voices; older children tend to move out of the range of the microphone. In addition, the mirror does not permit using rooms interchangeably for examination or observation.

The device is extremely simple, adaptable and inexpensive. If two adjoining rooms are to be used, an opening can be cut into the connecting door or wall. If the screen between the two rooms is installed as a removable panel, it can be replaced by plywood with a center of photographic glass when filming with a movie camera is desired. The architectural disposition of the two rooms is indicated in Fig. C-3. If only a single room is available, an observation alcove can be made by erecting a thin partition from floor to ceiling across one end of the room and incorporating a screen into the partition. A one-way-vision window also can be covered with a sliding panel and placed in an ordinary door connecting to a quiet corridor. This offers more or less brief glimpses of an examination with a minimum of disturbance and prearrangement, but the corridor cannot be a traffic artery.

The observation area should be as dark as possible. Enough light for ordinary recording purposes will enter through the screen. If only an observation station is constructed, the walls should be painted black or midnight blue. Dark curtains draped on the walls and thick carpeting on the floor serve to silence sounds made inadvertently by the observers. Care also should be taken so that light from windows or from lamps in the examination room will not strike directly through the screens; indirect lighting is better for this reason than direct lighting. Direct rays of light tend to reveal the observers' eye glasses and light-colored objects.

The principles of operation of the one-way-vision screen itself are simple. The surface of the mesh screen is painted white to produce a diffuse dazzle which makes the screen appear opaque. If the examining room is well lighted and the observation area darkened, the opaque effect from the examining room side is enhanced. At the same time the transparency of the screen to observers in the alcove is in no way interfered with.

To prepare a one-way-vision screen, ordinary 16-mesh wire screen can be used. Thin white enamel paint may be applied with painter's brush in several coats, if done with care so as not to clog the mesh. The paint should be permitted to dry between coats. No. 30 wire cloth has definite advantages, particularly if casein paint instead of ordinary enamel is used. The casein paint should be thinned down with water to the consistency of thin cream and then applied with an air brush. At intervals the air brush should be used to force only air through the screen in order to blow out any excess paint which may have clogged the mesh. This process should be repeated four or five times. Casein paint dries rapidly, and the successive coats may be applied in the course of one day. It is best to apply the paint before the screens are permanently mounted.

Appendix D

Audiovisual Aids

In their original work at the Clinic of Child Development at Yale University, Gesell and Amatruda developed an extensive library of short cinematic case studies and had plans to develop a systematic self-instruction series for the student. The films which were completed no longer are readily accessible, and are out of date by modern technical standards.

Three films were prepared at the Ohio State University by Dr. Knobloch, Dr. Pasamanick and Earl S. Sherard, Jr., M.D. They demonstrate both normal and abnormal patterns of development. When studied in conjunction with the text, particularly Chapters 3, 10 and 11, and Appendix A-6, they provide vivid, concrete illustrations of the behavior patterns that only can be approximated by verbal descriptions. They also demonstrate the techniques of the developmental examination.

DEVELOPMENTAL EVALUATION IN INFANCY

Part I. Normal Adaptive and Fine Motor Behavior

A single pattern on the 15-month developmental schedule, inserting the pellet into the bottle, is selected as a culminating pattern, and the evolution of each of seven patterns which must be integrated for its accomplishment is traced from 4 weeks. The seven patterns are ocular regard, active grasp, the development of approach, manipulation of the small object, interest in multiple objects, the concept of container and contained and the development of voluntary release. In the course of demonstrating their synthesis, essentially all the adaptive and fine motor patterns on the developmental schedules between 4 weeks and 15 months are illustrated. The film then indicates how principles involved in the evolution of this culminating pattern can be applied to the evolution of more advanced patterns, by tracing tower building from 52 weeks to 3 years of age.

Part II. Normal Gross Motor Behavior

A similar 15-month culminating pattern, assuming the erect posture unassisted and walking independently, is traced in the same fashion. The integration of six patterns is followed from 4 weeks to 15 months: head control, static; head control, dynamic; sitting, static; early locomotion, dynamic; standing, static; and standing, dynamic. The further evolution of the bipedal pattern is shown, and its relationship to cognitive behavior and the significance of a developmental approach are summarized briefly.

THE GESELL DEVELOPMENTAL
AND NEUROLOGIC EXAMINATION IN INFANCY

This film gives a dramatic cross-sectional view of normal development at each of four key ages, 16, 28, 40 and 52 weeks, and demonstrates the general techniques of infant evaluation. It supplements the above longitudinal film by synthesizing the behavior characteristic for each key age. At the same time, it shows how the behavior at each key age derives from immature patterns, and also foreshadows future development.

NORMAL AND ABNORMAL
NEUROLOGIC FUNCTION IN INFANCY

This film uses normal behavior at 40 weeks as a starting point and then shows eight infants with a variety of abnormalities who are chronologically or functionally approximately 40 weeks of age. The deviations range from abnormal neuromotor signs of minor degree to "cerebral palsy" and mental deficiency. The focus is on pointing out normal and abnormal neuromotor patterns; however, the film also indicates how these patterns must be evaluated in terms of their relationship with adaptive behavior and the general maturity level, in order to arrive at a diagnosis and prognosis.

Each film is 16-mm black-and-white optical sound, and is accompanied by a copy of the complete sound track. Films may be purchased or rented by addressing inquiries to The Department of Photography and Cinema, The Ohio State University, 156 West 19th Avenue, Columbus, Ohio 43210.

The rental fee for each title is $9.00, the purchase price as follows:

"Developmental Evaluation in Infancy"—Part I. 1500 feet (42 minutes), $145.00; Part II. 650 feet (18 minutes), $85.00; both parts, $220.00.

"Gesell Developmental and Neurologic Examination"—1200 feet (33 minutes), $150.00.

"Normal and Abnormal Neurologic Function in Infancy"—1100 feet (30 minutes), $150.00.

Appendix E

Bibliography

§1. SPECIFIC REFERENCES CITED IN THE TEXT

1. Alm I. Longterm prognosis for prematurely born children: Followup study of 999 premature boys born in wedlock and of 1002 controls. Acta Paediatr 42:1–116, 1953
2. Battaglia FC, Lubchenco LO. A practical classification of newborn infants by weight and gestational age. J Pediatr 71:159–163, 1967
3. Bayley N: Bayley Scales of Infant Development. New York, The Psychological Corporation, 1969
4. Bayley N. Value and limitations of infant testing. Children 5:129–133, 1958
5. Bender L. Schizophrenia in childhood. Nerv Child 1:138–140, 1942
6. Birch HG: The problem of "brain damage" in children in Brain Damage in Children, the Biological and Social Aspects. Edited by HG Birch. Baltimore, Williams & Wilkins, 1964, pp 3–12
7. Birch HG, Gussow JD: Disadvantaged Children. Health, Nutrition and School Failure. New York, Harcourt, Brace and World, and Grune & Stratton, 1970
8. Bowlby J: Maternal care and mental health. WHO Monogr Ser 179:11–14, 1952
9. Bowlby J, Ainsworth M, Boston M, Rosenbluth D. Effects of mother–child separation: Followup study. Br J Med Psychol 29:211–247, 1956
10. Brown JL. Prognosis from presenting symptoms of preschool children with atypical development. Amer J Orthopsychiat 30:382–390, 1960
11. Cattell P. The Measurement of Intelligence of Infants and Young Children. New York, The Psychological Coporation, 1960
12. Charles DC. Ability and accomplishment of persons earlier judged mentally deficient. Genet Psychol Monogr 47:3–71, 1953

13. Clements S: Minimal Brain Dysfunction in Children. NINDB Monograph No 3. Washington, DC, US Dept Health, Education and Welfare, 1966
14. Coleman MB, Lodge A, Barnet A, Cytryn L. A three year study of 5-hydroxytryptophan administration in Down's syndrome. Pediatr Res 7:192, 1973
15. Creak M (Chairman). Schizophrenic syndrome in childhood. Progress report of a working party. Cereb Palsy Bull 3:501–504, 1961
16. Doman RJ, Spitz EB, Zucman E, Delacato CH, Doman G. Children with severe brain injuries: Neurologic organization in terms of mobility. JAMA 174:257–262, 1960
17. Drillien CM: The Growth and Development of the Prematurely Born Infant. Baltimore, Williams & Wilkins, 1964
18. Drillien CM. A longituidnal study of the growth and development of prematurely and maturely born children: Part III. Mental development. Arch Dis Child 34:37–45, 1959
19. Drillien CM. A longitudinal study of the growth and development of prematurely and maturely born children: Part VII. Mental development 2–5 years. Arch Dis Child 36:233–240, 1961
20. Eighth Revision International Classification of Diseases, Public Health Service Publication No 1693, Volume 1, Tabular List. Washington, DC, US Government Printing Office
21. Eisenberg L: Psychoses: clinical features in The Child, His Psychological and Cultural Development, Volume 2, The Major Psychological Disorders and Their Treatment. Edited by AM Freedman, HI Kaplan. New York, Atheneum Press, 1972, pp 200–212
22. Eisenberg L, Kanner L. Early infantile autism 1943–1955. Am J Orthopsychiat 26:556–566, 1956
23. Frankenburg WK, Dodds JB. The Denver developmental screening test. J Pediatr 71:181–191, 1967
24. Furby L. Implications of within-group heritabilities for sources of between-group differences: IQ and racial differences. Dev Psychol 9:28–37, 1973
25. Gesell A. A History of Psychology in Autobiography, Vol IV. Edited by HS Langfeld, EG Boring, H Werner, RM Yerkes. Worcester, Mass, Clark University Press, 1952, pp 123–142
26. Gesell A, Amatruda CS: The Embryology of Behavior: The Beginnings of the Human Mind. New York, Harper & Brothers, 1945
27. Gesell A, Halverson HM, Thompson H, Ilg FL, Castner BM, Ames LB, Amatruda CS: The First Five Years of Life. New York, Harper & Brothers, 1940
28. Griffiths R: The Abilities of Babies. London, University of London Press Ltd, 1954
29. Heber R: Rehabilitation of Families at Risk for Mental Retardation: A Progress Report. Rehabilitation Research and Training Center in Mental Retardation, University of Wisconsin, Madison, 1971

30. Hirsch J. Behavior–genetic analysis and its biosocial consequences. Seminars Psychiat 2:89–105, 1970
31. Holowach J, Thurston DL, O'Leary J. Prognosis in childhood epilepsy. New Eng J Med 286:169–174, 1972
32. Hurley RL: Poverty and Mental Retardation: A Causal Relationship. New York, Random House, 1970
33. Illingworth RS: An Introduction to Developmental Assessment in the First Year. London, National Spastics Society, 1960
34. Illingworth RS. The predictive value of developmental tests in the first year, with special reference to the diagnosis of mental subnormality. J Child Psychol Psychiat 2:210–215, 1961
35. Jencks C: Inequality. A Reassessment of the Effect of Family and Schooling in America. New York, Basic Books, 1972
36. Kanner L. Autistic disturbances of affective contact. Nerv Child 2:217–250, 1943
37. Kanner L. Followup study of eleven autistic children originally reported in 1943. J Autism Child Schizo 1:119–145, 1971
38. Knobloch H, Calvin ME, Spencer F. The evaluation of atypical convulsive episodes in infancy. Pediatr Res 6:424, 1972
39. Knobloch H, Kerr Grant D. Etiologic factors in "early infantile autism" and "childhood schizophrenia." Am J Dis Child 102:535, 1961
40. Knobloch H, Pasamanick B. The developmental behavioral approach to the neurologic examination in infancy. Child Dev 33:181–198, 1962
41. Knobloch H, Pasamanick B: The distribution of intellectual potential in an infant population. The Epidemiology of Mental Disorder: A Symposium in Celebration of the Centennial of Emil Kraepelin. Edited by B Pasamanick. Washington, DC, American Association for the Advancement of Science, 1959, pp 249–272
42. Knobloch H, Pasamanick B. Environmental factors affecting human development before and after birth. Pediatr 26:210–218, 1960
43. Knobloch H, Pasamanick B: An evaluation of the consistency and predictive value of the 40 week Gesell Developmental Schedule in Child Development and Child Psychiatry. Edited by C Shagass, B Pasamanick. Washington, DC, American Psychiatric Association, 1960, pp 10–31
44. Knobloch H, Pasamanick B. Medical progress: Mental subnormality. New Eng J Med 266:1045–1051, 1092–1097, 1155–1161, 1962
45. Knobloch H, Pasamanick B. Predicting intellectual potential in infancy. Am J Dis Child 106:43–51, 1963
46. Knobloch H, Pasamanick B: Prediction from the assessment of neuromotor and intellectual status in infancy in Psychopathology of Mental Development. Edited by J Zubin. New York, Grune & Stratton, 1967, pp 387–400
47. Knobloch H, Pasamanick B: Treatment in mental subnormality in Current Pediatric Therapy–3. Edited by SS Gellis, BM Kagan. Philadelphia, WB Saunders, 1968, pp 18–24

48. Knobloch H, Pasamanick B, Sherard ES, Jr. A developmental screening inventory for infants. Pediatr. 38, Part II. 1095–1104, 1966

49. Knobloch H, Sotos JF, Sherard ES, Jr, Wehe RA. Prognostic and etiologic factors in hypoglycemia. J Pediatr 70:876–884, 1967

50. Koch R, Shaw KNF, Acosta PB, Fishler K, Schaeffler G, Wenz E, Wohlers A. An approach to management of phenylketonuria. J Pediatr 76:815–828, 1970

51. Krieger I, Sargent DA. A postural sign in the sensory deprivation syndrome in infants. J Pediatr 70:332–345, 1967

52. Langdon-Down J. Ethnic classification of idiots. London Hosp Rep 3:259, 1866

53. Lejeune J, Gautier M, Turpin R. Etudes des chromosomes somatiques des neuf enfants mongoliens. CR Acad Sci [D] (Paris) 248:1721, 1959

54. Lemkau P, Tietze C, Cooper M. Mental hygiene problems in an urban district. Ment Hyg 25:624–646, 1941

55. Lubchenco LO, Hansman C, Boyd E. Intrauterine growth in length and head circumference as estimated from live births at gestational ages from 26 to 42 weeks. Pediatr 37:403–408, 1966

55a. Matheney AP: Testing infant intelligence. Science 182:734, 1973

56. Maurer KM: Intellectual Status at Maturity as a Criterion for Selecting Items in Preschool Tests. University of Minneapolis Institute of Child Welfare Monograph Series No 21. Minneapolis, University of Minnesota Press, 1953

57. Moneysworth, The Consumer Newsletter: Babies: three thousand dollars a pound. 3:1–2, 1973

58. Nelson KB, Deutschberger J. Head size at one year as a predictor of four-year IQ. Dev Med Child Neurol 12:487–495, 1970

59. New York State Department of Mental Hygiene: Technical Report of the Mental Health Research Unit. Syracuse, NY, Syracuse University Press, 1955

60. Ounsted C, Lindsay J, Norman R: Biological Factors in Temporal Lobe Epilepsy. London, Heinemann, 1966, p 55

61. Pasamanick B, Knobloch H. Retrospective studies on the epidemiology of reproductive casualty: Old and new. Merrill-Palmer Quart Behav Dev 12:7–26, 1966

62. Powell GF, Brasel JA, Blizzard RM. Emotional deprivation and growth retardation simulating hypopituitarism: I. Clinical evaluation of the syndrome. New Eng J Med 276:1271–1278, 1967

63. Rettig S, Rawson HE, Knobloch H, Pasamanick B. A multidimensional computer analysis of some complications of pregnancy and their neuro-psychiatric sequelae. Fourth IBM Medical Symposium, Endicott, NY, 1962, p 132

64. Rider R, Harper P. Knobloch H, Fetter S. An evaluation of standards for the hospital care of premature infants. JAMA 165: 1233–1236, 1957

65. Rutter M. The influence of organic and emotional factors on the origins, nature and outcome of childhood psychosis. Dev Med Child Neurol 7:518–528, 1965

66. Rutter M, Greenfield G, Lockyer L. A five to fifteen year followup study of infantile psychosis. II. Social and behavioral outcome. Br J Psychiat 113:1183–1199, 1967
67. Seguin E. Traitment Moral, Hygiene et Education des Idiots et des Autres Enfants Arrieres ou Retardes dans leur Development. Paris, JB Bailliere, 1846
68. Sherard ES, Jr. personal communication
69. Skodak M, Skeels HM. A final followup study of one hundred adopted children. J Genet Psychol 75:85–125, 1949
70. Terman LM, Merrill MA: Measuring Intelligence. Boston, Houghton Mifflin, 1937
71. Terman LM, Merrill MA: Stanford-Binet Intelligence Scale, Manual for the Third Revision Form L-M. Boston, Houghton Mifflin, 1960
72. Thompson LJ. Learning disabilities: An overview. Am J Psychiat 130:393–399, 1973
73. Touwen BCL, Prechtl HFR: The Neurological Examination of Child with Minor Nervous Dysfunction. Philadelphia, JB Lippincott, 1970
74. Towbin A. Central nervous system damage in the human fetus and newborn infant. Am J Dis Child 119:529–542, 1970
75. Towbin A. Organic causes of minimal brain dysfunction. JAMA 217:1207–1214, 1971
76. Tredgold AF: Mental Retardation, 11th edition. Baltimore, Williams & Wilkins, 1970
77. Whitten CF, Pettit MG, Fischhoff J. Evidence that growth failure from maternal deprivation is secondary to undereating. JAMA 209:1675–1682, 1969
78. Wiener G. Scholastic achievement at age 12–13 of prematurely born infants. J Spec Ed 2:237–250, 1968
79. Wiener G, Rider RV, Oppel WC, Harper PA. Correlates of low birth weight. Psychological status at eight to ten years of age. Pediatr Res 2:110–118, 1968
80. Winick M, Rosso P. The effect of severe early malnutrition on cellular growth of human brain. Pediatr Res 3:181–184, 1969
81. Winick M, Rosso P. Head circumference and cellular growth of the brain in normal and marasmic children. J Pediatr 74:774–778, 1969
82. Yerushalmy J. The classification of newborn infants by birth weight and gestational age. J Pediatr 71:164–172, 1967
83. Yerushalmy J: Reiation of birth weight, gestational age, and the rate of intrauterine growth to perinatal mortality in Perinatal Mortality. Edited by EM Gold. Clin Obstet Gynec 13:107–129, 1970

§2. GENERAL REFERENCES

Barnett HL, Einhorn AH: Pediatrics, 14th edition. New York, Appleton-Century-Crofts, 1968

Cooke RE, Levin S: The Biologic Basis of Pediatric Practice. New York, McGraw-Hill, 1968

Farmer TW: Pediatric Neurology. New York, Harper & Row, 1968

Gellis SS, Feingold M, Rutman JY: Atlas of Mental Retardation Syndromes. Visual Diagnosis of Facies and Physical Findings. Washington, DC, US Government Printing Office, 1968

Hamerton JL: Human Cytogenetics (two volumes). New York, Academic Press, 1971

Holmes LB, Moser H, Halldorsson S, Mack C, Pant S, Matzilevich B: Mental Retardation: An Atlas of Diseases with Associated Physical Abnormalities. New York, Macmillan, 1971

Kanner L: Child Psychiatry, fourth edition. Springfield, Ill, Charles C Thomas, 1972

Knobloch H, Pasamanick B. Prospective studies on the epidemiology of reproductive casualty: methods, findings, and some implications. Merrill-Palmer Quart Behav Dev 12:27–43, 1966

McKusick VA: Mendelian Inheritance in Man, third edition. Baltimore, The Johns Hopkins Press, 1971

Milunsky A, Littlefield JW, Kanfer JN, Kolodny EH, Shih VE, Atkins L. Prenatal genetic diagnosis. New Eng J Med 283:1370–1381, 1441–1447, 1498–1504, 1970

Nelson WE, Vaughan VC, III, McKay RJ: Textbook of Pediatrics, ninth edition. Philadelphia, WB Saunders, 1969

Pasamanick B, Knobloch H. Retrospective studies on the epidemiology of reproductive casualty: old and new. Merrill-Palmer Quart Behav Dev 12: 7–26, 1966

Silverman WA: Dunham's Premature Infants. New York, Hoeber Medical Division, Harper & Row, 1964

Smith DW: Recognizable Patterns of Human Malformation. Genetic, Embryologic and Clinical Aspects. Vol VII, Major Problems in Clinical Pediatrics. Philadelphia, WB Saunders, 1970

Spock B: Baby and Child Care. New York, Pocket Books, 1968

Stanbury JB, Wyngaarden JB, Fredrickson DS: The Metabolic Basis of Inherited Disease, third edition. New York, McGraw-Hill, 1972

Steinberg AG, Bearn AG: Progress in Medical Genetics. New York, Grune & Stratton, 1972

Wilson SAK: Neurology (two volumes). Edited by AN Bruce. New York, Hafner, 1970

Warkany J: Congenital Malformations. Chicago, Year Book Medical Publishers, 1971

§3. SELECTED PUBLICATIONS OF THE YALE CLINIC OF CHILD DEVELOPMENT UNDER THE DIRECTION OF ARNOLD GESELL

Ames LB. The sequential patterning of prone progression in the human infant. Genet Psychol Monogr 19:409–460, 1937

Castner BM. The development of fine prehension in infancy. Genet Psychol Monogr 12:105–193, 1932
> A study of patterns of fine motor coordination as revealed by the pellet test.

Gesell A, Thompson H, Amatruda CS: An Atlas of Infant Behavior: A Systematic Delineation of the Forms and Early Growth of Human Behavior Patterns. Volume One: Normative Series. Gesell A, Keliher AV, Ilg FL, Carlson JJ: Volume Two: Naturalistic Series. New Haven, Yale University Press, 1934
> Volume One depicts the pattern phases of typical behavior of normative infants in the standard test situations at 4, 6, 8, 12, 16, 20, 24, 28, 32, 36, 40, 44, 48, 52 and 56 weeks of age. Volume Two reproduces naturalistic cinema excerpts of the daily life of normal infants, including sleep, waking, feeding, bath, play, bodily activities and social behavior.

Gesell A, Thompson H, Amatruda CS: Infant Behavior: Its Genesis and Growth. New York, McGraw-Hill, 1934
> An account of methods used in the developmental research of the Yale Clinic with genetic summaries of the developmental trends of infant behavior.

Gesell A, Thompson H, Amatruda CS: The Psychology of Early Growth including Norms of Infant Behavior and a Method of Genetic Analysis. New York, Macmillan, 1938
> A key to the delineations of the Atlas of Infant Behavior, listing in detail the various behavior patterns observed in the normative test situations.

Gesell A, Halverson HM, Thompson H, Ilg FL, Castner BM, Ames LB, Amatruda CS: The First Five Years of Life: A Guide to the Study of the Preschool Child. New York, Harper & Brothers, 1940

Gesell A, Amatruda CS: The Embryology of Behavior: The Beginnings of the Human Mind. New York, Harper & Brothers, 1945
> An ontogenetic account of the patterning of fetal and neonatal behavior from the standpoint of developmental morphology, based on clinical and cinematic studies of fetal infants, and illustrated by over 300 action photographs.

Gesell A: How a Baby Grows: A Story in Pictures. New York, Harper & Brothers, 1945
> A picture story portraying the growth of infant behavior with 800 action photographs; a simple introduction to a developmental point of view.

Gesell A, Halverson HM. The development of thumb opposition in the human infant. J Genet Psychol 48: 339–361, 1936
> Developmental and experimental study of the types and degrees of thumb opposition.

Gesell A, Ames LB. The ontogenetic organization of prone behavior in human infancy. J Genet Psychol 56:247–263, 1940
  Stages of development in the patterning of prone locomotion and upright posture.
Gesell A, Ames LB. Ontogenetic correspondences in the supine and prone postures of the human infant. Yale J Biol Med 15:565–573, 1943
Gesell A, Ames LB. The development of handedness. J Genet Psychol 70:155–175, 1947
Halverson HM. An experimental study of prehension in infants by means of systematic cinema records. Genet Psychol Monogr 10:107–286, 1931
Halverson HM. A further study of grasping. J Gen Psychol 7:34–64, 1932
Halverson HM. Complications of the early grasping reactions. Psychol Monogr 47:47–63, 1936
Halverson HM. Studies of the grasping responses of early infancy. J Genet Psychol 51: 371–449, 1937
  These four articles are quantitative experimental studies of the mechanisms of approach, grasp and release.
Ling B. A genetic study of sustained visual fixation and associated behavior in the human infant from birth to six months. J Genet Psychol 61:227–277, 1942
McGinnis J. Eye movements and optic nystagmus in early infancy. Genet Psychol Monogr 8:321–430, 1930
  An experimental study of early eye movements based on cinema records.

Index

Page numbers followed by the letter "t" indicate tabular material; those followed by "f" indicate illustrations.

Abortive grand mal seizures, 275
Action drawings, 25. *See also* Developmental stages
Adaptive behavior. *See* Developmental schedules; Glossary
and cortical integrity, 18
definition, 4–5
developmental sequences, 10f
in fetal infancy, 265t
film, 505
in final report of developmental examination, 448
and intellectual potential, 138–139, 431
and intelligence, 140
in neonatal period, 164
of normal and mentally deficient infants, 152t
and PKU, 175
questions for developmental screening inventory, 452t–453t
temporary and replacement patterns, 464–469
and validity of infant assessment, 144
Adaptive developmental quotients. *See also* Developmental quotients
by age, race and education of mother, 180t
by age, and socioeconomic status, 180t
Adaptive maturity level
and neuromotor diagnosis, 212, 444
Adjustable clinical table, 498, 501f
Adoption
agency versus independent, 371–372
case reports, 184, 371–372, 374–380
errors in, 371–372

Adoption *(continued)*
and handicapped children, 370
heredity and, 373
historic trends in, 369–371
probationary period, 370, 373–374, 381
race and, 370, 371
responsibility of physician in, 372–374
rights in, 369
risks in, 370–371
safety of, 381
Age(s). *See also* Corrected Chronologic Age; Gestational age
appearance of signs of environmental mental retardation, 191t
and behavior patterns, 6
and choice of examination sequences, 122
and developmental organization, 8, 9f–14f
and developmental quotient, 136–137
and developmental screening, 350–351
and diagnosis of autism, 335
and examination arrangements, 20f, 494f, 496f, 497f
key, 7–8, 25, 27. *See also* Developmental Stages
and mental retardation, 179–180
and prediction, 18
procedures for determination, 27
and retardation, 141
selection of questions for Developmental Screening Inventory, 461t
Air contrast studies, in differential diagnosis, 147

515

Cover design by Patrick H. Turner

74 75 76 77 78 10 9 8 7 6 5 4 3 2 1